Intraocular Inflammation and Uveitis

Section 9

2004–2005

(Last major revision 2003–2004)

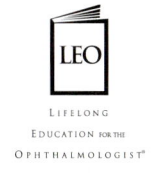

BASIC AND CLINICAL SCIENCE COURSE

AMERICAN ACADEMY
OF OPHTHALMOLOGY
The Eye M.D. Association

LEO
LIFELONG
EDUCATION FOR THE
OPHTHALMOLOGIST

The Basic and Clinical Science Course is one component of the Lifelong Education for the Ophthalmologist (LEO) framework, which assists members in planning their continuing medical education. LEO includes an array of clinical education products that members may select to form individualized, self-directed learning plans for updating their clinical knowledge. Active members or fellows who use LEO components may accumulate sufficient CME credits to earn the LEO Award. Contact the Academy's Clinical Education Division for further information on LEO.

The American Academy of Ophthalmology is accredited by the Accreditation Council for Continuing Medical Education to provide continuing medical education for physicians.

The American Academy of Ophthalmology designates this educational activity for a maximum of 30 category 1 credits toward the AMA Physician's Recognition Award. Each physician should claim only those hours of credit that he/she actually spent in the activity.

The American Medical Association has determined that non-U.S. licensed physicians who participate in this CME activity are eligible for AMA PRA category 1 credit.

The Academy provides this material for educational purposes only. It is not intended to represent the only or best method or procedure in every case, nor to replace a physician's own judgment or give specific advice for case management. Including all indications, contraindications, side effects, and alternative agents for each drug or treatment is beyond the scope of this material. All information and recommendations should be verified, prior to use, with current information included in the manufacturers' package inserts or other independent sources, and considered in light of the patient's condition and history. Reference to certain drugs, instruments, and other products in this course is made for illustrative purposes only and is not intended to constitute an endorsement of such. Some material may include information on applications that are not considered community standard, that reflect indications not included in approved FDA labeling, or that are approved for use only in restricted research settings. The FDA has stated that it is the responsibility of the physician to determine the FDA status of each drug or device he or she wishes to use, and to use them with appropriate patient consent in compliance with applicable law. The Academy specifically disclaims any and all liability for injury or other damages of any kind, from negligence or otherwise, for any and all claims that may arise from the use of any recommendations or other information contained herein.

Copyright © 2004
American Academy of Ophthalmology
All rights reserved
Printed in the United States of America

Basic and Clinical Science Course

Thomas J. Liesegang, MD, Jacksonville, Florida, *Senior Secretary for Clinical Education*
Gregory L. Skuta, MD, Oklahoma City, Oklahoma, *Secretary for Ophthalmic Knowledge*
Louis B. Cantor, MD, Indianapolis, Indiana, *BCSC Course Chair*

Section 9

Faculty Responsible for This Edition

E. Mitchel Opremcak, MD, *Chair*, Columbus, Ohio
Emmett T. Cunningham, Jr, MD, New York, New York
C. Stephen Foster, MD, Boston, Massachusetts
David Forster, MD, Falls Church, Virginia
Ramana S. Moorthy, MD, Indianapolis, Indiana
Marta Lopatynsky, MD, Morristown, New Jersey
 Practicing Ophthalmologists Advisory Committee for Education

Dr Cunningham is a vice president at Eyetech Pharmaceuticals, Inc.

The other authors state that they have no significant financial interest or other relationship with the manufacturer of any commercial product discussed in the chapters that they contributed to this publication or with the manufacturer of any competing commercial product.

Recent Past Faculty

H. Jane Blackman, MD
Brent E. Chalmers, MD
Scott Cousins, MD
William W. Culbertson, MD
David H. Fischer, MD
Rudolph M. Franklin, MD
Alan H. Friedman, MD
David Meisler, MD
Priscilla E. Perry, MD
Narsing A. Rao, MD
John D. Sheppard, Jr, MD
Paul Turgeon, MD
Robert S. Weinberg, MD
Sue Ellen Young, MD

In addition, the Academy gratefully acknowledges the contributions of numerous past faculty and advisory committee members who have played an important role in the development of previous editions of the Basic and Clinical Science Course.

American Academy of Ophthalmology Staff

Richard A. Zorab, *Vice President, Ophthalmic Knowledge*
Hal Straus, *Director, Publications Department*
Carol L. Dondrea, *Publications Editor*
Christine Arturo, *Acquisitions Editor*
Maxine Garrett, *Administrative Coordinator*

Cover design: Paula Shuhert Design
Cover photograph: Choroidal folds, by Patrick J. Saine, MEd, CRA, Dartmouth-Hitchcock Medical Center

**AMERICAN ACADEMY
OF OPHTHALMOLOGY**
The Eye M.D. Association

655 Beach Street
Box 7424
San Francisco, CA 94120-7424

Contents

General Introduction xi

Objectives 1
Introduction 3

PART I Immunology 5
Introduction to Immunology 7
   Glossary 7
   Abbreviations 8

1 Basic Concepts in Immunology 9
Definitions 9
   Adaptive Immune Response 9
   Innate Immune Response 10
   Similarities Between Adaptive and Innate Immune Responses 10
   Differences Between Adaptive and Innate Immune Responses 11
   Immunity Versus Inflammation .12
Components of the Immune System 13
   Leukocytes 13
   Lymphoid Tissues 16

2 Immunization and Adaptive Immunity: The Immune Response Arc 17
Overview of the Immune Response Arc 17
Phases of the Immune Response Arc 19
   Afferent Phase 19
   Processing Phase 22
   Effector Phase 25
Immune Response Arc and Primary or Secondary Immune
  Responses 27
   Concept of Immunologic Memory 27
Regional Immunity and Immunologic Microenvironments 28
   Regional Immunity 28
   Immunologic Microenvironments 28
Clinical Examples of the Concept of the Immune Response Arc 29

3 Ocular Immune Responses 33
Immune Responses of the Conjunctiva 33
   Features of the Immunologic Microenvironment 33
   Immunoregulatory Systems 36
Immune Responses of the Anterior Chamber, Anterior Uvea,
  and Vitreous 36

Features of the Immunologic Microenvironment. 36
Immunoregulatory Systems 37
Immune Responses of the Cornea 39
Features of the Immunologic Microenvironment. 39
Immunoregulatory Systems 39
Immune Responses of the Retina, RPE, and Choroid 40
Features of the Immunologic Microenvironment. 40
Immunoregulatory Systems 42

4 Mechanisms of Immune Effector Reactivity 43
Effector Reactivities of Innate Immunity 43
Bacteria-Derived Molecules That Trigger Innate Immunity 43
Other Triggers or Modulators of Innate Immunity 46
Innate Mechanisms for the Recruitment and Activation of
Macrophages 50
Effector Reactivities of Adaptive Immunity 54
Antibody-Mediated Immune Effector Responses 54
Lymphocyte-Mediated Effector Responses 63
Combined Antibody and Cellular Effector Mechanisms 70
Mediator Systems That Amplify Innate and Adaptive Immune
Responses. 74
Plasma-Derived Enzyme Systems 75
Vasoactive Amines 77
Lipid Mediators .77
Cytokines 80
Reactive Oxygen Intermediates 83
Reactive Nitrogen Products 85
Neutrophil-Derived Granule Products 86

5 Special Topics in Ocular Immunology 87
Immunoregulation of the Adaptive Immune Response 87
T- and B-cell Antigen Receptor Repertoire 87
Tolerance and Immunoregulation 87
Molecular Mimicry 89
HLA Associations and Disease 90
Normal Function of HLA Molecules 90
Allelic Variation 91
MHC and Transplantation 93
Disease Associations. 94
Immunotherapeutics 95
Nonsteroidal Anti-Inflammatory Drugs (NSAIDs) 96
Glucocorticosteroids. 96
Cytotoxic Chemotherapy 96
Cyclosporine 97

PART II Intraocular Inflammation and Uveitis 99

6 Clinical Approach to Uveitis 101
Symptoms of Uveitis 101
Signs of Uveitis 102

        Anterior Segment. 102
        Intermediate Segment 105
        Posterior Segment 106
    Classification of Uveitis 106
        Anterior Uveitis 106
        Intermediate Uveitis. 107
        Posterior Uveitis 107
        Panuveitis (Diffuse Uveitis) 107
    Review of the Patient's Health and Other Associated Factors 110
    Differential Diagnosis and Prevalence of Uveitic Entities 111
    Laboratory and Medical Evaluation 113
    Medical Management of Uveitis 114
        Mydriatic and Cycloplegic Agents 114
        Corticosteroids 115
        Immunomodulating and Immunosuppressive Agents 118
        Other Immunomodulatory Agents. 120
    Surgery 121
    Diagnostic Survey for Uveitis 122

7 Anterior Uveitis. **127**
    Acute Anterior Nongranulomatous Iritis and Iridocyclitis 127
        HLA-B27–Related Diseases 128
        Behçet Syndrome. 133
        Glaucomatocyclitic Crisis (Posner-Schlossman Syndrome) . . . 135
        Lens-Associated Uveitis. 135
        IOL-Associated Postoperative Inflammation 137
        Herpetic Disease 138
        Other Viral Diseases. 140
        Drug-Induced Uveitis 141
    Chronic Iridocyclitis 141
        Juvenile Rheumatoid Arthritis 141
        Fuchs Heterochromic Iridocyclitis (Fuchs Uveitis Syndrome) . . 144
        Idiopathic Iridocyclitis. 146

8 Intermediate Uveitis and Pars Planitis **147**
    Pars Planitis 147
        Clinical Characteristics 147
        Differential Diagnosis 148
        Ancillary Tests and Histopathology 148
        Prognosis 149
        Treatment 149
        Complications. 150
    Multiple Sclerosis 152

9 Posterior Uveitis **153**
    Infectious Diseases. 154
        Viral Disease 154
        Fungal Diseases 160

Protozoal Diseases 164
Helminthic Diseases. 170
Immunologic Diseases 173
Collagen Vascular Diseases 173
Retinochoroidopathies 176

10 Panuveitis **187**
Infectious Diseases. 187
Bacterial Disease 187
Helminthic Diseases. 195
Immunologic and Granulomatous Diseases 197
Sarcoidosis 197
Sympathetic Ophthalmia 200
Vogt-Koyanagi-Harada (VKH) Disease 203

11 Endophthalmitis **207**
Signs and Symptoms 207
Infectious Endophthalmitis 207
Postoperative Endophthalmitis 209
Posttraumatic Endophthalmitis 211
Endophthalmitis Associated With Filtering Blebs. 212
Endogenous Endophthalmitis 213
Prophylaxis 214
Diagnosis 215
Differential Diagnosis 215
Obtaining Intraocular Specimens 215
Cultures and Laboratory Evaluation of Intraocular Specimens . . . 216
Treatment 217
Surgical Management 217
Medical Management 217
General Considerations for Treatment 219
Outcomes of Treatment 219

12 Masquerade Syndromes **221**
Nonneoplastic Masquerade Syndromes 221
Retinitis Pigmentosa. 221
Ocular Ischemic Syndrome 221
Chronic Peripheral Rhegmatogenous Retinal Detachment 222
Endogenous Nocardial Endophthalmitis. 223
Endogenous Fungal Endophthalmitis. 223
Neoplastic Masquerade Syndromes 228
Primary Central Nervous System Lymphoma 228
Neoplastic Masquerade Syndromes Secondary to Systemic
Lymphoma 231
Neoplastic Masquerade Syndromes Secondary to Leukemia 231
Neoplastic Masquerade Syndromes Secondary to Uveal Lymphoid
Proliferations 231
Nonlymphoid Malignancies 232

Metastatic Tumors 233
Bilateral Diffuse Uveal Melanocytic Proliferation. 233

13 Complications of Uveitis. 235
Cataracts 235
Glaucoma 237
Hypotony 239
Cystoid Macular Edema 239
Vitreous Opacification and Vitritis 239
Retinal Detachment 240
Retinal and Choroidal Neovascularization 240

14 Ocular Involvement in AIDS 241
Virology of HIV 242
Pathogenesis 242
Natural History 243
Transmission 245
Diagnosis 245
Management of HIV Infection 246
Systemic Conditions. 246
Ophthalmic Complications 248
External Eye Manifestations 258
The Ophthalmologist's Role 261
Precautions in the Health Care Setting 261
Precautions in Ophthalmic Practice 261

Basic Texts 263
Related Academy Materials 265
Credit Reporting Form 267
Study Questions 271
Answers 279
Index 283

General Introduction

The Basic and Clinical Science Course (BCSC) is designed to meet the needs of residents and practitioners for a comprehensive yet concise curriculum of the field of ophthalmology. The BCSC has developed from its original brief outline format, which relied heavily on outside readings, to a more convenient and educationally useful self-contained text. The Academy updates and revises the course annually, with the goals of integrating the basic science and clinical practice of ophthalmology and of keeping ophthalmologists current with new developments in the various subspecialties.

The BCSC incorporates the effort and expertise of more than 80 ophthalmologists, organized into 14 section faculties, working with Academy editorial staff. In addition, the course continues to benefit from many lasting contributions made by the faculties of previous editions. Members of the Academy's Practicing Ophthalmologists Advisory Committee for Education serve on each faculty and, as a group, review every volume before and after major revisions.

Organization of the Course

The Basic and Clinical Science Course comprises 14 volumes, incorporating fundamental ophthalmic knowledge, subspecialty areas, and special topics:

1. Update on General Medicine
2. Fundamentals and Principles of Ophthalmology
3. Optics, Refraction, and Contact Lenses
4. Ophthalmic Pathology and Intraocular Tumors
5. Neuro-Ophthalmology
6. Pediatric Ophthalmology and Strabismus
7. Orbit, Eyelids, and Lacrimal System
8. External Disease and Cornea
9. Intraocular Inflammation and Uveitis
10. Glaucoma
11. Lens and Cataract
12. Retina and Vitreous
13. International Ophthalmology
14. Refractive Surgery

In addition, a comprehensive Master Index allows the reader to easily locate subjects throughout the entire series.

References

Readers who wish to explore specific topics in greater detail may consult the journal references cited within each chapter and the Basic Texts listed at the back of the book.

These references are intended to be selective rather than exhaustive, chosen by the BCSC faculty as being important, current, and readily available to residents and practitioners.

Related Academy educational materials are also listed in the appropriate sections. They include books, audiovisual materials, self-assessment programs, clinical modules, and interactive programs.

Study Questions and CME Credit

Each volume of the BCSC is designed as an independent study activity for ophthalmology residents and practitioners. The learning objectives for this volume are stated on page 1. The text, illustrations, and references provide the information necessary to achieve the objectives; the study questions allow readers to test their understanding of the material and their mastery of the objectives. Physicians who wish to claim CME credit for this educational activity may do so by mail, by fax, or online. The necessary forms and instructions are given at the end of the book.

Conclusion

The Basic and Clinical Science Course has expanded greatly over the years, with the addition of much new text and numerous illustrations. Recent editions have sought to place a greater emphasis on clinical applicability, while maintaining a solid foundation in basic science. As with any educational program, it reflects the experience of its authors. As its faculties change and as medicine progresses, new viewpoints are always emerging on controversial subjects and techniques. Not all alternate approaches can be included in this series; as with any educational endeavor, the learner should seek additional sources, including such carefully balanced opinions as the Academy's Preferred Practice Patterns.

The BCSC faculty and staff are continuously striving to improve the educational usefulness of the course; you, the reader, can contribute to this ongoing process. If you have any suggestions or questions about the series, please do not hesitate to contact the faculty or the editors.

The authors, editors, and reviewers hope that your study of the BCSC will be of lasting value and that each section will serve as a practical resource for quality patient care.

Objectives

Upon completion of BCSC Section 9, *Intraocular Inflammation and Uveitis*, the reader should be able to:

- Outline the immunologic and infectious mechanisms involved in the occurrence and complications of uveitis and related inflammatory conditions, including acquired immunodeficiency syndrome (AIDS)
- Identify general and specific pathophysiological processes that affect the structure and function of the uvea, lens, intraocular cavities, retina, and other tissues in acute and chronic intraocular inflammation
- Choose appropriate examination techniques and relevant ancillary studies
- Develop appropriate differential diagnoses for ocular inflammatory disorders
- Describe the principles of medical and surgical management of uveitis and related intraocular inflammation, including indications for and complications of immunosuppressive agents
- Describe criteria that can be applied to differentiate the masquerade syndromes from true uveitis

Introduction

This section of the BCSC is divided into two parts. Part II, Intraocular Inflammation and Uveitis, will come as no surprise to the reader opening a volume of the same name. Part II introduces the clinical approach to uveitis and devotes a chapter each to the different forms of uveitis, as classified anatomically, and to endophthalmitis. It then discusses the masquerade syndromes, both nonneoplastic and neoplastic. The following chapter discusses the complications of all forms of uveitis, and the final chapter of Part II covers the ocular involvement in AIDS, offering the most complete summary of this topic in the BCSC series.

The reader may, however, not expect to find one third of the book, Part I, Immunology, going into such great depth. Why are so many pages given to this topic? What relevance does it have to Part II? Progress in basic immunology, as well as in the regional immunology of the eye, has translated into major advances in recent years. Our understanding of the mechanisms by which uveitis and other intraocular diseases develop has helped clinicians to identify and establish uveitis entities and to develop specific treatments directed at altered immune processes. These clinically relevant advances include the discovery of unique immune responses in the intraocular cavities and subretinal space; the delineation of the association between HLA and various uveitis entities; and the detection of infectious agents by immunologic methods such as Western blot, ELISA, and others. Lymphocytic studies for cell surface markers and in vitro studies based on antibodies have helped in clearly separating those uveitis entities that are mediated by immune mechanisms, in particular those resulting from organ-specific antibodies, from those caused by altered lymphocyte functions. The latter mechanism appears to be prevalent in posterior uveitis, and altered cell-mediated immunity can be directed to retinal proteins or other ocular antigens in these intraocular inflammations. Such findings have led to the introduction of potential therapeutic modalities such as oral tolerance, a promising though still experimental approach.

The section on immunology has been rewritten and expanded to describe basic aspects of the human immune response, including responses specific to the ocular structures; the effector mechanisms of immunity, including antibody-mediated and lymphocyte-generated mechanisms; and the various pro- and anti-inflammatory cytokines and other effector molecules, including reactive oxygen species and nitric oxide products. Clinical examples are interspersed throughout the immunology text, discussing the clinical relevance of the issues covered in diagnosis and management of uveitis. A clear understanding of the immune mechanisms will enhance an appreciation of the clinical features and principles behind the management of uveitis triggered by either an infectious agent or another insult.

The authors would like to acknowledge Aize Kijlstra, PhD, and J. Wayne Streilein, MD, for their assistance in reviewing Part I.

PART I

Immunology

Introduction to Immunology

Chapters 1 through 5 discuss the human immune system and its ocular effects in detail. Many specific terms are used, and some may be defined only briefly in an early chapter and then explained in depth in a later chapter. Similarly, abbreviations that may be unfamiliar to the reader often are used after the term has been spelled out at first mention. The following glossary and list of abbreviations are designed to provide the reader with a handy reference to terminology used in Part I, especially those terms discussed in later chapters and abbreviations that appear far from their original descriptions, and not as comprehensive listings.

Glossary

Antibody A glycoprotein that is able to bind biochemically to a specific antigenic substance.

Antigen Foreign substance that activates an adaptive immune response.

Antigen-presenting cells Specialized cells that carry antigen to a lymph node, process it into fragments, and present the fragments to T-cell antigen receptors.

Chemotaxis Attraction generated in macrophages, neutrophils, eosinophils, and lymphocytes by substances released at sites of inflammatory reactions, such as lymphokines, complement, and various mediators.

Complement Effector molecules used to amplify inflammation for both innate and adaptive immunity.

Cytokine A generic term for any soluble polypeptide mediator synthesized and released by cells for the purposes of intercellular signaling and communication.

Epitope Each specific portion of an antigenic molecule to which the immune system responds.

Fc receptor The Fc domain of each immunoglobulin monomer contains the attachment site for effector cells and complement activation.

Hapten A small molecule, not antigenic by itself, that can react with antibodies when conjugated to a larger antigenic molecule.

Isotype Different subclasses of immunoglobulin.

Leukotriene A compound formed from arachidonic acid that functions as a regulator of allergic and inflammatory reactions, probably contributing significantly to inflammatory infiltration.

Lymphatics Common term for *afferent lymphatic channels*, which drain extracellular fluid to a regional lymph node, conveying immune cells and whole antigen, and *efferent lymphatic channels*, which drain to the circulatory system.

Mediator Substance released from cells as the result of the interaction of antigen with antibody or by the action of antigen with a sensitized lymphocyte.

Abbreviations

ACAID anterior chamber–associated immune deviation

ADCC antibody-dependent cellular cytotoxicity

ANCA antineutrophil cytoplasmic antibody

APC antigen-presenting cell(s)

CAM cell-adhesion molecule(s)

CTL cytotoxic T lymphocytes

DC dendritic cells

DH delayed hypersensitivity

HLA human leukocyte antigen

IFN interferon

IL interleukin

LC Langerhans cells

LPS lipopolysaccharide

MAC membrane attack complex

MALT mucosa-associated lymphoid tissue

MHC major histocompatibility complex

PAF platelet-activating factor(s)

PG prostaglandin

PMN polymorphonuclear leukocytes, or neutrophils

TGF transforming growth factor

Th T helper cell, as in *Th0, Th1*, etc.

TNF tumor necrosis factor

CHAPTER 1

Basic Concepts in Immunology

Definitions

In general, an immune response is a sequence of cellular and molecular events designed to rid the host of an offending stimulus, usually from a pathogenic organism, toxic substance, cellular debris, or neoplastic cell. Two broad categories of immune responses have been recognized: *adaptive* and *innate*. Simply put, adaptive immunity, also called *specific* or *acquired immunity*, can be conceptualized as "user programmable." Within an individual, adaptive responses react to specific environmental stimuli (ie, unique antigens) with a stimulus-specific (ie, antigen-specific) immunologic response. In contrast, innate immune responses, also called *natural immunity*, are "factory preprogrammed." All individuals are endowed with a genetically predetermined set of responses to a wide range of noxious environmental stimuli. Different stimuli can often trigger the same responses.

Adaptive Immune Response

Adaptive immunity is a host response set in motion by a specific environmental stimulus, or antigen. An antigen usually represents an alien substance completely foreign to the organism, and the immune system must generate, de novo, a specific receptor against it that must, in turn, recognize a unique molecular structure in the antigen for which no specific preexisting receptor was present. The organism attempts to defend itself by the following steps:

- Recognizing the unique foreign antigenic substance as distinguished from self
- Processing the unique antigen with receptors newly created by specialized tissues (the immune system)
- Generating unique antigen-specific immunologic effector cells (especially T and B lymphocytes) and unique antigen-specific soluble effector molecules, such as antibodies, which function to remove the specific stimulating antigenic substance from the organism while ignoring the presence of other, irrelevant antigenic stimuli

Thus, the adaptive immune system is not genetically predetermined but evolves as an ongoing way for an individual's T and B lymphocytes to continually generate new antigen receptors through recombination, rearrangement, and mutation of the germline genetic structure. This creates a vast repertoire of novel antigen receptor molecules that vary tremendously among individuals within a given species.

The immune response to a mutated virus is the classic example of this process. Viruses such as influenza virus are continuously mutating, thus developing new antigenic structures. The susceptible host could not possibly have evolved receptors needed to recognize each of these new viral mutations. However, each new mutation serves as an antigen that stimulates a specific adaptive immune response by the host to the virus. The adaptive response recognizes the virus in question and not other organisms, such as polio virus. Following environmental exposure, the adaptive immune response has been programmed to adapt to the new specific antigen.

Innate Immune Response

Innate immunity is a pattern recognition response by the organism to

- Identify various offensive stimuli (especially infectious agents, toxins, or cellular debris from injury) in an antigen-independent manner
- Respond in a stereotyped, preprogrammed fashion determined by the preexistence of receptors for the stimulus
- Generate generic biochemical mediators and cytokines that recruit nonspecific effector cells, especially macrophages and neutrophils, to remove the offending stimulus in a nonspecific manner through phagocytosis or enzymatic degradation

The stimuli of innate immunity interact with receptors that have been genetically predetermined by evolution to recognize and respond to molecular *motifs* on triggering stimuli. These motifs often include a specific amino acid sequence, certain lipoproteins, certain phospholipids, or other specific molecular patterns. The receptors of innate immunity are identical among all individuals within a species. In this way the receptors on monocytes, neutrophils, and sometimes parenchymal tissues resemble the receptors for neurotransmitters or hormones.

The innate immune response to acute infection is the classic example of this process. For example, in endophthalmitis, bacteria-derived toxins or host cell debris stimulate the recruitment of neutrophils and monocytes, leading to the production of inflammatory mediators and phagocytosis of the bacteria. The triggering mechanisms and subsequent effector response to *Staphylococcus* are nearly identical to those mounted against other organisms. Nonspecific receptors that recognize families of related toxins or molecules in the environment determine this response.

Similarities Between Adaptive and Innate Immune Responses

Receptor activation

Both responses use receptors present on white blood cells to recognize offending stimuli, but the *recognition receptors* are fundamentally different.

Inflammatory or noninflammatory responses

Both responses can trigger inflammation, but they usually operate at a subclinical level so that the individual is unaware of the response.

Nonspecific effector cells and molecules

Although only the adaptive immune response employs T and B lymphocytes as antigen-specific effector cells, both forms of immunity use neutrophils, eosinophils, and monocytes as nonspecific effector cells and the same chemical mediators as amplification systems.

Differences Between Adaptive and Innate Immune Responses

Triggering stimuli

Adaptive immunity is triggered by an antigen, usually in the form of a protein, although carbohydrates or lipids can sometimes be antigenic. Innate immunity is triggered by bacterial toxins and cell debris, often in the form of carbohydrate, phospholipid, and other nonprotein molecules.

Recognition receptors

The antigen receptors of adaptive immunity, such as antibody molecules and T-cell antigen receptor molecules, are specific for each antigen, recognizing unique molecular regions of an antigen called *epitopes*. The receptors used by innate immunity, such as scavenging receptors or toxin receptors, recognize conserved molecular patterns or motifs shared among various triggering stimuli.

Time of onset after triggering

Because adaptive immune responses are acquired, they require recognition, processing, and effector phases that need several days for activation. Therefore, onset is delayed. Innate immunity is preprogrammed, requiring only the direct activation of a cellular receptor to initiate an effector response, which induces release of mediators or recruitment of cells within hours.

Memory

Adaptive immune responses demonstrate memory, so that on second exposure to the same antigen, the release of effectors is more vigorous and rapid than during the original response. Innate responses are genetically preprogrammed to react stereotypically to each encounter. Memory implies that the secondary, or repeat encounter, immune response is regulated by mechanisms different from the primary, or initial virgin encounter, immune response, specifically by memory T and B cells.

Specificity

Adaptive immune responses demonstrate specificity for each unique offending antigen. Innate responses do not. Specificity is maintained through the use of antibodies and antigen-specific T and B cells that recognize specific biochemical information, such as linear amino acid sequences for T cells and three-dimensional geometry for B cells. Subtle biochemical changes (ie, amino acid substitutions) in the structure of the antigen remove specific recognition for memory responses but preserve overall antigenicity for a new primary response. In contrast, similar subtle changes in toxin structure or other stimuli for innate immunity do not necessarily alter the innate response if the changes do not involve the pattern recognition sites within the molecule.

Immunity Versus Inflammation

An immune response is the process for removal of an offending stimulus. When this response becomes clinically apparent within a tissue, it can be termed an *inflammatory response*. More precisely, an inflammatory response is a sequence of molecular and cellular events triggered by innate or adaptive immunity resulting in five characteristic cardinal clinical manifestations:

- Pain
- Hyperemia
- Edema
- Heat
- Loss of function

These clinical signs reflect two main physiologic changes within a tissue: cellular recruitment and altered vascular permeability. Inflammatory response is associated with the following typical pathological findings:

- Infiltration of effector cells mediated by and resulting in release of biochemical and molecular mediators/amplifiers of inflammation, such as cytokines (ie, interleukins and chemokines) and lipid mediators (ie, prostaglandins and platelet-activating factors)
- Presence of oxygen metabolites (ie, superoxide and nitrogen radicals)
- Presence of granule products as well as catalytic enzymes (ie, collagenases and elastases)
- Activation of plasma-derived enzyme systems (ie, complement components such as anaphylatoxins)

See Chapter 3 for a more detailed discussion.

In practice, many clinicians use the term *immune response* to mean adaptive immunity and the term *inflammation* to imply innate immunity. However, it is important to remember that both adaptive and innate immune responses usually function physiologically at a subclinical level without overt manifestations. For example, in most persons, ocular surface allergen exposure that occurs daily in all humans, or bacterial contamination during cataract surgery that occurs in most eyes, is usually cleared by innate or adaptive mechanisms without overt inflammation. Similarly, both adaptive and innate immunity can trigger inflammation, and the physiologic changes induced by each form of immunity may be indistinguishable. For example, the hypopyon of bacterial endophthalmitis, which results from innate immunity against bacterial toxins, and the hypopyon of lens-associated uveitis, which presumably results from an inappropriate adaptive immune response against lens antigens, cannot be clearly distinguished clinically or histologically.

Delves PJ, Roitt IM. Advances in immunology: the immune system. *N Engl J Med*. 2000; 343:37–49 (part 1); 108–117 (part 2).

Medzhitov R, Janeway C. Advances in immunology: innate immunity. *N Engl J Med*. 2000; 343:338–344.

Roitt IM, Delves PJ. *Roitt's Essential Immunology*. 10th ed. Malden, MA: Blackwell Science; 2001.

Components of the Immune System

Leukocytes

White blood cells, or *leukocytes*, are nucleated cells that can be distinguished from one another by the shape of their nuclei and the presence or absence of granules. They are further defined by uptake of various histologic stains.

Neutrophils

Neutrophils, also called *polymorphonuclear leukocytes (PMNs)*, are the most abundant granulocytes in the blood. They are efficient phagocytes that readily clear tissues and degrade ingested material. They act as important effector cells through the release of granule products and cytokines. Through specific receptors, such as complement receptors, PMNs can be recruited and triggered by immune mechanisms. Nonimmune mechanisms also recruit PMNs at sites of injury through poorly characterized receptor ligand interactions. Chapter 4 discusses PMN activation recruitment in greater detail.

PMNs dominate the infiltrate in experimental models and clinical examples of active bacterial infections of the conjunctiva, sclera (scleritis), cornea (keratitis), or vitreous (endophthalmitis). PMNs are also dominant in many models of active viral infections of the cornea (herpes simplex virus keratitis) and retina (herpes simplex virus retinitis) and in some human viral infections. PMNs also constitute the principal cell type in lipopolysaccharide-induced inflammation and after direct injection of most cytokines into various ocular tissues.

Eosinophils

Eosinophils, like PMNs, also contain abundant cytoplasmic granules and lysosomes. However, the biochemical nature of the granules in eosinophils consists of more basic and binding acidic dyes, and eosinophils differ from PMNs in the way they respond to certain triggering stimuli. Eosinophils have receptors for and become activated by many mediators; interleukin-5 (IL-5) is especially important. Eosinophil granule products, such as major basic protein or ribonucleases, are ideal for destroying parasites; not surprisingly, these cells accumulate at sites of parasitic infection. Eosinophils are numerous in skin infiltrates during the late-phase allergic response, in atopic lesions, and in lung infiltrates during asthma. T-cell production of IL-5 within the infiltrated site is probably an important regulator of eosinophil function locally, although many of the specific mechanisms for regulation of eosinophil recruitment, activation, and function remain unknown.

Eosinophils are abundant in the conjunctiva and tears in many forms of atopic conjunctivitis, especially vernal and allergic conjunctivitis. However, eosinophils are not considered major effectors for intraocular inflammation, except during helminthic infections of the eye, especially acute endophthalmitis caused by toxocariasis.

Basophils and mast cells

Basophils are the bloodborne equivalent of the tissue-bound mast cell. Mast cells exist in two major subtypes, connective tissue and mucosal, both of which can release preformed granules and synthesize certain mediators de novo. *Connective tissue mast cells* contain abundant granules with histamine and heparin, and they synthesize prostaglandin D_2 upon stimulation. In contrast, *mucosal mast cells* require T-cell cytokine help for granule formation, and they therefore normally contain low levels of histamine. Mucosal mast cells synthesize mostly leukotrienes after stimulation. The tissue location can alter the granule type and functional activity, but the regulation of these important differences is not well understood.

Basophils and mast cells differ from other granulocytes in several important ways. The granule contents are different from those of PMNs or eosinophils, and mast cells express high-affinity Fc receptors for the immunoglobulin IgE. *Fc,* from "fragment, crystallizable," refers to the region of immunoglobulin that mediates cell surface receptors. Mast cells act as major effector cells in IgE-mediated immune-triggered inflammatory reactions, especially allergy or immediate hypersensitivity. Mast cells may also participate in the induction of cell-mediated immunity, wound healing, and other functions not directly related to IgE-mediated degranulation (ie, release of cell contents). Thus, other stimuli, such as complement or certain cytokines, may also trigger degranulation.

The normal human conjunctiva contains significant numbers of mast cells localized in the substantia propria but not in the epithelium. In certain atopic and allergic disease states, such as vernal conjunctivitis, not only does the number of mast cells increase in the substantia propria, but the epithelium also becomes densely infiltrated. Careful anatomical studies have shown that the choroid and anterior uveal tract also contain significant densities of connective tissue–type mast cells, whereas the cornea has none.

Monocytes and macrophages

Monocytes, the circulating cells, and macrophages, the tissue-infiltrating equivalents, are important effectors in all forms of immunity and inflammation. Monocytes are relatively large cells (12–20 µm in suspension but up to 40 µm in tissues) that travel through many normal sites. Most normal tissues have at least two identifiable macrophage populations: tissue-resident macrophages and blood-derived macrophages. Although many exceptions exist, in general, tissue-resident macrophages represent monocytes that migrated into a tissue during embryologic development, thereby acquiring tissue-specific properties and specific cellular markers. In many tissues, resident macrophages have been given tissue-specific names: Kupffer cells in the liver, alveolar macrophages in the lung, or microglia in the brain and retina. Blood-derived macrophages usually represent monocytes that have recently migrated from the blood into a fully developed tissue site.

Macrophages serve the following three primary functions:

- Scavengers to clear cell debris and pathogens
- Antigen-presenting cells for T lymphocytes
- Inflammatory effector cells

In vitro studies seem to indicate that resting monocytes can be primed through various signals into efficient antigen-presenting cells and, upon additional signals, activated into effector cells. Effective activation stimuli include exposure to various bacterial toxins such as lipopolysaccharide, phagocytosis of antibody-coated or complement-coated pathogens, or exposure to mediators released during inflammation such as IL-1 or interferon-γ.

Only on full activation do macrophages become most efficient at the synthesis and release of inflammatory mediators and the killing and degradation of phagocytosed pathogens. At some sites of inflammation, macrophages undergo a morphologic change in size and histologic features into a cell called an *epithelioid cell*. Epithelioid cells can fuse into multinucleated *giant cells*. Macrophages are extremely important effector cells in both adaptive and innate immunity, with or without overt inflammation. They are often detectable in acute ocular infections, even if other cell types such as PMNs are more numerous. Chapter 4 discusses these issues in more detail.

Dendritic cells and Langerhans cells

Dendritic cells (DCs) are terminally differentiated, bone marrow–derived, circulating mononuclear cells that are distinct from the macrophage-monocyte lineage. They make up approximately 0.1%–1.0% of blood mononuclear cells. However, in tissue sites, DCs become large (15–30 µm) with cytoplasmic veils that form extensions two to three times the diameter of the cell, resembling the dendritic structure of neurons. In many nonlymphoid and lymphoid organs, DCs become a system of antigen-presenting cells. These sites recruit DCs by defined migration pathways, and DCs in each site share features of structure and function. DCs function as accessory cells important to the processing and presentation of antigens to T cells; the distinctive function of DCs is to initiate responses in quiescent lymphocytes. Thus, DCs may act as the most potent leukocytes for generating primary T-cell–dependent immune responses.

Epidermal Langerhans cells (LCs) are the best-characterized subset of DCs. LCs account for approximately 3%–8% of cells in most human epithelia, including the skin, conjunctiva, nasopharyngeal mucosa, vaginal mucosa, and rectal mucosa. LCs are identified on the basis of their many dendrites, electron-dense cytoplasm, and Birbeck granules. LCs are not active antigen-presenting cells, although activity develops after in vitro culture with certain cytokines. As a result, LCs transform and lose their granules and thus fully resemble blood and lymphoid DCs. Evidence suggests that LCs can leave the skin and move along the afferent lymph to draining lymphoid organs. LCs are important components of the immune system and play a role in antigen presentation, control of lymphoid cell traffic, differentiation of T cells, and induction of delayed hypersensitivity. Elimination of LCs from skin before antigen challenge inhibits the induction of the contact hypersensitivity response. In the conjunctiva and limbus, LCs are the only ones that constitutively express class II major histocompatibility molecules. Many kinds of irritation to the cornea can result in central migration of the peripheral LCs.

Lymphocytes

Lymphocytes are small (10–20 µm) cells with large dense nuclei also derived from stem-cell precursors within the bone marrow. However, unlike other leukocytes, lymphocytes require subsequent maturation in peripheral lymphoid organs. Originally characterized and differentiated according to a series of ingenious but esoteric laboratory tests, lymphocytes can now be subdivided by the detection of specific cell surface proteins (ie, *surface markers*). These markers are in turn related to the functional and molecular activity of individual subsets. Three broad categories of lymphocytes have been identified: T cells; B cells; and non-T, non-B lymphocytes. These subsets are discussed in greater detail below.

Gallin JI, Snyderman R, eds. *Inflammation: Basic Principles and Clinical Correlates.* 3rd ed. Philadelphia: Lippincott; 1999.

Lymphoid Tissues

Primary lymphoid tissues

The bone marrow is the site for replenishment and maturation of all leukocyte and lymphoid precursors. Thus, pluripotential stem cells differentiate into various myeloid or lymphoid precursor cells, which then differentiate into monocyte precursors, T- and B-lymphocyte precursors, and so on. B lymphocytes mature within the bone marrow, whereas immature T lymphocytes exit the bone marrow and mature within the thymus. Mature B and T lymphocytes then exit into the blood, where they enter secondary lymphoid tissues. Granulocytes and monocytes exit the bone marrow directly as functional effectors, although some monocyte subpopulations can further differentiate in peripheral tissues.

Secondary lymphoid tissues

The central lymphoid structures—lymph nodes and spleen—are very important to the adaptive immune response. Mature but naive lymphocytes, those that have not been exposed to antigens, enter lymph nodes through specialized postcapillary venules and take up residence in specialized areas (follicles for B cells and the paracortical region for T cells) until antigen exposure occurs. The lymphocytes can recirculate and travel between different nodes. Certain sites, termed *peripheral lymphoid structures,* especially mucosa and skin, are important for initial interaction with antigen because of their location as barrier to the outside world.

CHAPTER 2

Immunization and Adaptive Immunity: The Immune Response Arc

To understand the clinically relevant features of the adaptive immune response, the reader can consider the sequence of events that follows immunization with antigen using the skin, which is the classic experimental method of introducing antigen to the adaptive immune response. Several general immunologic concepts, especially the concept of the immune response arc, the primary adaptive immune response, and the secondary adaptive immune response, are involved in this process.

Overview of the Immune Response Arc

Interaction between antigen and the adaptive immune system at a peripheral site, such as the skin, can be subdivided, using the concept of the immune response arc, into three phases:

- Afferent
- Processing
- Effector

Each is analogous to the three phases of the neural reflex arc (Fig 2-1). For example, in the neural response to the patellar deep tendon reflex, the *afferent response* begins with the recognition of a stimulus (the activation of the stretch receptor by percussion of the patellar tendon), followed by transformation of the stimulus into a neural signal that is conveyed along an afferent neuron into the central nervous system. In the central nervous system, complex neural *processing* occurs. Finally, along an efferent neuron, the neural signal is conveyed back to the site (quadriceps muscle), which is activated to contract (ie, an *effector response*).

Similarly, in the adaptive immune response, antigen is recognized during the *afferent* phase of the immune response, when the antigenic information is conveyed through the lymphatics and antigen-presenting cells (APCs) to the lymph node. There, *processing* of the antigenic signal occurs, resulting in release of immune messengers (antibodies, B cells, and T cells) into efferent lymphatics and venous circulation. The intent of the

18 • Intraocular Inflammation and Uveitis

NEURAL REFLEX ARC

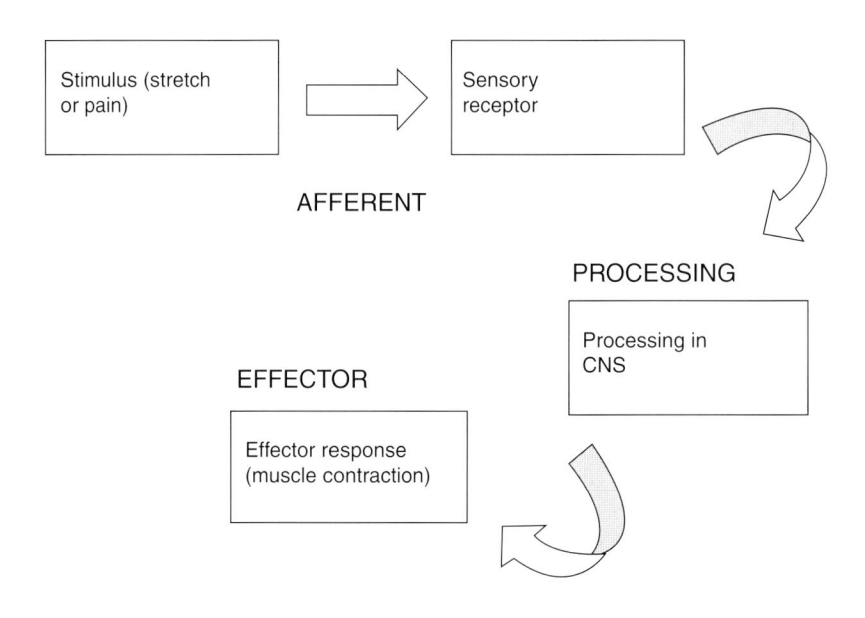

IMMUNE RESPONSE ARC

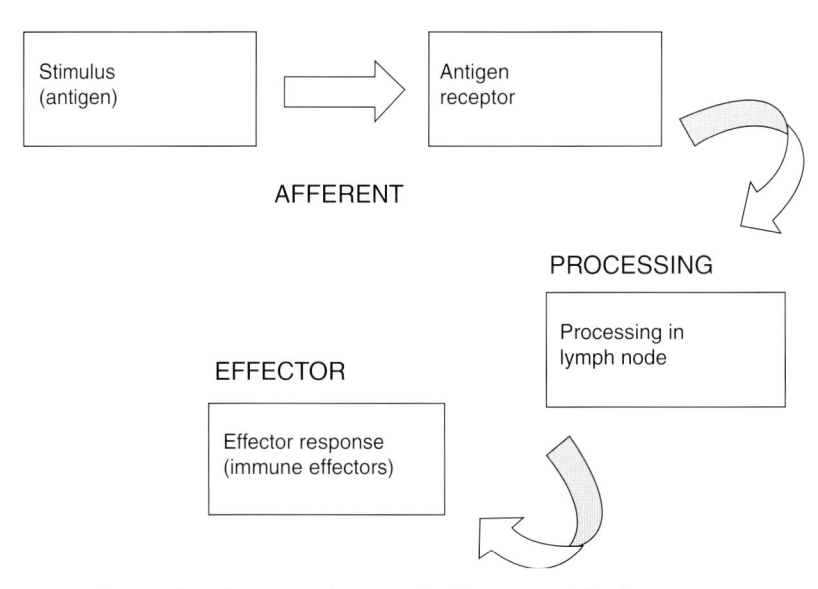

Figure 2-1 Comparison between the neural reflex arc and the immune response arc.

immune system is conveyed back to the original site, where an *effector response* occurs (ie, immune complex formation or delayed hypersensitivity reaction). The following discussion covers the important aspects of each phase in more detail.

Phases of the Immune Response Arc

Afferent Phase

The initial recognition, transport, and presentation of antigenic substances to the adaptive immune system constitute the afferent phase of the immune response arc. Traditionally, the term *antigen* was reserved for those foreign substances that combined with antibody, and the term *immunogen* was used for those substances capable of activating an adaptive immune response. Today, most immunologists tend to use *antigen* to refer to both situations. The term *epitope* refers to each specific portion of an antigenic molecule to which the immune system can respond. A complex three-dimensional protein probably has multiple antigenic epitopes against which different antibodies might bind, as well as many other sites that remain invisible to the immune system. In addition, such a protein often can be enzymatically digested into many different peptide fragments, some of which contain molecular information to serve as antigenic epitopes for T-cell recognition and some of which are not recognized at all by the immune system.

Afferent lymphatic channels

Also simply called *lymphatics,* afferent lymphatic channels are veinlike structures that drain extracellular fluid (ie, lymph) from a site into a regional node. Lymphatics serve two major purposes: to convey immune cells and to carry whole antigen from the site to a lymph node.

Antigen-presenting cells

APCs are specialized cells that take up antigen at a site, carry it to the lymph node, and then process the antigen, which is almost always in the form of a protein, into fragments (ie, intracellular enzymatic digestion into peptides of 7–11 amino acids), place the peptide antigen fragments into a specialized antigen-binding groove within human leukocyte antigen (HLA) molecules, and present antigen peptide fragments within the pocket of the HLA molecules to T-cell antigen receptors, thereby beginning the activation process of adaptive immunity. Different HLA molecules vary in their capacity to bind various peptide fragments within the groove, and thus the HLA type determines the repertoire of peptide antigens capable of being presented to T cells. APCs from one individual cannot present to T cells derived from a second individual unless the two individuals share a common HLA haplotype that can bind the antigen in question. See Chapter 5 for a discussion of HLA molecules. Table 5-1 gives a short history of research on the HLA system.

Class II MHC molecules (ie, HLA-DR, -DP, or -DQ) serve as the antigen-presenting platform for *CD4,* or *helper,* T cells (Fig 2-2). All APCs for CD4 T cells must express the class II MHC molecule, and the antigen receptor on the helper T cell can recognize

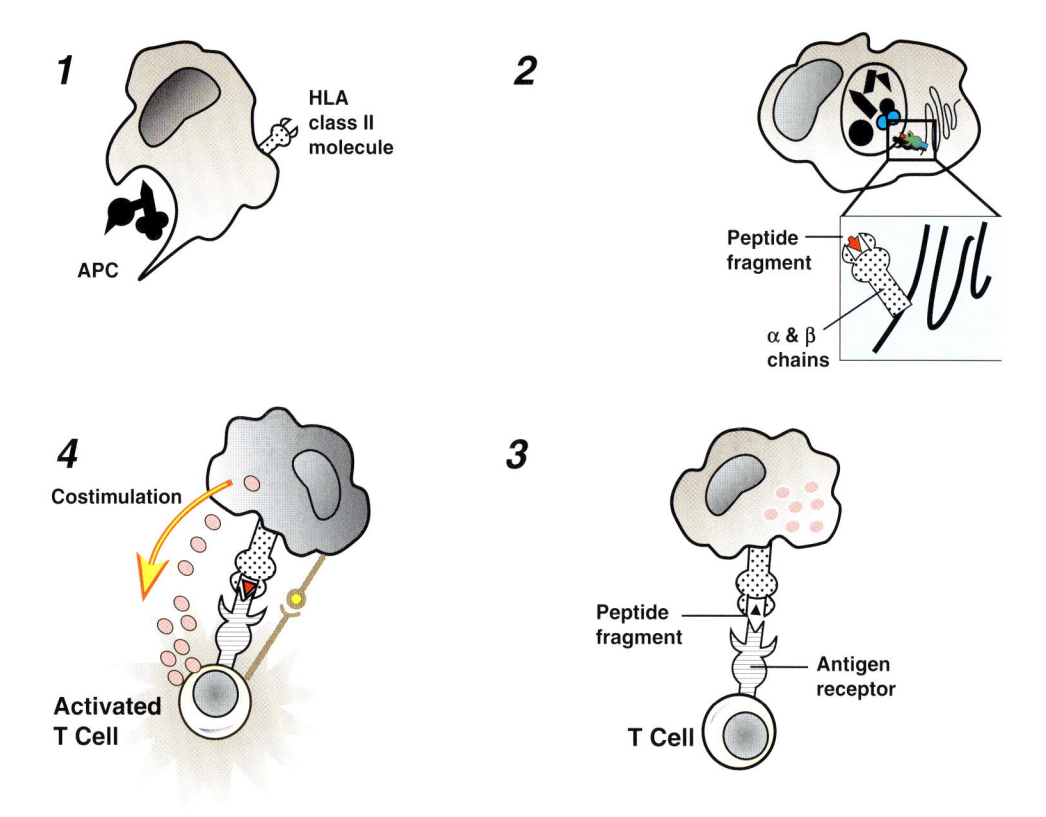

Figure 2-2 Class II–dependent antigen-processing cells (APCs). **1,** APCs endocytose exogenous antigens into the endosomal compartment. **2,** There, the antigen is digested into peptide fragments and placed into the groove formed by the α and β chains of the class II human leukocyte antigen (HLA) molecule. **3,** The CD4 T-cell receptor recognizes the fragment–class II complex. **4,** With the help of costimulatory molecules such as CD28/B7 interactions and cytokines, the CD4 T cell becomes primed, or partially activated. *(Illustration by Barb Cousins, modified by Joyce Zavarro.)*

peptide antigens only if they are presented with class II molecules simultaneously. However, only certain cell types express class II MHC on their plasma membrane. Macrophages and dendritic cells are the two most important class II APCs. B cells can also function as class II–dependent APCs, especially within a lymph node. Any cell that is induced to express MHC class II molecules also can potentially serve as an APC, although this topic is beyond the scope of this discussion. In general, class II–dependent APCs are best for processing extracellular protein antigens that have been endocytosed from the external environment, such as bacterial or fungal antigens.

Class I MHC molecules (ie, HLA-A, -B, or -C) serve as the antigen-presenting platform for *CD8,* or *suppressor,* T cells (Fig 2-3). Class I molecules are present on almost all nucleated cells, indicating that most cells have the potential to stimulate CD8 T cells. The CD8 T-cell antigen receptor must recognize its own class I type before it can respond to tumor or viral antigens on the appropriate target cell, and therefore CD8 T cells from

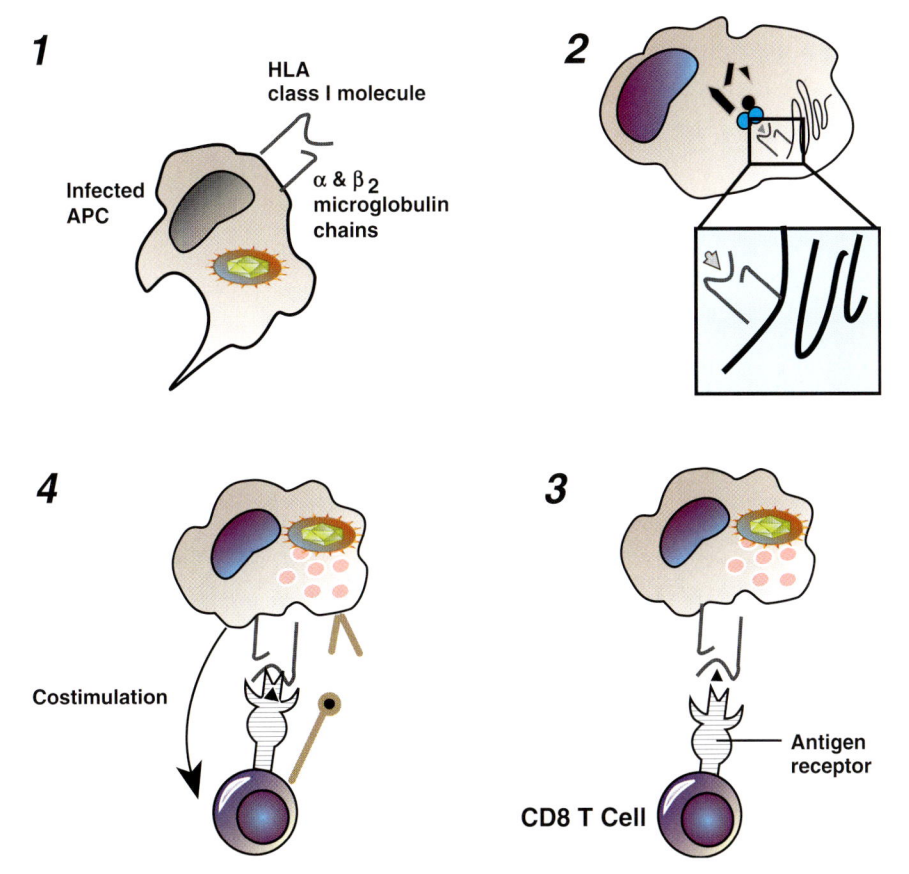

CHAPTER 2: Immunization and Adaptive Immunity: The Immune Response Arc • 21

Figure 2-3 Class I–dependent antigen-processing cells (APCs). **1,** APC is infected by a virus, which causes the cell to synthesize virus-associated peptides that are present in the cytosol. **2,** The viral antigen must be transported (through specialized transporter systems) into the endosomal compartment, where the antigen encounters class I human leukocyte antigen (HLA) molecules. The fragment is placed into the pocket formed by the α chain of the class I HLA molecule. Unlike class II molecules, the second chain, called β_2-microglobulin, is constant among all class I molecules. **3,** The CD8 T-cell receptor recognizes the fragment–class I complex. **4,** With the help of costimulatory molecules such as CD28/B7 interaction and cytokines, the CD8 T cell becomes primed, or partially activated. A similar mechanism is used to recognize tumor antigens that are produced by cells after malignant transformation. *(Illustration by Barb Cousins, modified by Joyce Zavarro.)*

one individual will not respond to a target cell from another individual if the class I MHC molecules do not correspond. In general, class I APCs are best for processing peptide antigens that have been synthesized by the host cell itself, including most tumor peptides or viral peptides after host cell infection.

Several other important topics that greatly influence the afferent phase are beyond the scope of this book. The immunology texts listed as references can be consulted for more detail concerning the following:

- The nature of antigen
- The immunologic microenvironment of different tissues (eg, anatomical and functional differences among sites in APCs, growth factors, immunoregulatory molecules, blood–tissue barriers)
- Expression of HLA molecules on tissues other than leukocytes

Processing Phase

The conversion of the antigenic stimulus into an immunologic response through priming of naive B and T lymphocytes within the lymph nodes and spleen occurs during the processing phase of the immune response arc. This process is also called *activation* or *sensitization* of lymphocytes. Processing involves regulation of the interaction between antigen and naive lymphocytes, B cells or T cells that have not yet encountered their specific antigen, followed by their subsequent activation (Fig 2-4). Immunologic processing has been the topic of extensive research, and the details are beyond the scope of this book. This discussion focuses on a few key concepts.

Preconditions necessary for processing

Helper T lymphocytes are the key regulatory and functional cell type for immune processing. Most helper T cells express CD4 molecule on the cell membrane. As mentioned above, T cells have an antigen receptor that detects antigen only when a trimolecular complex is formed consisting of APC-HLA molecule, processed antigen fragment, and T cell–T cell antigen receptor. The CD4 molecule stabilizes binding and enhances signaling between the HLA complex and the T-cell receptor. When helper T cells specific for an antigen become primed and partially activated, they acquire new functional properties, including cell division, cytokine synthesis, and cell membrane expression of *accessory molecules* such as cell-adhesion molecules or costimulatory molecules. The synthesis and release of immune cytokines, especially IL-2, by T cells is crucial for progression of initial activation and functional differentiation of T cells. The primed T cell produces IL-2, a potent mitogen, which can then stimulate the same cell to become further activated in an autocrine fashion.

Helper T-cell differentiation

At the stage of initial priming CD4 T cells are usually classified as *T helper 0,* or *Th0,* cells. However, CD4 T cells can differentiate into functional subsets based on differences of gene activation and secretion of specific panels of cytokines. One subset, called *T helper 1,* or *Th1,* becomes capable of secreting interferon-γ (IFN-γ), tumor necrosis factor β, and IL-12 but *not* IL-4, IL-5, and IL-10. The other subset, *T helper 2,* or *Th2,* becomes capable of secreting IL-4, IL-5, and IL-10 but not Th1 cytokines.

These subsets are important because the different cytokines produced by Th1 or Th2 profoundly influence immune processing, B-cell antibody synthesis, and cell-mediated effector responses (see below). For example, cytokines such as IFN-γ produced by Th1 cells block the differentiation and activation of Th2 cells, and vice versa. The regulation determining whether a Th1 or a Th2 response develops in response to exposure to a

Immune Processing

B Cell

IgM	IgG1 or 3	IgG4	IgE	IgA
Complement, ADCC	Agglutinize	Allergen	Secretory

CD4 T Cells

Helper "Th1"

Cytokines synthesized:
IL-2
IFN-γ
TNF-β
IL-12

Functions:
Inhibits Th2
Helps IgG1, IgG3

Helper "Th2"

Cytokines synthesized:
IL-4
IL-5
IL-10

Functions:
Inhibits Th1
Helps IgE, IgA

Lymph Node

CD8 T Cells

Suppressor

Cytokines synthesized:
TGF-β
Others

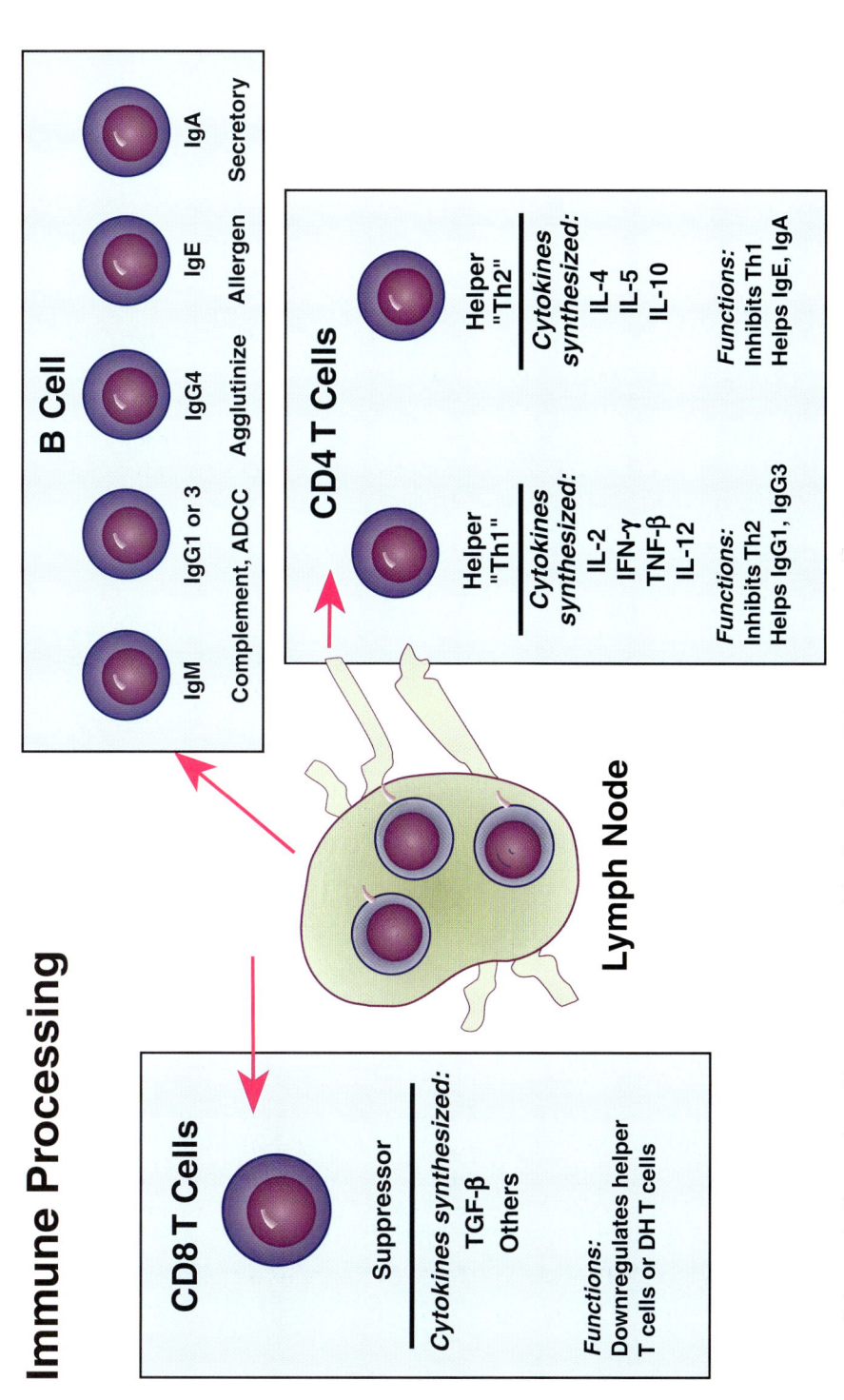

Functions:
Downregulates helper T cells or DH T cells

Figure 2-4 Schematic illustration of immune processing of antigen within the lymph node. On exposure to antigen and antigen-processing cells (APCs) within the lymph node, the three major lymphocyte subsets—B cells, CD4 T cells, and CD8 T cells—are activated to release specific cytokines and perform specific functional activities. B cells are stimulated to produce one of the various antibody isotypes, whose functions include complement activation, antibody-dependent cellular cytotoxicity, agglutinization, allergen recognition, or release into secretions. (See Chapter 4 for a detailed discussion.) CD4 T cells become activated into T helper 1 (Th1) or T helper 2 (Th2) subsets. Th1 cells function to help B cells to secrete immunoglobulin G1 (IgG1) and IgG3; to inhibit Th2; and to release cytokines such as interleukin-2 (IL-2), interferon-γ (IFN-γ), tumor necrosis factor β (TNF-β), and interleukin-12 (IL-12). Th2 cells function to help B cells to secrete IgE and IgA; to inhibit Th1 cells; and to synthesize cytokines such as IL-4, IL-5, and IL-10. CD8 T cells become activated into suppressor T cells that function by inhibiting other CD4 T cells, often by secreting cytokines such as TNF-β. *(Illustration by Barb Cousins, modified by Joyce Zavarro.)*

particular antigen is not entirely understood, but presumed variables include cytokines preexisting in the microenvironment, the nature or amount of antigen, and the type of APC. For example, IL-12 that is produced by macrophage APCs might preferentially induce Th1 responses.

> Von Andrien UH, MacKay CR. Advances in immunology: T-cell function and migration—two sides of the same coin. *N Engl J Med*. 2000;343:1020–1034.

B-cell activation

One of the major regulatory functions for helper T cells concerns B-cell activation. B lymphocytes are responsible for producing antibodies, which are glycoproteins able to bind biochemically to a specific antigenic substance. B cells begin as naive lymphocytes bearing on the cell surface antibodies IgM and IgD, which serve as the B-cell antigen receptor. Through these surface antibodies, B cells can detect epitopes on intact antigens and thus do not require antigen processing by APCs. After appropriate stimulation of the B-cell antigen receptor, helper T cell–B cell interaction occurs, leading to further B-cell activation and differentiation. B cells acquire new functional properties, such as cell division, cell surface expression of accessory molecules, and the ability to synthesize and release large quantities of antibodies. Most important, activated B cells acquire the ability to change antibody class from IgM to another class (eg, to IgG1, IgA, or another immunoglobulin). This shift requires a molecular change of the immunoglobulin heavy chain class at the genetic level, which is regulated by specific cytokines released by the helper T cell. For example, treatment of an antigen-primed B cell with the cytokine IFN-γ induces a switch from antibody IgM to IgG1. Treatment with IL-4 induces a switch from IgM to IgE switch. Chapter 4 discusses the importance of the different antibody classes in immune reactivity.

Role of suppressor T cells

The regulation of the B-cell and helper T-cell response has recently been clarified, and the roles of antigen receptors, tolerance, and immune microenvironments are discussed in Chapter 5. The immunoregulatory role of suppressor T cells has become partially clarified, especially through the induction of immunosuppressive cytokine synthesis by regulatory T cells. Classically, suppressor T cells were observed to express the CD8 marker and to become activated during the initial phases of processing. More recently, certain CD4 T cells have also been observed to have suppressive functions. In many cases, both CD8 and CD4 suppressors appear to operate by the release of immunosuppressive cytokines such as transforming growth factor–β, which can inhibit or alter the helper or effector function of other T cells. Other classic mechanisms of suppressor T-cell function, such as complicated antigen-specific T-cell circuits and release of antigen-specific suppressor molecules, have received less attention. The mechanism for activation of suppressor T cells is under investigation, but immunization of antigens orally or through an anterior chamber injection are two immune response arcs that preferentially induce suppressor T cells (see below). The relationship between CD8 suppressor T cells and CD8 cytotoxic effector cells is unclear; these two probably represent different subpopulations of CD8 T cells.

Effector Phase

During the effector phase, the adaptive immune response (eg, get rid of offending foreign antigen) is physically carried out. Antigen-specific effectors exist in two major subsets:

- T cells
- B cells plus their antibodies

A third population of *non-T, non-B effector lymphocytes,* formerly called *null cells,* is sometimes also grouped with immune effectors, although these cells are not antigen-specific and might be considered part of the innate immune system.

In general, effector lymphocytes require two exposures to antigen:

- The initial exposure, often called *priming* or *activation,* occurring in the lymph node
- A second exposure, often called *restimulation,* happening in the peripheral tissue in which the initial antigen contact occurred

This second exposure is usually necessary to fully exploit the effector mechanism within a local tissue. All of these effector mechanisms are described in much more detail in Chapter 4.

Subsets of effector T lymphocytes can be distinguished into two main types by functional differences in experimental assays or by differences in cell surface expression of marker molecules (Fig 2-5). *Delayed hypersensitivity (DH) T cells* usually express CD4 marker and release specific cytokines such as IFN-γ and tumor necrosis factor β. They function by homing into a tissue, recognizing antigen and APCs, becoming fully activated, and releasing cytokines and mediators that then recruit other nonspecific, antigen-independent effector cells such as neutrophils, basophils, or monocytes. As for helper T cells, Th1 and Th2 types of DH effector cells have been identified.

Cytotoxic T lymphocytes are the other type of major effector T cell. Cytotoxic T lymphocytes express CD8 marker and serve as effector cells for killing tumors or virally infected host cells through release of cytotoxic cytokines or specialized pore-forming molecules. The subset of effector lymphocytes formerly called null cells but now grouped as non-T, non-B lymphocytes includes natural killer cells, lymphokine-activated cells, and killer cells.

Antibodies, or *immunoglobulins,* are soluble antigen-specific effector molecules of adaptive immunity. After appropriate antigenic stimulation with T-cell help, B cells secrete IgM antibodies, and later other isotypes, into the efferent lymph fluid draining into the venous circulation. Antibodies then mediate a variety of immune effector activities by combining with antigen in the blood or in tissues.

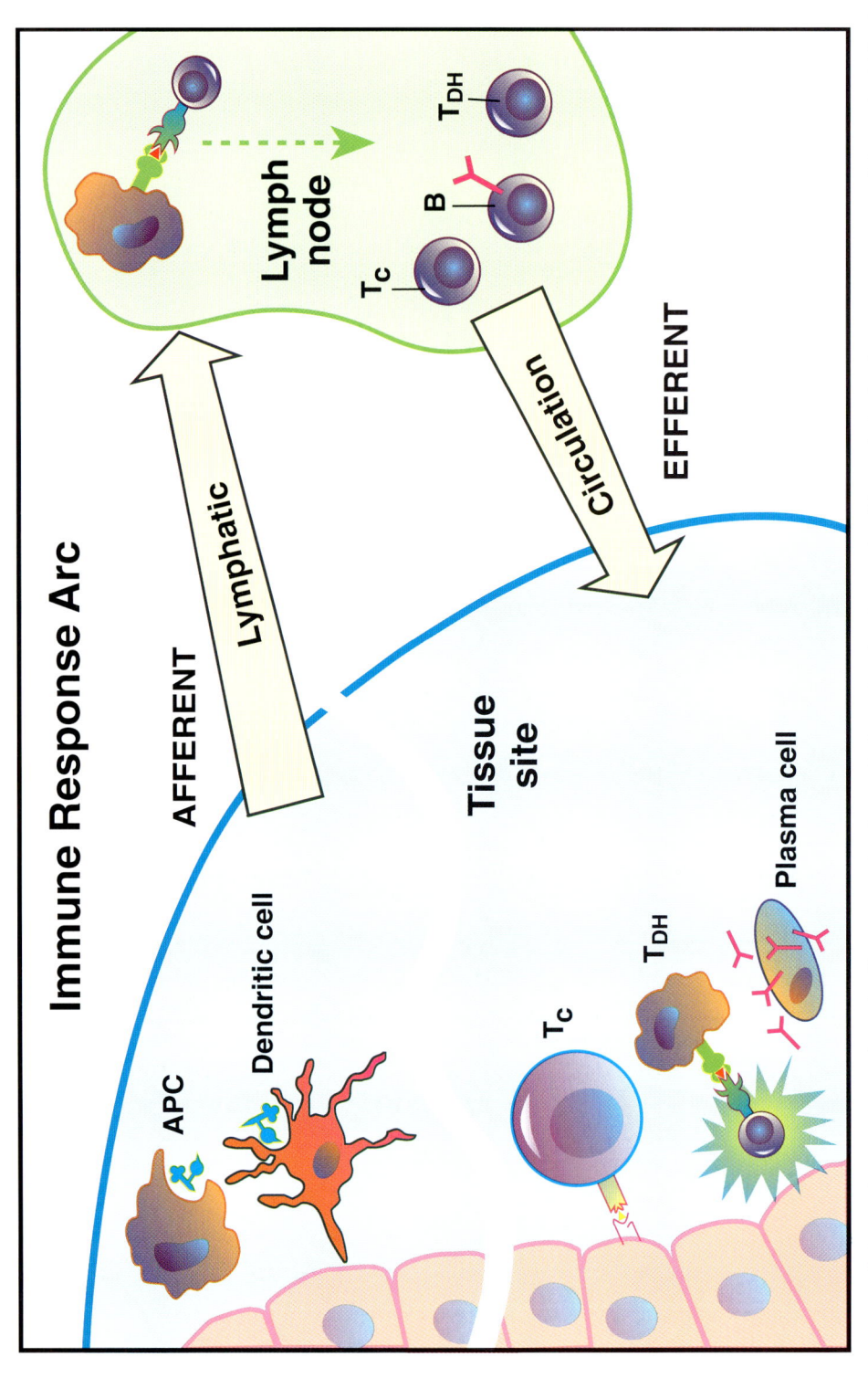

Figure 2-5 Schematic representation of effector mechanisms during adaptive immunity. Not only is the immune response initiated within the tissue site, but ultimately the immune response arc is completed when effectors encounter antigen within the tissue after release into the circulation from the lymph node. The three most important effector mechanisms of adaptive immunity include cytotoxic T cells (T_C), delayed hypersensitivity T cells (T_{DH}), and antibody-producing B cells, especially plasma cells. APC, antigen-processing cells. *(Illustration by Barb Cousins, modified by Joyce Zavarro.)*

Immune Response Arc and Primary or Secondary Immune Responses

Concept of Immunologic Memory

Immunologic memory is probably the most distinctive feature of adaptive immune responses and is in many ways synonymous with the idea of protective immunization. Classically, immunologic memory was the concept used to explain why serum antibody production for a specific antigen increased markedly after reexposure to that antigen but not after exposure to a different antigen. Later it was learned that the concept of memory applied not only to antibody production by B cells but also to T lymphocytes.

Differences in primary and secondary responses

Memory implies that the second encouner with an antigen is regulated differently from the first encounter. Differences in the primary and secondary immune response arc, especially in the processing and effector phases, offer partial explanation. During the processing phase of the primary response, antigen must find the relatively rare specific B cell (perhaps 1 in 100,000) and T cell (perhaps 1 in 10,000), then stimulate these cells from a completely resting and naive state, a sequence that requires days. The secondary processing response for T and B cells is shorter for at least three reasons:

- Upon removal of antigen, T and B lymphocytes activated during the primary response may gradually return to a resting state, but they retain the capacity to become reactivated within 12–24 hours of antigen exposure. That is, they are now memory cells rather than naive cells.
- Because stimulated lymphocytes divide, the population of potential antigen-responsive T or B cells will have increased manyfold, and these cells will have migrated to other sites of potential encounters with antigen.
- In some cases, such as in mycobacterial infection, low doses of antigen may remain in the node or site, producing a chronic, low-level, continuous antigenic stimulation of T and B cells.

For antibody responses, another memory function dependent on antibody requires even less time and operates primarily at the level of the effector phase. IgM produced during the effector phase of the primary response and released into the blood is often too large to passively leak into a peripheral site. However, during the secondary response, antibody class switching has occurred so that IgG or other isotypes that have passively leaked into a site or have been actively produced there can immediately combine with an antigen, causing the secondary response triggered by antibody to be very rapid *(immediate hypersensitivity)*.

Homing

Memory also requires that lymphocytes demonstrate a complex migratory pattern called *homing*. Thus, lymphocytes pass from the circulation into various tissues from which they subsequently depart and then pass by way of lymphatics to reenter the circulation. Homing involves the variable interaction between lymphocytes and endothelial cells using multiple *cell-adhesion molecules,* which are discussed in Chapter 4. Usually, the major types of lymphocytes that migrate into tissue sites are memory lymphocytes that express higher levels of certain cell-adhesion molecules, such as the integrins and immunoglobulin superfamily, than do naive cells. Naive lymphocytes tend to migrate to lymphoid tissues, where they have the chance of meeting their cognate antigen. Inflammation, however, changes the rules and serves to break down homing patterns. At inflammatory sites, the volume of lymphocyte migration is far greater and selection much less precise, although migration of memory cells or activated lymphocytes still exceeds that of naive cells.

Regional Immunity and Immunologic Microenvironments

Regional Immunity

The idea that each organ and tissue site has its own particular immune response arc, which may vary significantly from the classic cutaneous response, is called *regional immunity.* Regional immunity of the tissue site can characterize all three phases—afferent, processing, and efferent—of the responses involved. For instance, the immune response arc for oral immunization (eg, polio vaccine) differs from intramuscular immunization (eg, mumps/measles/rubella vaccine), which differs from cutaneous vaccination (eg, bacille Calmette-Guérin vaccine). Regional immunity also affects the transplantation of donor tissue, such as a kidney or cornea. Such transplantations require the recipient to produce afferent, processing, and effector responses to the transplant, all modified by the unique location. Chapter 3 describes regional immune concepts relevant to the eye. See also BCSC Section 8, *External Disease and Cornea,* for a discussion of the regional immunity of the cornea in Part XI, Corneal Transplantation.

Immunologic Microenvironments

Regional immunologic differences occur because different tissue sites are composed of different *immunologic microenvironments.* The concept of immunologic microenvironment incorporates a broad range of anatomical and physiological differences among tissues or organs that regulate the immune response:

- The presence of well-formed lymphatics
- Specialized immunologic structures (Peyer's patches or conjunctival follicles)
- Blood–tissue barriers to macromolecules or cell migration
- Type of resident APC
- Constitutive synthesis of immunoregulatory cytokines or molecules by the parenchymal cell types
- Many other factors

The analysis of immunologic microenvironments has become important for understanding the immunology of transplantation, infection, or autoimmunity for gene therapy or many organ systems.

Clinical Examples of the Concept of the Immune Response Arc

The concept of the immune response arc is a powerful tool to understand clinically relevant immunologic phenomena. The two examples of cutaneous immunity (see the following Clinical Examples) illustrate this feature. Throughout the discussion in Chapters 3, 4, and 5, such clinical examples are interspersed with the text to provide similar illustrations.

Male DK, Cooke A, Owen M, et al. *Advanced Immunology*. 3rd ed. St Louis: Mosby; 1996.
Roitt IM, Delves PJ. *Roitt's Essential Immunology*. 10th ed. Malden, MA: Blackwell Science; 2001.

CLINICAL EXAMPLES

Primary response to poison ivy toxin The first encounter with the poison ivy resin urushiol and contact on the epidermal surface of an exposed extremity, such as the forearm, trigger the immunologic mechanisms of poison ivy dermatitis. The *afferent phase* of this primary response begins when the toxin permeates into the epidermis, where much of it binds to extracellular proteins, forming a protein–toxin conjugate technically called a *hapten*. Some of the toxin is taken up by APCs (especially Langerhans cells), and over the next 4–18 hours the toxin-stimulated LCs leave their normal location in the basal epidermis and migrate along afferent lymphatics into the draining lymph nodes. During this time, the toxin is internalized into endocytic compartments and processed by the LCs so that it can be recognized by helper T cells within the node. Some of the free toxin or hapten is also carried by lymph into the node.

In the lymph node, the *processing phase* begins. The urushiol-stimulated LCs interact with T cells, seeking over the next 3–5 days the rare T cell that has the correct specific antigen receptor. Once located, the naive T cell becomes primed. It is induced to undergo cell division, to acquire new functions such as cytokine secretion, and to upregulate certain surface molecules and receptors of the plasma membrane. These primed cells ultimately either function as helper cells or become effector cells that leave the node through efferent lymphatics, accumulate in the thoracic duct, and then enter venous blood, where they recirculate.

Free toxin or hapten not taken up by APCs experiences a different fate during the processing phase. It enters a zone of the lymph node populated by B cells. These naive B cells express membrane-bound antibody (IgM and IgD) that serves as antigen receptor. If a chance encounter occurs between the correct antibody and the toxin, the B cell becomes partially activated. However, completion of the B-cell activation requires further interaction with helper T cells, which release cytokines, inducing B cells to undergo cell division and to increase production of antibodies, thus releasing antitoxin antibody into the lymph fluid and ultimately the venous circulation.

The *effector phase* begins when the primed T cells, primed B cells, or antibody leave the lymphatics and enter the peripheral site of the original antigen encounter. By 5–7 days after exposure, much of the urushiol toxin might have already been removed through nonspecific clearance mechanisms such as desquamation of exposed epidermis, washing of involved skin, and subclinical effects of innate immunity. When toxin-stimulated APCs do remain at the site, primed T cells become further activated into effector cells, releasing inflammatory mediators to recruit other leukocyte populations. This represents the contact hypersensitivity type of delayed hypersensitivity. Rarely, if adequate free toxin is present, IgG antitoxin immune complexes can form and mediate inflammation (see below). However, if most of the antigen is already cleared, then the primed T cell may enter the skin but become inactive, retaining memory. Or the T cell may exit the skin through afferent lymphatics to reenter the lymph node. Similarly, antibody or antibody-producing B cells may remain in the skin or reach the lymph nodes.

Secondary response to poison ivy toxin The immunologic mechanisms work much faster after the second encounter with poison ivy toxin. The *afferent phase* of this secondary response begins when the toxin permeates the epidermis. Again, some of the toxin is taken up by the LCs and internalized over the next 4–18 hours into endocytic compartments and processed in a way that can be recognized by T cells. If a memory T cell is present at the cutaneous site, then the *processing* and *effector phases* occur within 24 hours at the site, as the memory T cell becomes activated upon interacting with the LC. In addition, some LCs leave the skin, enter the draining node, and encounter memory T cells there.

Processing during the secondary response is much quicker, and within 24 hours restimulated memory cells enter the circulation and migrate to the toxin-exposed cutaneous site. Because abundant toxin remains, additional T cell–LC stimulation occurs, inducing vigorous T-cell cytokine production. The inflammatory mediators, in turn, recruit neutrophils and monocytes, leading to a severe inflammatory reaction within 12–36 hours after exposure, causing the typical epidermal blisters of poison ivy. Because the response is delayed by 24 hours, it is considered delayed hypersensitivity and, in this case, a specific form of delayed hypersensitivity called *contact hypersensitivity*.

Primary and secondary response to tuberculosis The primary and secondary immune response arcs can occur at different sites, as with the immunologic mechanisms of the first and second encounter with *Mycobacterium tuberculosis* antigens. The *afferent phase* of the primary response occurs after the inhalation of the live organisms, which proliferate slowly within the lung. Alveolar macrophages ingest the bacteria and transport the organisms to the hilar lymph nodes, where the *processsing phase* begins. Over the next few days, as T and B lymphocytes are primed, the hilar nodes become enlarged because of the increased number of dividing T and B cells as well as generalized increased trafficking of other lymphocytes through the node. The *effector phase* begins when the primed T cells recirculate and enter the infected lung. T cells interact with macrophage-ingested bacteria, and cytokines are released that activate neighboring macrophages to fuse into giant cells, forming caseating granulomas. Meanwhile, some of the effector T cells home to other lymph nodes throughout the body, where they become inactive memory T cells, trafficking and recirculating throughout the secondary lymphoid tissue.

A secondary response using the immune response arc of the skin is the basis of the tuberculin skin test to diagnose TB. The *afferent phase* of the secondary response begins when purified protein derivative (PPD) reagent, antigens purified from mycobacteria, is injected into the dermis, where the PPD is taken up by dermal macrophages. The secondary *processing phase* begins when these PPD-stimulated macrophages migrate into the draining lymph node, where they encounter memory T cells from the previous lung infection, leading to memory T-cell reactivation. The secondary *effector phase* commences when these reactivated memory T cells recirculate and home back into the dermis and encounter additional antigen/macrophages at the site, causing the T cells to become fully activated and release cytokines. Within 24–72 hours, these cytokines induce infiltration of additional lymphocytes and monocytes as well as fibrin clotting. This process produces the typical indurated dermal lesion of the tuberculosis skin test, called the *tuberculin form* of delayed hypersensitivity.

CHAPTER 3

Ocular Immune Responses

Just as regional differences in immune responses occur because of differences in the immunologic microenvironments of various tissue sites, regional differences can be identified for specific locations within and around the eye. Immune responses in health and disease are affected by differences in the immunologic microenvironment (Table 3-1) in such areas as

- Conjunctiva
- Anterior chamber, anterior uvea (iris and ciliary body), and vitreous
- Cornea and sclera
- Retina/retinal pigment epithelium (RPE)/choriocapillaris

Immune Responses of the Conjunctiva

Features of the Immunologic Microenvironment

The conjunctiva shares many of the features typical of mucosal sites. It is composed of two layers: an epithelial layer and a connective tissue layer called the *substantia propria*. The conjunctiva is well vascularized and has good lymphatic drainage to preauricular and submandibular nodes. The tissue is richly invested with Langerhans cells, other dendritic cells, and macrophages to serve as potential antigen-presenting cells (APCs). Conjunctival follicles that enlarge after certain types of ocular surface infection or inflammation represent collections of T cells, B cells, and APCs. Observation of the function of similar sites, such as Peyer's patches of the intestine, suggests that follicles might represent a site for localized immune processing of antigens that permeate through the thin overlying epithelium to be processed by T cells and B cells locally within the follicle.

The conjunctiva, especially the substantia propria, is richly infiltrated with potential effector cells, predominately mast cells. All antibody isotypes are represented, and presumably local production as well as passive leakage occurs. IgA is the most abundant antibody in the tear film. Soluble molecules of the innate immune system are also represented, especially complement. The conjunctiva appears to support most adaptive and innate immune effector responses, especially antibody-mediated and lymphocyte-mediated responses, although IgE-mediated mast cell degranulation is one of the most common and important. Chapter 4 discusses these mechanisms in greater detail. See also Part IV of BCSC Section 8, *External Disease and Cornea*.

Table 3-1 Comparison of Immune Microenvironments in Various Normal Ocular Sites

	Conjunctiva	Cornea/Sclera	Anterior Chamber, Anterior Uvea, Vitreous	Subretina/RPE/Choroid
Anatomical features	Lymphatics, follicles	Lymphatics at limbus, none centrally Macromolecules diffuse through stroma	No lymphatics, antigen clearance through trabecular meshwork Partial blood–uveal barrier	No lymphatics Blood–retina barrier Uveal circulation permeable
Resident APC	Dendritic and Langerhans cells, macrophages	Langerhans cells at limbus No APC in central cornea No APC in sclera Epithelium/endothelium can be induced to express class II MHC	Many dendritic cells and macrophages in iris and ciliary body Hyalocytes are macrophage-derived	Microglia in the retina Dendritic cells and macrophages in choriocapillaris RPE can be induced to express class II MHC
Specialized immune compartments for localized immune processing	?? Follicles	None	None	None
Resident effector cells	Mast cells, T cells, B cells, plasma cells, rare PMN	Centrally—none Sclera—none	Rare to no T cells or B cells, rare mast cells	Retina—normally no lymphocytes Choroid—mast cells, some lymphocytes
Resident effector molecules	All antibody isotypes, especially IgE, IgG subclasses, IgA in tears Complement and kininogen precursors present	Peripherally Igs but minimal IgM Centrally minimal antibody, some complement present Sclera: low antibody concentration, minimal IgM	Kallikrein but not kininogen precursors Some complement present, but less than in blood Minimal Igs in iris, some IgG in ciliary body and aqueous humor	Retina—minimal to no Igs Choroid—IgGs and IgA
Immunoregulatory systems	Mucosa-associated lymphoid tissue	Immune privilege—Fas ligand, avascularity, lack of central APC	Immune privilege—anterior chamber-associated immune deviation, immuno-suppressive factors in aqueous, Fas ligand	Immune privilege—?? mechanisms

CLINICAL EXAMPLE

Immune response to viral conjunctivitis Conjunctivitis caused by adenovirus infection is a common ocular infection (see BCSC Section 8, *External Disease and Cornea*). Although details of the immune response after conjunctival adenovirus infection remain unknown, they can be inferred from knowledge of viral infection at other mucosal sites and from animal studies. After infection with adenovirus, the epithelial cells begin to die within 36 hours. Innate immune mechanisms that can assist in limiting infection become activated soon after infection. For example, infected cells produce cytokines such as interferons that limit spread of infectious virus and recruit nonspecific effector cells such as macrophages and PMNs.

However, the adaptive immune response to adenovirus infection is considered more important in viral clearance. The primary adaptive response begins when macrophages and dendritic cells presumably become infected or take up cell debris and viral antigens. Both APCs and extracellular antigenic material are conveyed to the preauricular and submandibular nodes along lymphatics, where vigorous helper T-cell and antibody responses are activated, producing lymphadenopathy. Local immune processing may also occur within the follicle if virus invades the epithelial capsule. During the early effector phase of the primary B-cell response, IgM antibodies are released into the blood that will *not* be very effective in controlling surface infection, although they will prevent widespread viremia. However, IgM-bearing B cells eventually infiltrate the conjunctival stroma and may release antibody locally in the conjunctiva. Later, during the primary effector response, class switching to IgG or IgA may occur to mediate local effector responses, such as neutralization or complement-mediated lysis of infected cells.

The most active effector response later in acute viral infection comes from natural killer cells and CD8 cytotoxic T lymphocytes (CTLs), which kill infected epithelium. However, adenovirus can block the expression of class I MHC on infected cells and thereby escape being killed by CTLs. Adaptive immunity can also activate macrophages by antiviral DH mechanisms later during infection, and DH response to viral antigens is thought to contribute to the development of the corneal subepithelial infiltrates that occur in some patients late in adenovirus infection.

The secondary response of the conjunctiva, assuming a prior primary exposure to the same virus at some other mucosal site, differs in that antibody-mediated effector mechanisms dominate. Because of MALT, antivirus IgA is present not only in blood but also in tears as a result of differentiated IgA-secreting B cells in the lacrimal gland, the substantia propria, and follicles. Thus, recurrent infection is often prevented by preexisting neutralizing antibodies that had disseminated into tears or follicles following the primary infection. However, if the inoculum of recurrent virus overwhelms this antibody barrier, or if the virus has mutated its surface glycoproteins recognized by antibodies, then epithelial infection does occur. Additional immune processing can occur in the follicle and draining nodes. Specific memory effector CTLs are effective in clearing infection within a few days.

Nathanson N, ed. *Viral Pathogenesis*. Philadelphia: Lippincott; 1996.

Pepose JS, Holland GN, Wilhelmus KR, eds. *Ocular Infection and Immunity*. St. Louis: Mosby; 1996.

Immunoregulatory Systems

The most important immunoregulatory system for the conjunctiva is called *mucosa-associated lymphoid tissue (MALT)*. The concept MALT refers to the interconnected network of mucosal sites (the epithelial lining of the respiratory tract, gut, and genitourinary tract and the ocular surface and its adnexae) that share certain specific immunologic features:

- Rich investment of APCs
- Specialized structures for localized antigen processing (ie, Peyer's patches or tonsils)
- Unique effector cells (ie, intraepithelial T cells and abundant mast cells)

However, the most distinctive aspect of MALT is the distribution and homing of effector T and B cells induced by immunization at one mucosal site to all MALT sites because of the shared expression of specific cell-adhesion molecules on postcapillary venules of the mucosal vasculature. MALT immune response arcs tend to favor T helper 2 (Th2)-dominated responses that result in production of predominantly IgA and IgE antibodies. Immunization of soluble antigens through MALT, especially in the gut sites, often produces oral tolerance, presumably by activating Th2-like regulatory T cells that suppress Th1–delayed hypersensitivity (DH) effector cells.

Immune Responses of the Anterior Chamber, Anterior Uvea, and Vitreous

Features of the Immunologic Microenvironment

Numerous specialized anatomical features of the anterior region affect ocular immune responses. The anterior chamber is a fluid-filled cavity; circulating aqueous humor provides a unique medium for intercellular communication between cytokines, or immune cells, and resident tissue cells of the iris, ciliary body, and corneal endothelium. Although aqueous humor is relatively protein-depleted compared to serum (about 0.1%–1.0% of serum total protein), even normal aqueous humor contains a complex mixture of biological factors, such as immunosuppressive cytokines, neuropeptides, and complement inhibitors, that can influence immunologic events within the eye.

A partial blood–ocular barrier is present. Fenestrated capillaries in the ciliary body allow a size-dependent concentration gradient of plasma macromolecules to permeate the interstitial tissue; smaller plasma-derived molecules are present in higher concentration than are larger molecules. The tight junctions between the pigmented and the non-pigmented ciliary epithelium provide a more exclusive barrier, preventing interstitial macromolecules from permeating directly through the ciliary body into the aqueous humor. Nevertheless, low numbers of plasma macromolecules bypass the nonpigmented epithelium barrier and may permeate by diffusion anteriorly through the uvea to enter the anterior chamber through the anterior iris surface.

The inner eye does not contain well-developed lymphatics. Rather, clearance of soluble substances depends on the aqueous humor outflow channels; clearance of particulates depends on endocytosis by trabecular meshwork endothelial cells or macrophages. Nevertheless, antigen inoculation into the anterior chamber results in efficient communication with the systemic immune response. Intact soluble antigens gain entrance to the venous circulation, where they communicate with the spleen.

The iris and ciliary body contain a rich investment of macrophages and dendritic cells that serve as APCs and possible effector cells. Immune processing is unlikely to occur locally, but APCs leave the eye by the trabecular meshwork and home to the spleen, where processing occurs that favors a Th2 response and preferential activation of CD8 suppressor T cells. Few resident T cells and some mast cells are present in the normal anterior uvea. B cells, eosinophils, and polymorphonuclear neutrophils (PMNs) appear to be absent. Very low concentrations of IgG, complement components, and kallikrein occur in normal eyes.

The vitreous has not been characterized as carefully as the anterior chamber, but the vitreous probably manifests most of the same properties with several notable exceptions. The vitreous gel can electrostatically bind charged protein substances and may thus serve as an antigen depot as well as a substrate for leukocyte cell adhesion. Because the vitreous contains type II collagen, it may serve as a depot of potential autoantigen in some forms of uveitis related to arthritis in which type II collagen in the joint is an autoantigen. See also BCSC Section 12, *Retina and Vitreous.*

Immunoregulatory Systems

The anterior uvea has an immunoregulatory system that has been described as *immune privilege.* The modern conception of immune privilege refers to the observation that tumor implants or allografts unexpectedly survive better within an immunologically privileged region, whereas a similar implant or graft is rapidly rejected by immune mechanisms within the skin or other nonprivileged sites. Other immune-privileged sites are the subretinal space, the brain, and the testes. Although the nature of the antigen involved is probably important, immune privilege of the anterior uvea has been observed with a wide variety of antigens, including alloantigens (ie, transplantation antigens), tumor antigens, haptens, soluble proteins, autoantigens, bacteria, and viruses.

Immune privilege is mediated by influences on both the afferent and the effector phases of the immune response arc. Immunization using the anterior segment as the afferent phase of a primary immune response arc results in a unique generation of immunologic effectors. Immunization as with lens protein or other autoantigens through the anterior chamber does not result in the same pattern of systemic immunity as does immunization by skin, contrary to intuitive assumptions. Immunization by an anterior chamber injection in experimental animals results in an altered form of systemic immunity to that antigen called *anterior chamber–associated immune deviation (ACAID).*

Following injection of antigen into the anterior chamber, the afferent phase begins when specialized macrophages residing in the iris recognize and take up the antigen. The APC function of these uveal macrophages has been altered by exposure to immunoregulatory cytokines normally present within aqueous humor and uveal tissue, especially transforming growth factor β2 (TGF-β2). The process by which aqueous humor factors convert macrophages into ACAID-inducing APCs is unknown. The TGF-β–exposed antigen-stimulated ocular macrophages leave by the trabecular meshwork and Schlemm's canal to enter the venous circulation, where they preferentially migrate to the spleen. Here, the antigen signal is processed, with activation of not only helper T cells and B cells but also suppressor T cells. the CD8 suppressor cells serve to alter CD4 helper T-cell responses in the spleen and to downregulate CD4 T-cell DH responses to the specific *immunizing* antigen at all body sites. Thus, the resulting effector response is characterized by a selective suppression of antigen-specific DH and a selectively diminished production of complement-fixing isotypes of antibodies. The other antibody isotypes and cytotoxic T-cell precursors are the same as those occurring after conventional cutaneous immunization.

Several other mechanisms for ACAID have been proposed. A small percentage of intact antigen can leave the eye to enter the blood, where it tends to be processed within the spleen. Low doses of intravenous antigens produce a form of immunosuppression that has been called *low-zone tolerance*. Various mechanisms for immunoregulatory T-cell activation within the eye have been suggested as well.

Especially important to the clinician is the capacity of a tissue site to sustain the secondary effector phase of the immune response arc, because the primary immune response arc in autoimmune diseases might have occurred outside of the eye. In this regard, the secondary effector phase of the anterior segment is also immunosuppressive and has been termed the *effector blockade*. Because various immunoregulatory systems are normally present within the eye, intact immunologic effectors that are functional elsewhere—in the skin, for example—are *partially* blocked from activation and function within the anterior segment. Thus, Th1 DH T cells, cytotoxic T cells, natural killer cells, and complement activation appear to function less effectively in the anterior uvea than elsewhere. For instance, the anterior uvea is *relatively* resistant to induction of a secondary purified protein derivative DH response after primary immunization with mycobacteria in the skin. Mechanisms for effector blockade are multifactorial but include production of the following:

- Immunosuppressive cytokines, produced by ocular tissues
- Immunosuppressive neuropeptides, produced by ocular nerves
- Functionally unique APCs
- Complement inhibitors in aqueous humor
- Other factors

Recently, investigators have demonstrated the expression of a molecule called *Fas ligand* (FasL, or CD95 ligand) on iris and corneal endothelium. FasL is normally expressed in the thymus and a few other immune-privileged sites such as the testes. FasL is a potent trigger of programmed cell death, or *apoptosis,* of lymphocytes. Thus, FasL can induce apoptotic killing of infiltrating T cells, thereby preventing T-cell effector function. The loss of these protective mechanisms is presumed to occur prior to the development of uveitis.

The vitreous cavity has not been so well characterized immunologically, but preliminary experimental evidence suggests that an ACAID-like primary immune response arc probably applies to the vitreous as well, especially in an eye that has undergone vitrectomy. The existence of effector blockade in the vitreous is controversial, but this form of immunosuppression might be stimulated by vitrectomy. Other rationales for performing vitrectomy in eyes with uveitis are

- To remove any depot of antigen, including type II collagen, trapped in the gel
- To remove the gel substrate for cell-adhesion molecules to recruit and adhere leukocytes
- To allow circulation of immunosuppressive factors in aqueous humor

> **CLINICAL EXAMPLE**
>
> **Therapeutic potential of immune privilege** It is unknown whether ACAID has practical consequences for clinical diseases, although ACAID is thought to play a role in immunologic tolerance to lens crystallins after cataract surgery and in immunologic acceptance of corneal transplantation. ACAID can influence the immune response to ocular autoantigens. Animals immunized through the anterior chamber with the retinal autoantigens S-antigen or interphotoreceptor retinol-binding protein develop ACAID, and they are then protected from experimental autoimmune uveitis in the contralateral eye after subsequent conventional cutaneous immunization. Recently, ACAID has been reproduced by infusion of monocytes that were first treated extracorporeally with TGF-β and antigen, suggesting a potential clinically relevant method for immunotherapy.
>
> Ferguson TA, Griffith TS. A vision of cell death: insights into immune privilege. *Immunol Rev.* 1997;156:167–184.

Immune Responses of the Cornea

Features of the Immunologic Microenvironment

The cornea is unique in that the periphery and the central portions of the tissue represent distinctly different immunologic microenvironments (Fig 3-1). Obviously, only the limbus is vascularized. Whereas the limbus is richly invested with Langerhans cells, the peripheral, paracentral, and central cornea are normally devoid of APCs. However, various stimuli such as mild trauma, certain cytokines (eg, IL-1), or infection can recruit APCs to the central cornea. Plasma-derived enzymes (ie, complement), IgM, and IgG are present in moderate concentrations in the periphery, but only low levels of the IgGs are present centrally.

Corneal cells also appear to synthesize various antimicrobial and immunoregulatory proteins. Effector cells are absent or scarce in the normal cornea, but PMNs, monocytes, and lymphocytes can readily migrate through the stroma if appropriate chemotactic stimuli are activated. Lymphocytes, monocytes, and PMNs can also adhere to the endothelial surface during inflammation, giving rise to keratic precipitates or the classic Khodadoust line of endothelial rejection (Fig 3-2). Localized immune processing probably does not occur in the cornea. See also BCSC Section 8, *External Disease and Cornea*.

Immunoregulatory Systems

The cornea also demonstrates a form of immune privilege different from that observed in the anterior uvea. Immune privilege of the cornea is multifactorial. Normal limbal physiology is a major component, especially the maintenance of avascularity and lack of APCs in the mid and central cornea. The absence of APCs and lymphatics partially inhibits afferent recognition in the central cornea, and the absence of postcapillary venules centrally can limit the efficiency of effector recruitment, although both effector cells and molecules can ultimately infiltrate even avascular cornea. Another factor is the presence of intact immunoregulatory systems of the anterior chamber (ie, ACAID), to which the corneal endothelium is exposed.

40 • Intraocular Inflammation and Uveitis

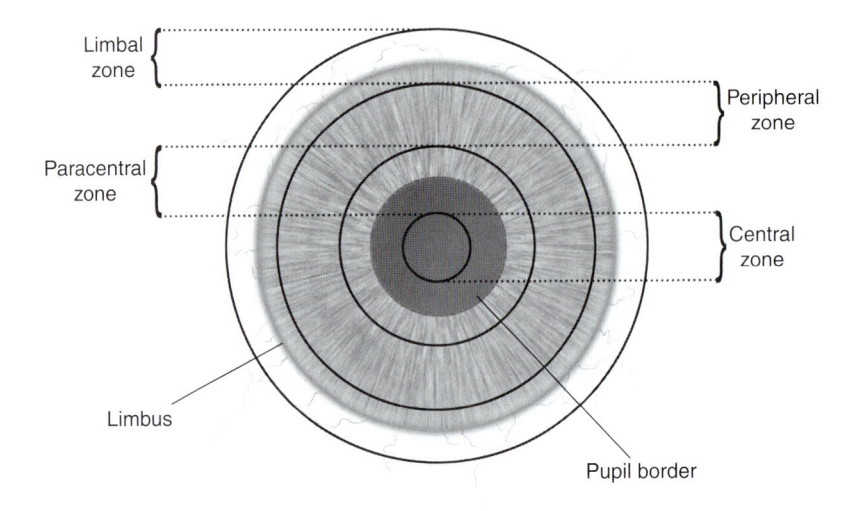

Figure 3-1 Topographic zones of the cornea. *(Illustration by Christine Gralapp.)*

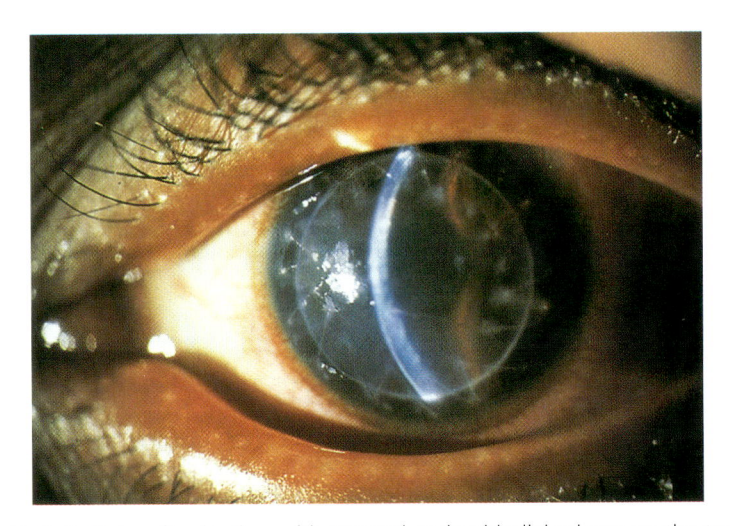

Figure 3-2 Endothelial graft rejection with stromal and epithelial edema on the trailing aspect of the migrating Khodadoust line.

Immune Responses of the Retina, RPE, and Choroid

Features of the Immunologic Microenvironment

The immunologic microenvironments of the retina, RPE, choriocapillaris, and choroid have not been well characterized. The retinal circulation demonstrates a blood–ocular barrier at the level of tight junctions between adjacent endothelial cells. The vessels of the choriocapillaris are highly permeable to macromolecules, allowing transudation of most plasma macromolecules into the extravascular spaces of the choroid and chorio-

> **CLINICAL EXAMPLE**
>
> **Corneal allograft rejection** Penetrating keratoplasty, the transplantation of foreign corneal allografts, enjoys an extremely high success rate (>90%) even in the absence of systemic immunosuppression. This rate compares favorably to the transplantation rates of other donor tissues. The mechanisms of corneal graft survival have been attributed to immune privilege. In experimental models, factors contributing to rejection include the following:
>
> - Presence of central corneal vascularization
> - Induction of MHC molecule expression by the stroma, which is normally quite low
> - Contamination of the donor graft with donor-derived APCs prior to transplantation
> - MHC disparity between the host and the donor
> - Preimmunization of the recipient to donor transplantation antigens
>
> In addition, loss of immunoregulatory systems of the anterior chamber can apparently influence corneal allograft immunity, and the expression of FasL on corneal endothelium has been observed to greatly influence allograft protection. Rapid replacement of donor epithelium by host epithelium removes this layer as an antigenic stimulus. Once activated, however, antibody-dependent DH and CTL-related mechanisms can target transplantation antigens in all corneal layers.
>
> Streilein JW. Regulation of ocular immune responses. *Eye.* 1997;11:171–175.

capillaris. The tight junctions between the RPE cells probably provide the true physiological barrier between the choroid and the retina. Well-developed lymphatics are absent, although both the retina and the choroid have abundant potential APCs. In the retina, resident microglia (bone marrow–derived cells related to monocytes) are interspersed within all layers and can undergo physical changes and migration in response to various stimuli. The choriocapillaris and choroid are richly invested with certain potential APCs, especially macrophages and dendritic cells.

RPE can be induced to express class II MHC molecules, suggesting that RPE may also interact with T cells. The presence of T lymphocytes or B lymphocytes within the normal posterior segment has not been carefully addressed, but effector cells appear to be absent from the normal retina. The density of mast cells is moderate in the choroid, especially around the arterioles, but lymphocytes are present only in very low density. Eosinophils and neutrophils appear to be absent. Under various clinical or experimental conditions, however, high densities of T cells, B cells, macrophages, and PMNs can infiltrate the choroid, choriocapillaris, and retina. The RPE and various cell types within the retina and the choroid (ie, pericytes) can synthesize many different cytokines (eg, TGF-β) that may alter the subsequent immune response. Local immune processing does not appear to occur. See also BCSC Section 12, *Retina and Vitreous.*

Immunoregulatory Systems

Recently, it has been demonstrated that a form of immune privilege is present after subretinal injection of antigen. The mechanism is unclear but is probably similar to ACAID. This observation may be important because of growing interest in retinal transplantation and gene therapy. The capacity of the choriocapillaris and choroid to function as unique environments for the afferent or effector phases has not yet been evaluated.

> **CLINICAL EXAMPLES**
>
> **Retinal transplantation** Transplantation of retina or RPE is being investigated as a method for regeneration of retinal function in various disorders. In experimental animals, subretinal transplantation of fetal retinal tissue or various kinds of RPE allografts often show longer survival than the same grafts implanted elsewhere, even without systemic immunosuppression. The afferent phase recognition of alloantigens is likely performed by retinal microglia or recruited blood-derived macrophages from the choriocapillaris.
>
> The subretinal cytokine environment remains unknown since transplantation is performed in the setting of retinal diseases, such as retinitis pigmentosa or macular degeneration, in which the blood–retina barrier is altered and retinal cell/RPE injury is present. However, injured RPE can still synthesize either immunosuppressive or inflammatory cytokines. The site of immune processing is unknown, but the spleen or some other secondary compartment outside of the eye is probably involved. When rejection does occur, the effector mechanisms are also unclear. In mice with fetal retinal grafts, immune rejection occurs by an unusual slowly progressive cytotoxic mechanism not involving typical antibody-mediated cytolysis or DH T cells. In humans and nonhuman primates, rejection of RPE allografts has occurred in both subacute and chronic forms.
>
> **Retinal gene therapy** Retinal gene therapy is the therapeutic use of intentional transfection of photoreceptors or RPE with a replication-defective virus that has been genetically altered to carry a replacement gene of choice. This gene becomes expressed in any cell infected by the virus. Immune clearance of the virus has been shown to cause loss of expression of the transferred gene in other body sites. If immune privilege protects the viral vector or the protein synthesized by the transferred gene from immune clearance, then subretinal gene therapy might enjoy greater success in the eye than elsewhere. This topic is currently under intense investigation.

CHAPTER 4

Mechanisms of Immune Effector Reactivity

Immunologists have long been fascinated with all three phases of the adaptive immune response as well as related issues such as developmental biology and the ontogeny of lymphoid precursors. From the clinician's perspective, however, the effector phase is the most important aspect of both innate and adaptive immune responses, since patients who present with inflammation presumably have already experienced the afferent and processing phases of adaptive immunity or they are in the midst of the triggering mechanisms of innate immunity. In the following discussion, immune effector responses are subdivided into three categories:

- *Innate immune effector responses:* bacterial triggers, nonspecific effector molecules, neutrophil activation, macrophage activation
- *Adaptive immune effector responses:* antibody-dependent responses, lymphocyte-dependent responses, combination antibody/cellular responses
- *Amplification mechanisms relevant to both immune responses:* inflammatory mediators, cytokines, related topics

Effector Reactivities of Innate Immunity

Whereas adaptive immune responses use a complex afferent and processing system to activate effector responses, innate immune responses generally use more direct triggering mechanisms. Four of the most important triggering or response mechanisms to initiate an effector response of innate immunity are reviewed here (Table 4-1).

Bacteria-Derived Molecules That Trigger Innate Immunity

Bacterial lipopolysaccharide

Bacterial lipopolysaccharide (LPS), also known as *endotoxin,* is an intrinsic component of most gram-negative bacterial cell walls. One of the most important triggering molecules of innate immunity, LPS consists of three components:

- Lipid A
- Lipopolysaccharide
- A protein core

Lipid A is responsible for most of the inflammatory effects of LPS.

Table 4-1 Effector Reactivities of the Innate Immune Response in the Eye

Bacteria-derived molecules that trigger innate immunity
Lipopolysaccharide (LPS)
Other cell wall components
Exotoxins and secreted toxins

Nonspecific soluble molecules that trigger or modulate innate immunity
Plasma-derived enzymes
Acute phase reactants
Local production of cytokines by parenchymal cells within a tissue site

Innate mechanisms for recruitment and activation of polymorphonuclear cells
Cell adhesion and transmigration
Activation mechanisms
   Phagocytosis of bacteria

Innate mechanisms for recruitment and activation of macrophages
Cell adhesion and transmigration
Activation mechanisms
   Scavenging
   Priming
   Activation

LPS is an important cause of morbidity and mortality during infections with gram-negative bacteria and is the major cause of shock, fever, and other pathophysiological responses to bacterial sepsis. The pleiotropic effects of LPS include activation of monocytes and polymorphonuclear neutrophils (PMNs), leading to upregulation of genes for various cytokines (IL-1, IL-6, tumor necrosis factor [TNF]); degranulation; activation of complement through the alternative pathway; and direct impact on vascular endothelium. The cellular effects of LPS are the result of interactions with specific cell receptors, such as CD18/CR3, an LPS scavenger receptor on macrophages and lymphocytes. In addition, a circulating LPS-binding protein has been identified. Binding by the LPS-binding protein complex with the CD14 molecule on the macrophage surface leads to activation.

Other bacterial cell wall components

The bacterial cell wall and membrane are complex, with numerous polysaccharide, lipid, and protein structures that can initiate the innate immune response whether or not they act as antigens for adaptive immunity. Such toxins may include

- Muramyl dipeptide
- Lipoteichoic acids, in gram-positive bacteria
- Lipoarabinomannan, in mycobacteria
- Other poorly characterized soluble factors, such as heat shock proteins, common to all bacteria

Killed lysates of many types of gram-positive bacteria or mycobacteria have been demonstrated to directly activate macrophages, making them useful as adjuvants. Some of these components have been implicated in various models for arthritis and uveitis. In many cases, the molecular mechanisms are probably similar to LPS.

> **CLINICAL EXAMPLE**
>
> **LPS-induced uveitis** Humans are intermittently exposed to low doses of LPS that are released from the gut, especially during episodes of diarrhea and dysentery, and exposure to LPS may play a role in dysentery-related uveitis, arthritis, and Reiter syndrome. Systemic administration of a low dose of LPS in rabbits, rats, and mice produces a mild acute uveitis; this effect occurs at doses of LPS lower than those that cause apparent systemic shock. In rabbits, a breakdown of the blood–ocular barrier occurs because of leakage of plasma proteins through uveal vessels and loosening of the tight junctions between the nonpigmented ciliary epithelium. Rats and mice develop an acute PMN and monocytic infiltrate in the iris and ciliary body within 24 hours.
>
> The precise mechanism of LPS-induced ocular effects after systemic administration is unknown. One possibility is that LPS circulates and binds to the vascular endothelium or other sites within the anterior uvea. Alternatively, LPS might cause activation of uveal macrophages or circulating leukocytes, leading them to preferentially adhere to the anterior uveal vascular endothelium. Degranulation of platelets is among the first of histologic changes in LPS uveitis, probably mediated by eicosanoids, platelet-activating factors, and vasoactive amines. The subsequent intraocular generation of several mediators, especially leukotriene B_4, thromboxane B_2, prostaglandin E_2, and IL-6, correlates with the development of the cellular infiltrate and vascular leakage.
>
> Not surprisingly, direct injection of LPS into various ocular sites can initiate a severe localized inflammatory response. For example, intravitreal injection of LPS triggers a dose-dependent infiltration of the uveal tract, retina, and vitreous with PMNs and monocytes. Injection of LPS into the central cornea causes development of a ring infiltrate as a result of the infiltration of PMNs circumferentially from the limbus.

Exotoxins and other secretory products of bacteria

Various bacteria are known to secrete products such as *exotoxins* into the microenvironment in which the bacterium is growing. Many of these products are enzymes that, although not directly inflammatory, can cause tissue damage that subsequently results in inflammation. Examples include

- Collagenases
- Hemolysins such as streptolysin O, which can kill PMNs by causing cytoplasmic and extracellular release of their granules
- Phospholipases such as the *Clostridium perfringens* α-toxins, which kill cells and cause necrosis by disrupting cell membranes

Intravitreal injection of a cytolytic toxin derived from *Bacillus cereus* can cause direct necrosis of retinal cells. In addition, the metabolic byproducts of bacterial physiology can result in nonspecific tissue alterations that predispose to inflammation, such as altered tissue pH.

Some bacteria secrete small formyl peptide molecules related to the tripeptide *N*-formylmethionylleucylphenylalanine (FMLP). These formyl peptides are potent triggering stimuli for innate immunity. FMLP interacts with specific receptors on leukocytes, resulting in their recruitment into the site. In vitro FMLP activates PMNs, causes degranulation, and stimulates chemotaxis. Injection of FMLP into the cornea, conjunctiva, or vitreous produces infiltration with PMNs and monocytes, which can be prevented by pretreatment with corticosteroids, cyclooxygenase inhibitors, and competitive inhibitors of FMLP.

Gallin JI, Snyderman R, eds. *Inflammation: Basic Principles and Clinical Correlates.* 3rd ed. Philadelphia: Lippincott Williams & Wilkins; 1999.

Medzhitov R, Janeway C. Innate immunity. *N Engl J Med.* 2000;343:338–344.

Other Triggers or Modulators of Innate Immunity

As discussed in earlier chapters, the adaptive immune response employs one main family of soluble effector molecules: antibodies specific for antigen. Although no similar mechanism exists for innate immunity, various *nonspecific* soluble protein molecules are used by the innate immune response.

Plasma-derived enzyme systems, especially *complement*, are discussed below under amplification systems since they are effector molecules used to amplify inflammation for both innate and adaptive immunity. However, it is important to emphasize that complement, especially when activated through the alternative pathway, is a major effector molecule for innate immunity. Thus, stimuli that activate the alternative pathway, such

CLINICAL EXAMPLE

Role of bacterial toxin production and severity of endophthalmitis The effect of toxin production by various bacterial strains on the severity of endophthalmitis has recently been evaluated in experimental studies. It has been known for nearly a century that intraocular injection of LPS is highly inflammatory and accounts for much of the enhanced pathogenicity of gram-negative infections of the eye. Using clinical isolates or bacteria genetically altered to diminish production of various types of bacterial toxins, investigators have recently demonstrated that toxin elaboration by the living organism in gram-positive or -negative endophthalmitis greatly influences inflammatory cell infiltration and retinal cytotoxicity. This research suggests that sterilization with antibiotic therapy alone, in the absence of antitoxin therapy, may not prevent activation of innate immunity, ocular inflammation, and vision loss in eyes infected by toxin-producing strains.

Booth MC, Atkuri RV, Gilmore MS. Toxin production contributes to severity of *Staphylococcus aureus* endophthalmitis. In: Nussenblatt RB, Whitcup SM, Caspi RR, et al, eds. *Advances in Ocular Immunology.* New York: Elsevier; 1994:269–272.

Jett BD, Parke DW 2nd, Booth MC, et al. Host/parasite interactions in bacterial endophthalmitis. *Zentralb Bakteriol.* 1997;285:341–367.

as microbial cell walls, plastic surfaces of IOLs, or traumatized tissues, are potential triggering mechanisms of innate immunity.

Another important family of molecules for innate immunity is the group of *acute phase reactants,* such as C-reactive protein and α_2-macroglobulin. Although generally synthesized by the liver and released into blood, many of these molecules are also made by macrophages or produced locally in tissues. α_2-Macroglobulin is especially interesting: It is a natural scavenging molecule, capable of binding various types of proteins and substances presumably for clearance from the host. α_2-Macroglobulin is present in aqueous humor during uveitis and is synthesized by various ocular parenchymal cells of the eye as well. Enzyme systems in tears, such as lysozyme and lactoferrin, also play a role in ocular surface defenses.

Finally, various traumatic or toxic stimuli within ocular sites can trigger innate immunity. For example, trauma or toxins interacting directly with nonimmune ocular parenchymal cells, especially iris or ciliary body epithelium, retinal pigment epithelium, retinal Müller cells, or corneal or conjunctival epithelium, can result in a wide range of mediator, cytokine, and eicosanoid synthesis (see Table 4-7 later in the chapter), and this mechanism probably should be considered a form of innate immunity. Thus, phagocytosis of staphylococcus by corneal epithelium, microtrauma to ocular surface epithelium by contact lenses, chafing of iris or ciliary epithelium by an IOL, or laser treatment of the retina can stimulate ocular cells to produce mediators that assist in the recruitment of innate effector cells such as PMNs or macrophages.

CLINICAL EXAMPLE

Uveitis-glaucoma-hyphema (UGH) syndrome One cause of postoperative inflammation following cataract surgery, UGH syndrome is related to the physical presence of certain IOL styles. Although UGH syndrome was more common when rigid anterior chamber lenses were used during the early 1980s, it has also been reported with posterior chamber lenses. The pathogenesis of UGH syndrome appears to be related to various mechanisms for activation of innate immunity. One of the most likely mechanisms is cytokine and eicosanoid synthesis triggered by mechanical chasing or trauma to the iris or ciliary body. Plasma-derived enzymes, especially complement or fibrin, can enter the eye through vascular permeability altered by surgery or trauma and can then be activated by the surface of IOLs, especially those composed of polymethylmethacrylate (PMMA). Adherence of bacteria and leukocytes to the surface has also been implicated. Toxicity caused by contaminants on the lens surface during manufacturing has become rare. Recent research suggests that surface modification of IOLs, such as coating with heparin, might diminish the capacity of IOL materials to activate innate immune effector mechanisms. Nevertheless, even many noninflamed eyes with IOLs can demonstrate histologic evidence of low-grade foreign-body reactions around the haptics.

Pepose JS, Holland GN, Wilhelmus KR, eds. *Ocular Infection and Immunity.* St Louis: Mosby; 1996.

Innate Mechanisms for the Recruitment and Activation of Neutrophils

Neutrophils, referred to here as *polymorphonuclear neutrophils,* or *PMNs,* are among the most efficient effectors of innate immunity following trauma or acute infection. PMNs are categorized as either *resting* or *activated,* based on secretory and cell membrane activity. Cellular recruitment of resting, circulating PMNs by the innate immune response occurs rapidly in a tightly controlled process requiring two main mechanisms:

- PMN adhesion to the vascular endothelium through cellular adhesion molecules (CAMs) on leukocytes as well as on endothelial cells in postcapillary venules
- Transmigration of the PMNs through the endothelium and its extracellular matrix, mediated by various chemotactic factors

For resting PMNs to escape from blood vessels, an essential adhesion with activated vascular endothelial cells must occur, which is triggered by various innate stimuli such as LPS, physical injury, thrombin, histamine, or leukotriene release as well as other agonists.

The initial phase involves *neutrophil rolling,* a process by which PMNs bind loosely but reversibly to nonactivated endothelial cells (Fig 4-1). Involved are molecules on both cell types belonging to at least three sets of CAM families:

- The *selectins,* especially L-, P-, and E-selectin
- The *integrins,* especially leukocyte function–associated antigen 1 (LFA-1) and Mac-1
- Molecules in the immunoglobulin (Ig) superfamily, especially intercellular adhesion molecule 1 (ICAM-1) and ICAM-2

The primary events are mediated largely by members of the selectin family and occur within minutes of stimulation. The ligands for selectin molecules are as yet poorly characterized oligosaccharides found in the cell membranes. Nonactivated PMNs express L-selectin, which mediates a weak bond to endothelial cells. Upon exposure to the activating factors mentioned above, endothelial cells become activated, expressing in turn at least two other selectins (E and P) by which they can bind to the PMNs and help stabilize the interaction by a process called *adhesion.* Subsequently, other factors such as platelet-activating factor (PAF), various cytokines, and bacterial products can induce the up-regulation of the β-integrin family. As integrins are expressed, the selectins are shed, and PMNs then bind firmly to endothelial cells through the immunoglobulin superfamily molecules.

Subsequent to adhesion, various chemotactic factors are required to induce *transmigration* of PMNs across the endothelial barrier and extracellular matrix into the tissue site. Chemotactic factors are short-range signaling molecules that diffuse in a declining concentration gradient from the source of production within a tissue to the vessel itself. PMNs have receptors for these molecules, and they are induced to undergo membrane changes so they can migrate in the direction of highest concentration. A large number of such factors have been identified:

- Complement products (C5a)
- Fibrin split products

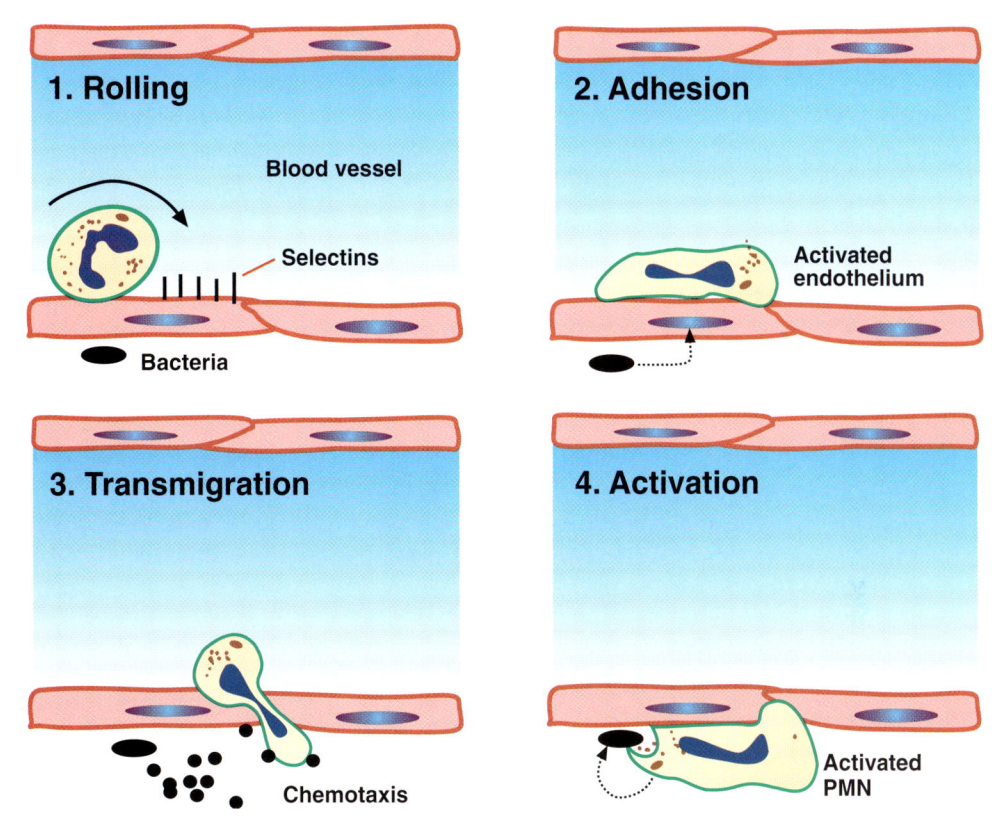

Figure 4-1 Four steps of polymorphonuclear neutrophil (PMN) migration and activation. **1,** In response to innate stimuli, such as bacterial invasion of tissue, *rolling* PMNs within the blood vessel bind loosely but reversibly to nonactivated endothelial cells by selectins. **2,** Exposure to innate activating factors activates endothelial cells, which in turn express E- and P-selectins, β-integrins, and immunoglobulin superfamily molecules to enhance and stabilize the interaction by a process called *adhesion*. **3,** Chemotactic factors triggered by the infection induce *transmigration* of PMNs across the endothelial barrier into the extracellular matrix of the tissue. **4,** Finally, PMNs are fully *activated* into functional effector cells upon stimulation by bacterial toxins and phagocytosis. *(Illustration by Barb Cousins, modified by Joyce Zavarro.)*

- Certain neuropeptides, such as substance P
- Bacteria-derived formyl tripeptides, such as FMLP
- Leukotrienes
- α-Chemokines, such as IL-8
- Many others

Another function of certain chemotactic factors is that they may also enhance endothelial cell activation to upregulate CAM and to synthesize additional chemotactic factors.

Activation of PMNs into functional effector cells begins during adhesion and transmigration but is fully exploited upon interaction with specific signals within the injured or infected site. Perhaps the most effective triggers of activation are bacteria and their toxins, especially LPS. Other innate or adaptive mechanisms (especially complement) and chemical mediators (such as leukotrienes and PAF) can also contribute to PMN activation. Unlike monocytes or lymphocytes, PMNs do not leave a tissue to recirculate but remain and die.

Phagocytosis

Phagocytosis of bacteria and other pathogens is a selective receptor-mediated process, and the two most important receptors are the *antibody Fc receptors* and the *complement receptors*. Thus, those pathogens in complexes with antibody or with activated complement components are specifically bound to the cell surface membrane–expressed Fc or complement (C) receptors and are effectively ingested. Other, less well characterized receptors may also mediate attachment to phagocytes. Particle ingestion is an energy-requiring process that is modulated by several biochemical events within the cells. Concomitant processes that occur in the cells during ingestion include

- Membrane synthesis
- Lysosomal enzyme synthesis
- Generation of metabolic products of oxygen and nitrogen
- Migration of the various types of granules toward the phagosome

Ultimately, several granules fuse with the phagosomes, a process that may occur prior to complete invagination, spilling certain granule contents outside of the phagocyte. Phagocytes are endowed with multiple means of destroying microorganisms, especially antimicrobial polypeptides that reside within cytoplasmic granules, reactive oxygen radicals generated from oxygen during the respiratory burst, and reactive nitrogen radicals, which are discussed later in this chapter. Although these mechanisms are primarily designed to destroy pathogens, released contents such as lysosomal enzymes may contribute to amplification of inflammation and tissue damage.

Innate Mechanisms for the Recruitment and Activation of Macrophages

Monocyte-derived macrophages are the second important type of effector cell for the innate immune response following trauma or acute infection. The various molecules involved in monocyte adhesion and transmigration from blood into tissues are probably similar to those discussed with PMNs, although they have not been studied as thoroughly. However, the functional activation of macrophages is more complex. Macrophages exist in different levels or stages of metabolic and functional activity, each representing different "programs" of gene activation and synthesis of macrophage-derived cytokines or mediators:

- Resting (immature or quiescent)
- Primed
- Activated

A fourth category of macrophages, often called *stimulated, reparative,* or *inflammatory,* is used by some authorities to refer to those macrophages that are not quite fully activated. This multilevel model is clearly oversimplified, but it does provide a framework for conceptualizing different levels of macrophage activation in terms of acute inflammation (Fig 4-2).

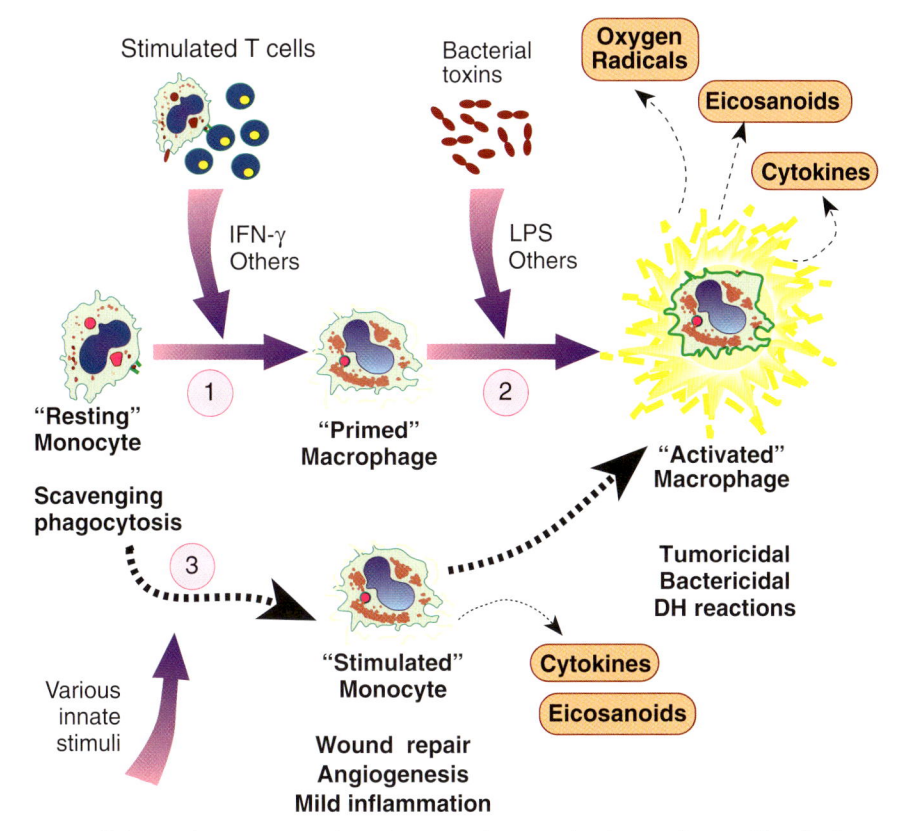

Figure 4-2 Schematic representation of macrophage activation pathway. Classically, *resting monocytes* are thought to be the principal noninflammatory scavenging phagocyte. **1,** Upon exposure to low levels of interferon-γ from T cells, monocytes become primed, upregulating class II major histocompatibility complex molecules and other functions. *Primed monocytes* function in antigen presentation. **2,** *Fully activated macrophages,* after exposure to bacterial lipopolysaccharide and interferon, are tumoricidal and bactericidal and mediate severe inflammation. **3,** *Stimulated monocytes* are incompletely activated, producing low levels of cytokines and eicosanoids but not reactive oxygen intermediates. These cells participate in wound healing, angiogenesis, and low-level inflammatory reactions. *(Illustration by Barb Cousins, modified by Joyce Zavarro.)*

Resting and scavenging macrophages

Host cell debris is cleared from a tissue site by phagocytosis in a process called *scavenging*. Resting macrophages are the classic scavenging cell, capable of phagocytosis and uptake of the following:

- Dead cell membranes by recognition of phosphatidyl serine
- Chemically modified extracellular protein through acetylated or oxidized lipoproteins
- Sugar ligands through mannose receptors
- Naked nucleic acids as well as bacterial pathogens

> **CLINICAL EXAMPLE**
>
> **Phacolytic glaucoma** Mild infiltration of scavenging macrophages centered around retained lens cortex or nucleus fragments occurs in nearly all eyes with lens injury, including those subjected to routine cataract surgery. This infiltrate is notable for the *absence* of prominent neutrophil infiltration or significant nongranulomatous inflammation. An occasional giant cell may be present, but granulomatous changes are not extensive.
>
> Phacolytic glaucoma is a variant of scavenging macrophage infiltration in which glaucoma occurs in the setting of a hypermature cataract that leaks lens protein through an *intact* capsule. Lens protein–engorged scavenging macrophages are present in the anterior chamber, and glaucoma develops as these cells block the trabecular meshwork outflow channels. Other signs of typical lens-associated uveitis are conspicuously absent. Experimental studies suggest that lens proteins may be chemotactic stimuli for monocytes.

Resting monocytes express scavenging receptors of at least three types but synthesize very low levels of proinflammatory cytokines. In general, scavenging can occur in the absence of inflammation.

Primed macrophages

Resting macrophages become primed by exposure to certain cytokines. Upon priming, thse cells become positive for major histocompatability complex (MHC) class II antigen and capable of functioning as APCs to T cells. Priming implies activation of specialized lysosomal enzymes such as cathepsins D and E for degrading proteins into peptide fragments, upregulation of certain specific genes such as class II MHC and costimulatory molecules such as B7.1, and increased cycling of proteins between endosomes and surface membrane. Prototypically, primed macrophages resemble dendritic cells. They can exit tissue sites by the afferent lymphatics to reenter the lymph node. Classically, T-cell–derived IFN-γ was thought to be the most important priming signal. It is now known, however, that many cytokines not necessarily of T-cell origin can also prime macrophages, and the cellular response to the priming stimulus has tissue-specific variations.

Activated and stimulated macrophages

Activated macrophages are classically defined as macrophages producing the full spectrum of proinflammatory and cytotoxic cytokines; thus, they are the cells that mediate and amplify acute inflammation (delayed hypersensitivity), tumor killing, and major antibacterial activity. *Epithelioid cells* and *giant cells* represent the terminal differentiation of the activated macrophage. Activated macrophages synthesize numerous mediators to amplify inflammation:

- Inflammatory or cytotoxic cytokines such as IL-1, IL-6, TNF-α
- Reactive oxygen or nitrogen intermediates
- Lipid mediators
- Other products

Traditionally, full activation was observed to require stimulation by two signals: IFN-γ from delayed hypersensitivity (DH) T cells plus LPS from gram-negative bacteria. Nevertheless, the level of macrophage activation can vary tremendously and can be regulated much more precisely than is implied by the monolithic term *activated*.

It is now thought that macrophages can be partially activated by many different innate stimuli, such as

- Cytokines not derived from T cells, such as the chemokines
- Bacterial cell walls or toxins from gram-positive or acid-fast organisms
- Complement activated through the alternative pathway
- Foreign bodies composed of potentially toxic substances such as talc or beryllium
- Exposure to certain surfaces such as some plastics

Thus, macrophages that are partially activated to produce some inflammatory cytokines, but perhaps not fully activated to antimicrobial or tumoricidal function, are sometimes termed *stimulated* or *reparative* macrophages. Such partially activated macrophages also contribute to fibrosis and wound healing through synthesis of mitogens such as platelet-

CLINICAL EXAMPLE

Propionibacterium acnes *endophthalmitis* Infection of the capsular bag and residual lens material with the anaerobic organism *P acnes* has been found to cause some cases of chronic postoperative uveitis after cataract surgery and IOL implantation. This bacterium, presumably introduced at the time of surgery, replicates very slowly and fails to produce a significant purulent infection. Thus, the initial infection is noninflammatory and clinically inapparent. However, some clinical event, such as additional surgery with the Nd:YAG laser or other unknown trigger, results in inflammation apparently related to enhanced replication or release of the bacterium. Granulomatous inflammation ultimately develops that spreads to involve the residual lens and vitreous.

No clear explanation for the pattern of inflammation in the *P acnes* syndrome is presently known. Some investigators speculate that the infective plaque of organisms is growing, initially, within an anaerobic environment formed by a sequestered pocket of capsular flap and IOL, and the bacteria are thus isolated from the immune response. After release of the toxins, especially cell wall components, macrophages are directly activated through innate immunity to initiate a subacute inflammatory reaction. Activated macrophages then produce mediators and cytokines that amplify the inflammation.

derived growth factors, metalloproteinases, and other matrix degradation factors and angiogenesis through synthesis of angiogenic factors such as vascular endothelial growth factor.

Effector Reactivities of Adaptive Immunity

Although most adaptive (or innate) immune responses are protective and occur subclinically, when adaptive immune responses do cause inflammation, these responses have classically been called *immune hypersensitivity reactions*. The traditional classification for describing the four mechanisms of adaptive immune-triggered inflammatory responses was elaborated by Coombs and Gell in 1962, and a fifth category, *stimulatory hypersensitivity*, was added later (Table 4-2). Although this system is still useful, it was developed before T cells had been discovered, in a time when understanding was limited to antibody-triggered mechanisms. In addition, it is unlikely that any effector mechanism in a disease process is purely one type. For example, all antibody-dependent mechanisms require a processing phase using helper T cells, which may also contribute to effector responses. Finally, the term *hypersensitivity* may obscure the concept that many of these same mechanisms are often protective and noninflammatory. Thus, in some ways, this traditional classification is inadequate. This discussion introduces an expanded classification system that incorporates modern concepts for immune effector reactivities and, when appropriate, points out where the classic Coombs and Gell system applies (Table 4-3).

Male DK, Cooke A, Owen M, et al. *Advanced Immunology*. 3rd ed. St Louis: Mosby; 1996.
Roitt IM, Delves PJ. *Roitt's Essential Immunology*. 10th ed. Malden, MA: Blackwell Science; 2001.

Antibody-Mediated Immune Effector Responses

Structural and functional properties of antibody molecules

Structural features of immunoglobulins. Five major classes (M, G, A, E, and D) of immunoglobulin exist in nine different subclasses, or *isotypes* (IgG1, IgG2, IgG3, IgG4, IgM, IgA1, IgA2, IgE, and IgD). The basic immunoglobulin structure is composed of four covalently bonded glycoprotein chains forming a monomer of approximately 150,000–180,000 daltons (Fig 4-3). This monomer is about two and a half to three times the size of albumin. Each antibody monomer contains two identical *light chains*, either kappa (κ) or lambda (λ), and two identical *heavy chains* from one of the nine structurally distinct

Table 4-2 Types of Hypersensitivity (Coombs and Gell)

Type I	Anaphylactoid
Type II	Cytotoxic antibodies
Type III	Immune complex reactions
Type IV	Cell-mediated
Type V	Stimulatory

Table 4-3 Effector Reactivities of the Adaptive Immune Response in the Eye

Predominantly antibody-mediated soluble effectors
  Intravascular circulating antibodies that form circulating immune complexes with bloodborne antigen (Type III)
  Passive leakage of antibody into a tissue followed by complex formation with tissue-bound antigen causing
    Complement-mediated cell lysis (Type II)
    Complement activation with inflammation (a variant of Type III)
    Novel cytotoxic mechanisms
    Stimulation of cell activities (Type V)
  Local infiltration of circulating B cells into a tissue with local secretion of antibody and other cell activities (a variant of Type III)

Predominantly lymphocyte-mediated (cellular) effectors
  Delayed hypersensitivity T cells (Type IV)
    Th1 type of delayed hypersensitivity
    Th2 type of delayed hypersensitivity
  Cytotoxic lymphocytes
    Cytotoxic T lymphocytes
    Natural killer cells
    Lymphokine-activated killer cells

Combined antibody and cellular effector mechanisms
  Antibody-dependent cellular cytotoxicity (ADCC) with killer cells or macrophages
  Acute IgE-mediated mast cell degranulation (Type I)
  Chronic mast cell degranulation and Th2 delayed hypersensitivity

subclasses of immunoglobulins. Thus, the heavy chain type defines the specific isotype (Table 4-4). IgM can form pentamers or hexamers in vivo, and IgA can form dimers in secretions, so that the molecular size of these two classes in vivo is much larger than the others.

Each monomer has analogous regions called *domains*. Certain domains carry out specific functions of the antibody molecule. In particular, the *Fab region* on each molecule contains the antigen recognition/combining domain, called the *hypervariable region*. The opposite end of the molecule, on the heavy chain portion, contains the attachment site for effector cells *(Fc portion)* as well as the site of other effector functions, such as complement activation (eg, as for IgG3) or binding to secretory component so it can be transported through epithelia and secreted into tears (eg, as for IgA). Table 4-4 summarizes important structural differences of immunoglobulin isotypes.

Functional properties of immunoglobulins. All immunoglobulin isotypes do not mediate the effector functions of antibody activity equally. For example, human IgM and IgG3 are good complement activators, but IgG4 is not. Only IgA1 or IgA2 can bind secretory component and thus be actively passed into mucosal secretions after transport through the epithelial cell from the subepithelial location, where it is synthesized by B cells. Other isotypes must remain in the subepithelial tissue. A partial list of isotype-specific functions is included in Table 4-4. The importance of these differences is that two antibodies with identical capacity to bind to an antigen, but of different isotype, will have different effector and inflammatory outcomes.

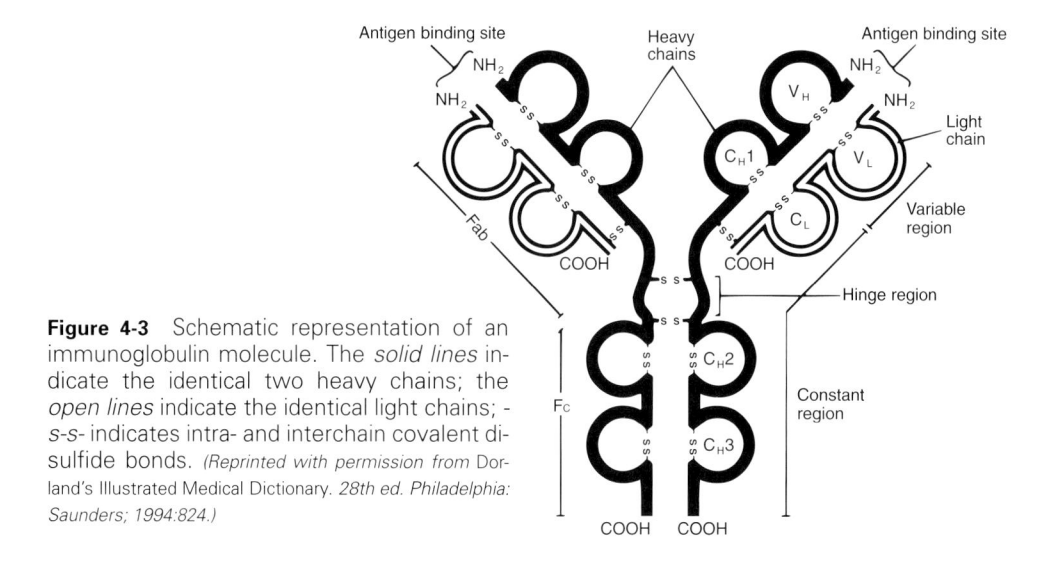

Figure 4-3 Schematic representation of an immunoglobulin molecule. The *solid lines* indicate the identical two heavy chains; the *open lines* indicate the identical light chains; -s-s- indicates intra- and interchain covalent disulfide bonds. *(Reprinted with permission from Dorland's Illustrated Medical Dictionary. 28th ed. Philadelphia: Saunders; 1994:824.)*

Terminology

Various regions of an antibody can themselves be antigenic. These antigenic sites are called *idiotopes* to be distinguished from *epitopes,* the antigenic sites on foreign molecules. Antibodies to idiotopes are called *idiotypes.* Anti-idiotypic antibodies might be important feedback mechanisms for immune regulation.

The concept of *monoclonal antibodies* has become very important in research and diagnostic medicine. After immunization with a particular antigen, a high frequency of B cells producing antibodies specific for that antigen will be present in the spleen or lymph nodes. Although one B cell synthesizes antibody of one antigenic specificity, different B cells responding to different epitopes of the same antigen produce specific antibodies to each different epitope. The population of all antigen-specific antibodies to the various epitopes is termed *polyclonal,* as these antibodies derive from different B cell clones or progeny from one initial parental B cell, each producing antibodies of different specificities.

For example, myeloma cells are immortal tumor cells that have the cellular machinery for making unlimited production of one antibody without additional helper stimulation by T cells, antigen, or cytokines. If activated B cells from an immunized host and myeloma cells are fused by various laboratory manipulations, then a population of *hybridomas* is formed. Each hybridoma makes an unlimited amount of the original B cell's single antibody, yet it is immortal and therefore easy to grow and care for in the laboratory. Thus, the antibody is *monoclonal,* since it represents the product of one specific parental B cell fused to the myeloma tumor. The population of hybridomas produced by this fusion can be screened for selection of the ones that may be synthesizing the monoclonal antibody of interest.

Table 4-4 Structural and Functional Properties of Immunoglobulin Isotypes

Immunoglobulin Isotype (Heavy Chain)	% of Total Serum Igs	Structural Properties - Relative Size	Structural Properties - Other Structural Features	Activates Complement	Functional Properties - Fc Receptor Binding Preferences	Functional Properties - Other Functions
IgD δ	<1%	Monomer	Mostly on surface of B cells	No		B-cell antigen receptor
IgM μ	5%	Pentamer or hexamer	Mostly on B cells or intravascular	Strong (classic pathway)		B-cell antigen receptor; agglutinization; neutralization; intravascular cytolysis
IgG1 γ	50%	Monomer	Intravascular, in tissues, crosses placenta	Moderate (classic pathway)	Monocytes	Cytolysis
IgG2 γ	18%	Monomer	Same as IgG1	Weak (classic pathway)	PMN monocytes, killer lymphocytes	ADCC
IgG3 γ	6%	Monomer	Same as IgG1	Strong (classic pathway)	PMN monocytes, killer lymphocytes	ADCC, agglutinization, cytolysis
IgG4 γ	3%	Monomer	Same as IgG1	No		Neutralization
IgE ε	<<1%	Monomer	Mostly in skin or mucosa, bound to mast cells	No	Mast cells	Mast cell degranulation
IgA1 α	15%	Mostly monomer in serum, dimer in secretions	In mucosal secretions, binds secretory component in subepithelial tissues for transepithelial transport and protection from proteolysis	Moderate (alternative pathway)		Mucosal immunity, neutralization
IgA2 α	3%	Same as IgA1	Same as IgA1	Same as IgA1		

Intravascular circulating antibodies that form circulating immune complexes with bloodborne antigen

Systemic release of antibody into the circulation or into external secretions occurs frequently after immunization, and antibody interactions with antigen solubilized in plasma or secretions are important effector mechanisms in this setting (Fig 4-4).

Neutralization, opsonization, and agglutinization When antibody combines with a live pathogen such as virus or bacteria, it can block, or *neutralize*, the ability of the pathogen to bind to host cell receptors, thereby preventing infection of host cells. This process can occur in the blood or in external secretions such as tears. The role of this process in preventing reinfection with adenovirus is discussed in the Clinical Example: Immune response to viral conjunctivitis in Chapter 3. When antibody coats a soluble pathogen or antigen in blood, the antibody can enhance phagocytosis or reticuloendothelial clearance by macrophage-like cells in the spleen or liver in a process called *opsonization*. Opsonization is usually facilitated by Fc receptor recognition by the phagocyte. In some cases, such as certain bacterial cell wall antigens, an antigen contains multiple identical antigenic sites on one molecule so that more than one antibody can bind each molecule. In these cases, the antibody/antigen complex may *agglutinize*, causing the complex to precipitate out of solution.

Deposition of circulating soluble immune complexes Usually, when antigen is soluble within blood, as during viremia or bacteremia, soluble immune complexes formed between antigen and antibody are efficiently removed from the circulation by binding to erythrocytes, then cleared by the reticuloendothelial system. However, in some cases, soluble immune complexes can passively deposit within the blood vessels, kidneys, and other vascular structures, usually facilitated by predisposing stimuli that cause altered

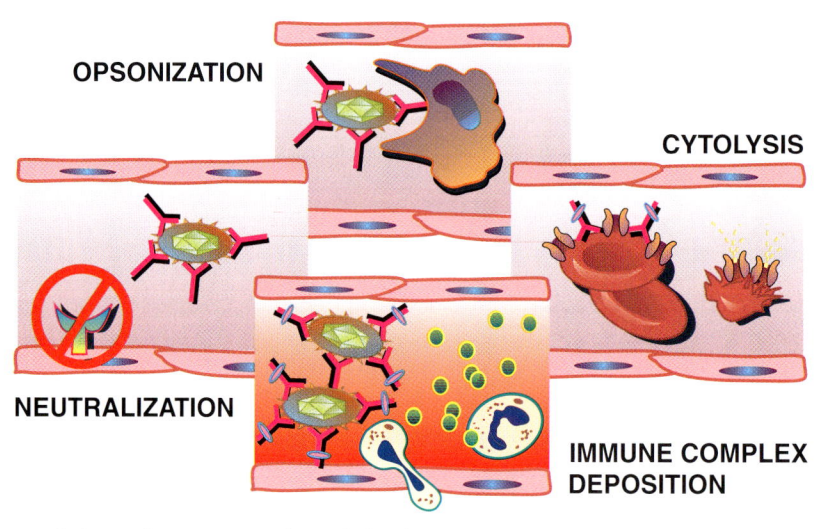

Figure 4-4 Schematic representation of the four most important antibody effector mechanisms in the blood. *(Illustration by Barb Cousins, modified by Joyce Zavarro.)*

vascular permeability (eg, mast cell degranulation). This mechanism must be differentiated from the in situ formation of immune complexes within a tissue, which is discussed below. Tissue deposition of circulating immune complexes can trigger an inflammatory response by activating complement, one variant of Coombs and Gell Type III.

The classic clinical setting in which circulating immune complexes caused a systemic disease was *serum sickness,* a disease occurring in the preantibiotic and presteroid era that was caused by a late primary or secondary immune response following intravenous treatment with animal serum for a patient suffering from infection or inflammation. Massive intravascular immune complex formation caused severe systemic vasculitis and chronic inflammation in many organs. Now, serum sickness occurs rarely after certain infections such as Lyme disease or in rare individuals treated with certain drugs, such as antibiotics. In these cases, the drug binds to self-proteins to form a drug/protein *neoantigen,* or *hapten,* that inadvertently initiates an immune response. Deposition of circulating immune complexes may occur in some forms of systemic vasculitis, but their causative role has been deemphasized recently.

Passive leakage of antibody into peripheral tissues followed by complex formation with tissue-bound antigen

Antibody in serum, especially of the IgG subclasses, can passively leak into peripheral tissues, particularly those with fenestrated capillaries, leading to formation of a local complex of antibody with tissue-associated antigens. Figure 4-5 illustrates the antibody effector mechanisms discussed below.

Complement-mediated cell lysis, or immune cytolysis If an antigen is associated with the external surface of the plasma membrane, antibody binding might activate the complement cascade to induce cell lysis through formation of specialized porelike structures called the *membrane attack complex* (ie, Coombs and Gell Type II). Hemolytic anemia of a newborn as a result of Rh incompatibility is the classic example of this process. Others include Hashimoto thyroiditis, glomerulonephritis of Goodpasture syndrome, and autoimmune thrombocytopenia. This mechanism does not appear to be very important in uveitis or ocular inflammation, although it may play a role in killing virus-infected cells during viral conjunctivitis.

> **CLINICAL EXAMPLE**
>
> **Anterior uveitis is probably not caused by circulating immune complexes**
> Following observations that uveitis developed in some animal models of serum sickness, investigators in the 1970s and 1980s sought to confirm a role for circulating immune complexes as a cause of anterior uveitis. Although elevated levels of immune complexes were detected in many patients, a convincing correlation with disease activity was never established. Now, most immunologists and clinicians think that the ocular deposition of circulating immune complexes is *not* an important pathogenic mechanism for uveitis in humans.

CYTOLYSIS

CELL DEGENERATION

STIMULATORY

ANTIBODY DEPOSITION

ARTHUS REACTION

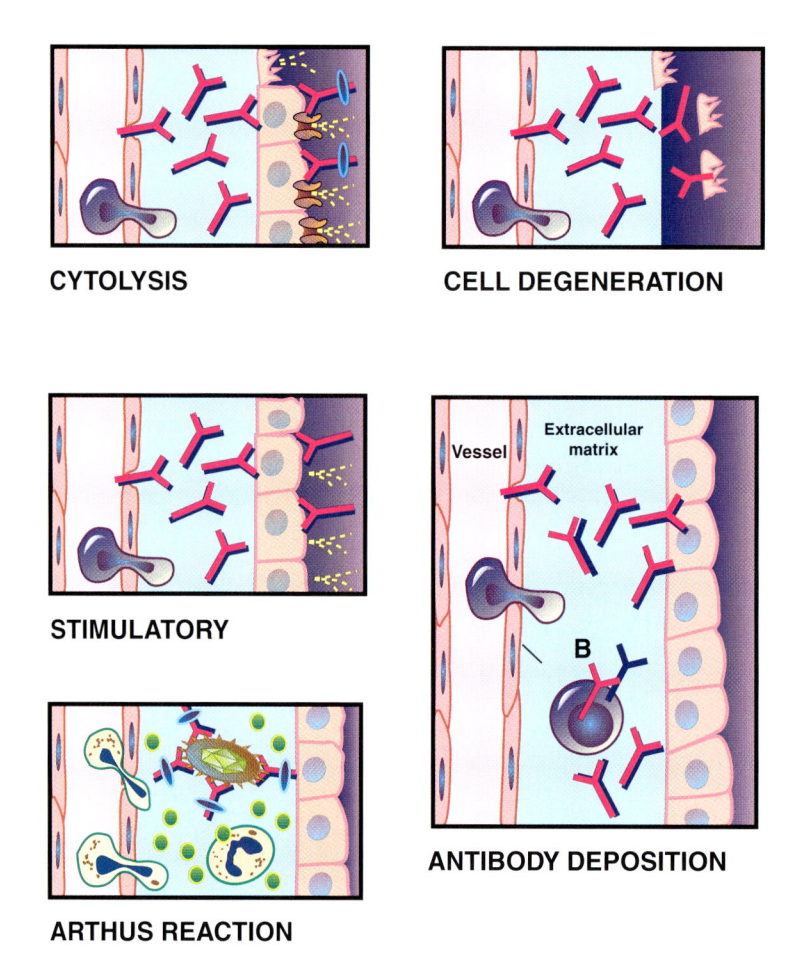

Figure 4-5 Schematic representation of the most important antibody effector mechanisms caused by passive leakage of antibody into tissues. *(Illustration by Barb Cousins, modified by Joyce Zavarro.)*

Tissue-bound immune complexes and the acute Arthus reaction When free antibody passively leaks from the serum into a tissue, it can combine with tissue-bound antigens trapped in the extracellular matrix or with cell-associated antigens such as a viral protein expressed on the surface of an infected cell. These in situ, or locally formed, complexes sometimes activate the complement pathway to produce complement fragments called *anaphylatoxins* (a second variant of Coombs and Gell Type III). This mechanism should be differentiated from the deposition of circulating immune complexes, which are preformed in the blood. Typically, the histology is dominated by neutrophils and monocytes. The resultant lesion, called the *acute Arthus reaction,* can be produced experimentally by injection of antigen into a tissue site of an animal previously immunized in a way to optimize antibody rather than T-cell production. In general, many types of glomerulonephritis and vasculitis are thought to represent this mechanism. See the Clinical Example: Retinal vasculitis in systemic lupus erythematosus in this chapter.

CLINICAL EXAMPLES

Retinal vasculitis in systemic lupus erythematosus Although rare, retinal vasculitis can develop in patients with systemic lupus erythematosus (SLE) (see Chapter 9). Observation of the probable mechanism for vasulitis elsewhere in SLE suggests that local immune complex formation plays a role in this development. DNA and histones released from injured cells can become trapped in the basement membrane of the blood vessel wall, perhaps as a result of electrostatic binding by matrix proteins. Circulating cationic anti-DNA IgG autoantibodies permeate into the vessel wall, bind the autoantigen, and activate complement. These cationic IgG antibodies are thought to have a stronger affinity for anionic extracellular matrix and therefore permeate tissues efficiently.

Complement fragments, or *anaphylatoxins*, initiate an Arthus reaction. The observed vascular sheathing in the retinal vessels is presumed to be caused by infiltration of neutrophils and macrophages in response to complement activation. However, helper T-cell responses and innate mechanisms may also contribute. In addition to DNA, other potential autoantigens in SLE include collagen and phospholipids.

Alternatively, molecular mimicry between basement membrane components and DNA may occur. The mechanism for the initiation of afferent events causing the induction of aberrant autoimmunity to DNA and other antigens is unknown. A similar effector mechanism has been postulated for scleritis in rheumatoid arthritis.

Cancer-associated retinopathy Cancer-associated retinopathy is a paraneoplastic syndrome in which some patients with carcinoma, especially small cell carcinoma of the lung or occasionally cutaneous melanoma, develop antibodies against a tumor-associated antigen that happens to cross-react with an ocular autoantigen. For example, some small cell carcinomas aberrantly synthesize recoverin, a normal protein in photoreceptors. The immune system inappropriately recognizes and processes recoverin and produces an antibody effector response, releasing antirecoverin antibodies into the circulation. These antibodies passively permeate the retina, are taken up by photoreceptors, and cause slowly progressive photoreceptor degeneration by a novel, poorly understood cytotoxic mechanism. Current research speculates that induction of programmed cell death may be caused by intracellular antibody/antigen complex formation after photoreceptor uptake of antirecoverin antibodies.

Novel cytotoxic mechanisms Circulating antibodies can cause tissue injury by mechanisms different from cytolysis or complement activation, using pathogenic mechanisms not yet elucidated. For example, some autoantibodies in systemic lupus erythematosus appear to be taken up by renal cells, leading to loss of function, and these may cause some cases of nephritis in the absence of immune complex activation. In paraneoplastic syndromes, autoantibodies to various tissues can develop and mediate *cellular degener-*

ation or other manifestations. See the Clinical Example: Cancer-associated retinopathy in this chapter.

Stimulatory antibodies Tissue- or cell-bound immune complexes that stimulate receptors on target cells are known as *stimulatory antibodies*. In some cases, antibody leaking into tissues or binding to cells in the blood can cross-react with and bind to a receptor or molecule expressed on the surface of normal parenchymal cells, thereby activating the receptor as if the antibody were the natural ligand for that receptor (Coombs and Gell Type V). For example, in Graves disease, antibodies to the thyroid-stimulating hormone receptor activate the thyroid gland as if the patient had taken an overdose of thyroid-stimulating hormone. Immunologists have used this information to develop many antibodies to activate cell receptors in the absence of the natural ligand and to develop antibodies with enzymatic or other metabolic functions. In other cases, the autoantibody can block function of the receptor, as in myasthenia gravis, wherein antiacetylcholine antibodies cause internalization of the normal receptor without activation, thereby depleting functional receptors from the nerve ending. Many other examples of stimulatory, or metabolically active, antibodies have been identified. See the Clinical Example: Scleritis or retinal vasculitis in Wegener granulomatosis in this chapter.

CLINICAL EXAMPLE

Scleritis or retinal vasculitis in Wegener granulomatosis Necrotizing scleritis is a common feature in Wegener granulomatosis, and retinal vasculitis can, rarely, develop in some of these patients as well (see Chapter 9). Although the mechanism for scleritis and retinal vasculitis in Wegener granulomatosis is unknown, the primary pathogenesis can be inferred from experimental studies of systemic disease to be a vasculitis mediated in part by stimulatory autoantibodies. The autoantigen is thought to be the PMN-derived serine protease *proteinase-3*. The initial effector process is thought to require the translocation of proteinase-3 from cytoplasmic granules to the cell surface after PMN exposure to various innate activational stimuli, such as a predisposing infection or systemic cytokine release. Then, antineutrophil cytoplasmic antibodies can bind surface proteinase-3, further activating and stimulating the PMNs. This process, in turn, causes the PMNs to bind to endothelium and to release granules and other mediators that injure the vessel wall. The endothelial cells then synthesize cytokines to recruit additional inflammatory cells, especially T cells, which amplify the process. The mechanism for the initiation of afferent events causing the induction of aberrant autoimmunity to proteinase-3 is unknown. However, the processing phase must also include proteinase-specific helper T cells, which are responsible for providing cytokine help to B cells; and DH effector cells presumably contribute to granuloma formation in tissue sites.

   Kallenberg CG, Brouwer E, Mulder AH, et al. ANCA—pathophysiology revisited. *Clin Exp Immunol*. 1995;100:1–3.

Infiltration of B cells into tissues and local production of antibody

B-cell infiltration B cells can infiltrate the site of an immunologic reaction in response to persistent antigenic stimulus, leading to a clinical picture of moderate to severe inflammation. If the process becomes chronic, plasma cell formation occurs, representing fully differentiated B cells that have become dedicated to antibody synthesis. In both of these cases, local production of antibody specific for the inciting antigen(s) occurs within the site. If the antigen is known, as for certain presumed infections, local antibody formation can be used as a diagnostic test.

Differentiation between local production of antibody and passive leakage from the blood involves calculation of the *Goldmann-Witmer coefficient*, which is generated by comparison of the ratio of intraocular fluid/serum antibody concentration for the specific antibody in question to the intraocular fluid/serum ratio of total immunoglobulin levels. Theoretically, a coefficient above 1.0 would indicate local production of antibodies within the eye. In practice, however, positive quotients above 3.0 are used most often to improve specificity and positive predictive value. See the Clinical Example: Diagnosis of atypical necrotizing retinitis in this chapter.

Local antibody production within a tissue and chronic inflammation. Persistence of antigen within a site coupled with infiltration of specific B cells and local antibody formation can produce a chronic inflammatory reaction with a complicated histologic pattern, often demonstrating lymphocytic infiltration, plasma cell infiltration, and granulomatous features (a third variant of Coombs and Gell Type III). This process is sometimes called the *chronic Arthus reaction*. This mechanism may contribute to the pathophysiology of certain chronic autoimmune disorders, such as rheumatoid arthritis, which feature formation of pathogenic antibody. See the Clinical Example: Phacoantigenic endophthalmitis in this chapter.

Lymphocyte-Mediated Effector Responses

Delayed hypersensitivity T lymphocytes

Delayed hypersensitivity (DH, or Coombs and Gell Type IV) represents the prototypical adaptive immune mechanism for lymphocyte-triggered inflammation. It is especially

---

CLINICAL EXAMPLE

Diagnosis of atypical necrotizing retinitis The sensitivity, specificity, and accuracy of aqueous humor antibody levels (intraocular antibody synthesis) were compared in the diagnoses of atypical retinitis ultimately caused by *Toxoplasma gondii*, varicella-zoster virus, herpes simplex virus, cytomegalovirus, and noninfectious causes. In general, the authors found that results were best (78% diagnostic accuracy) when the highest quotient greater than 1.0 was used for diagnosis even in the face of multiple positive quotients. False-positive quotients for cytomegalovirus were the most frequent confounding finding, causing four of six false diagnoses.

Davis JL, Feuer W, Culbertson WW, et al. Interpretation of intraocular and serum antibody levels in necrotizing retinitis. *Retina*. 1995;15:233–240.

> **CLINICAL EXAMPLE**
>
> **Phacoantigenic endophthalmitis** This condition is a form of lens-associated uveitis with three distinct zones of inflammation centered around the lens:
> - An inner zone of neutrophils invading the lens substance
> - A secondary zone of macrophages, epithelioid cells, or giant cells (or a combination thereof) surrounding the capsule injury site
> - An outer zone of fibrotic reparative or granulation tissue infiltrated with nongranulomatous inflammation and plasma cells, presumably secreting specific antibodies into ocular fluids
>
> Antibody-mediated autoimmunity has been well demonstrated in rats immunized against whole lens proteins. The mechanism for the initiation of afferent events causing the induction of aberrant autoimmunity to lens crystallins is unknown. The adaptive immune system of unaffected patients has already been exposed to crystallins in a "tolerizing" manner (see Chapter 5).
>
> Since lens-associated uveitis almost always occurs in a severely traumatized or congenitally abnormal eye, it has been suggested that the disease is initiated in eyes with an atypical immunologic microenvironment that allows a secondary afferent response to override tolerance. The effector phase appears to be dominated by complement-fixing antibodies specific for lens crystallins, which are either produced locally by B cells or plasma cells within the eye or leaked passively from the blood. Presumably, generation of the anaphylatoxin C5a by complement-activating immune complexes *within the lens substance* explains the neutrophil infiltration into the lens. Diffusion of anaphylatoxins into the anterior chamber probably results in a chemotactic gradient, yielding a zonal pattern. Activated macrophages must also contribute, since epithelioid and giant cells that are subsets of activated, differentiated macrophages are classic features. The mechanism for giant cell formation has not been totally resolved, but phagocytosis of immune complexes coated with complement can contribute to macrophage activation and induce giant cell formation. Injury to retina or other tissues is probably exacerbated by toxic oxygen radicals. It has been suggested that T-cell and innate effector mechanisms may also be involved.

powerful in secondary immune responses. Previously primed DH CD4 T cells leave the lymph node, home into local tissues where antigen persists, and become activated by further restimulation with the specific priming antigen and class II MHC–expressing APCs. Fully activated DH T cells secrete mediators and cytokines, leading to the recruitment and activation of macrophages or other nonspecific leukocytes (Fig 4-6). The term *delayed* for this type of hypersensitivity refers to the fact that this reaction becomes maximal 12–48 hours after antigen exposure.

Analysis of experimental animal models and the histopathological changes of human inflammation suggest that different subtypes of DH might exist. One of the most important determinants of the pattern of DH reaction is the subtype of DH CD4 T effector cells that mediate the reaction. Just as helper T cells can be differentiated into two

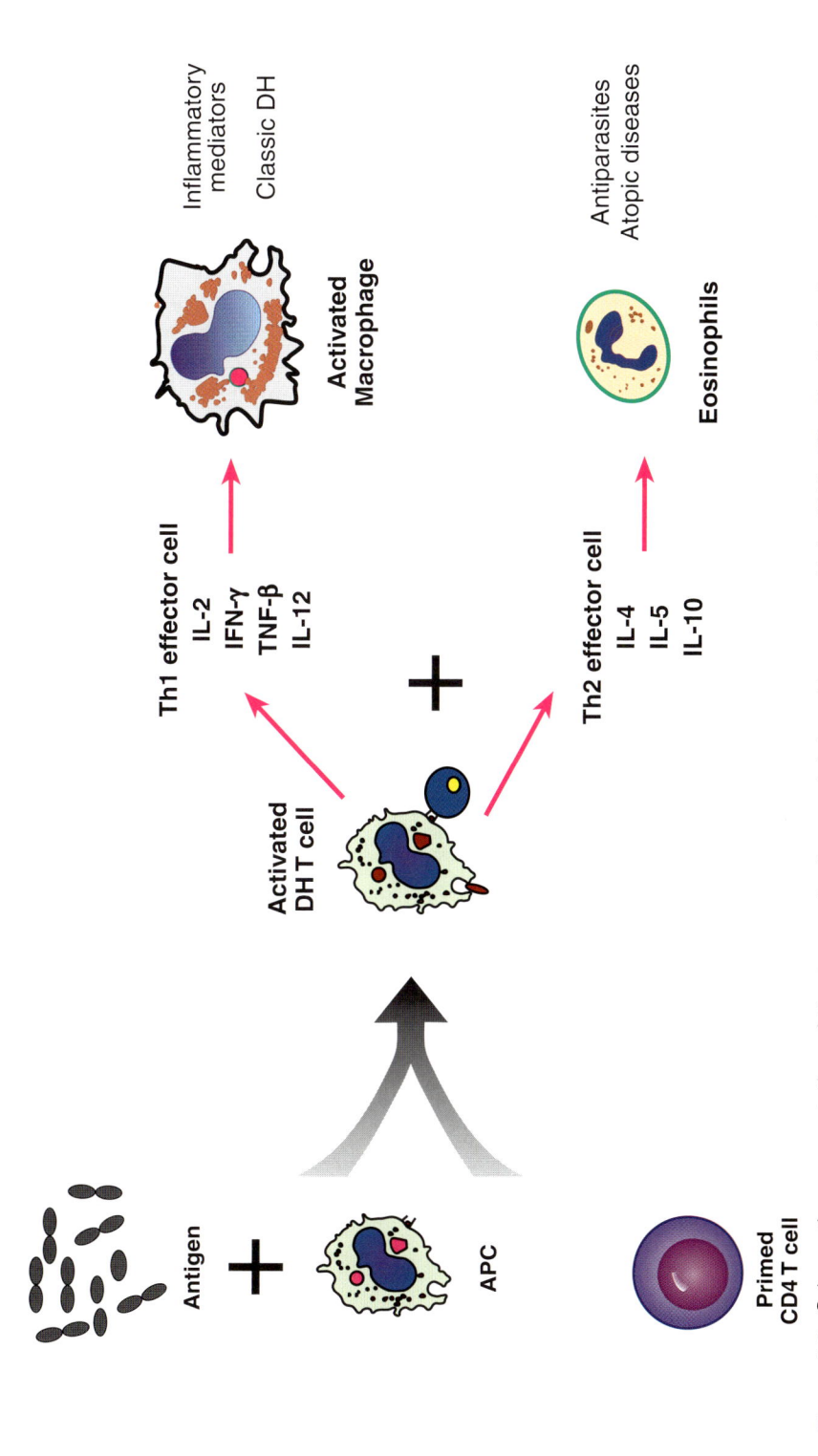

Figure 4-6 Schematic representation of the two major forms of delayed hypersensitivity (DH). CD4 T cells, having undergone initial priming in the lymph node, enter the tissue site, where they again encounter antigen-presenting cells (APC) and antigen. Upon restimulation, they become activated into either Th1 or Th2 effector cells. Th1 cells are the classic DH effector cells associated with most severe forms of inflammation. Th2 cells are thought to be less intensively inflammatory, but they have been associated with parasite-induced granulomas and atopic diseases. *(Illustration by Barb Cousins, modified by Joyce Zavarro.)*

groups—Th1 and Th2 subsets—according to the spectrum of cytokines secreted, DH T cells can also be grouped by the same criteria. Experimentally, the Th1 subset of cytokines, especially IFN-γ, also known as *macrophage-activating factor*, and TNF-β, activates macrophages to secrete inflammatory mediators and kill pathogens, amplifying inflammation. Thus, Th1-mediated DH mechanisms are thought to produce the following:

- The classic delayed hypersensitivity reaction (ie, the purified protein derivative skin reaction)
- Immunity to intracellular infections (ie, to mycobacteria or pneumocystis)
- Immunity to fungi
- Most forms of severe T-cell–mediated autoimmune diseases
- Chronic transplant rejection

The Th2 subset of DH cells secretes IL-4 and IL-5 and other cytokines. IL-4 can induce B cells to synthesize IgE, and IL-5 can recruit and activate eosinophils within a site. IL-4 can also induce macrophage granulomas in response to parasite-derived antigens. Thus, Th2-mediated DH mechanisms are thought to play a major role in the following:

- Response to parasite infections
- Late phase responses of allergic reactions
- Asthma
- Atopic dermatitis or other manifestations of atopic diseases

The inciting antigen and the immunologic microenvironment of the tissue site are other important variables in determining the pattern of DH, affecting the afferent and efferent phases, respectively. Some of these variables probably influence the development of a Th1 versus Th2 pattern of cytokine production as well. Some soluble antigens, especially in mucosal sites, can induce a type of DH with features of immediate hypersensitivity and basophil infiltration called *cutaneous basophil hypersensitivity*. Most epidermal toxins, especially heavy metals, plant toxins, or chemical toxins, cause monocyte infiltration and epidermal desquamation of the skin, the *contact hypersensitivity* type of Th1 DH. Deposition of certain insoluble antigens (bacterial or fungal debris) or immunization with soluble proteins using adjuvants causes the classic *tuberculin* type of Th1 DH that is characterized by fibrin deposition and monocyte and lymphocyte infiltration.

Persistence of certain infectious agents, especially bacteria within intracellular compartments of APCs or certain extracellular parasites, can cause destructive induration with granuloma formation and giant cells, the *granulomatous* form of DH. However, immune complex deposition (see the subhead "Lens-Associated Uveitis" in Chapter 7) or innate immune mechanisms in response to heavy metal or foreign-body reactions can also cause granulomatous inflammation in which the inflammatory cascade (resulting in DH) is triggered in the absence of specific T cells. Unfortunately, for most clinical entities in which T-cell responses are suspected, especially autoimmune disorders such as multiple sclerosis or arthritis, the precise immunologic mechanism remains highly speculative.

Cytotoxic lymphocytes

Cytotoxic T lymphocytes (CTLs) CTLs are a subset of antigen-specific T cells, usually bearing the CD8 marker, that are especially good at killing tumor cells and virus-infected

CLINICAL EXAMPLES

Toxocara granuloma (Th2 DH) *Toxocara canis* is a nematode parasite that infects up to 2% of all children and may occasionally produce vitreoretinal inflammatory manifestations. Although the ocular immunology of this disorder is not clearly delineated, animal models and a study of the immunopathogenesis of human nematode infections at other sites suggest the following scenario. The primary immune response begins in the gut after ingestion of viable eggs, which mature into larvae within the intestine. The primary processing phase produces a strong Th2 response, leading to a primary effector response that includes production of IgM, IgG, and IgE antibodies as well as Th2-mediated DH T cells. Hematogenous dissemination of a few larvae may result from accidental avoidance of immune effector mechanisms, leading to choroidal or retinal dissemination followed by invasion into the retina and vitreous. There, a Th2-mediated T-cell effector response recognizes larva antigens and releases Th2-derived cytokines to induce eosinophil and macrophage infiltration, causing the characteristic eosinophilic granuloma seen in the eye. In addition, antilarval B cells can infiltrate the eye and are induced to secrete various immunoglobulins, especially IgE. Finally, eosinophils, in part by attachment through Fc receptors, can recognize IgE or IgG bound to parasites and release cytotoxic granules containing the antiparasitic cationic protein directly in the vicinity of the larvae using a mechanism similar to antibody-dependent cellular cytotoxicity.

> Grencis RK. Th2-mediated host protective immunity to intestinal nematode infections. *Philos Trans R Soc Lond Biol Sci.* 1997;352:1377–1384.

Sympathetic ophthalmia (Th1 DH) Sympathetic ophthalmia is a bilateral panuveitis that follows penetrating trauma to one eye (see Chapter 10 for a more detailed discussion). This disorder represents one of the few human diseases in which autoimmunity can be directly linked to an initiating event. In most cases, penetrating injury activates the afferent phase. It is unclear whether the injury causes a de novo primary immunization to self-antigens, perhaps because of externalization of sequestered uveal antigens through the wound and exposure to the afferent immune response arc of the conjunctiva/extraocular sites, or if it instead somehow changes the immunologic microenvironment of the retina, RPE, and uvea so that a secondary afferent response is initiated that serves to alter preexisting tolerance to retinal and uveal self-antigens.

It is generally thought that the inflammatory effector response is dominated by a Th1-mediated DH mechanism generated in response to uveal or retinal antigens. CD4 T cells predominate early in the disease course, although CD8, or suppressor, T cells can be numerous in chronic cases. Activated macrophages are also numerous in granulomas, and Th1 cytokines have been identified in the vitreous or produced by T cells recovered from the eyes of affected patients. Although the target antigen for sympathetic ophthalmia is unknown, cutaneous immunization in experimental animals with certain retinal antigens (arrestin, rhodopsin, interphotoreceptor retinol–

binding protein), RPE-associated antigens, and melanocyte-associated tyrosinase can induce autoimmune uveitis with physiology or features suggestive of sympathetic ophthalmia. Th1-mediated DH is thought to mediate many forms of ocular inflammation. Table 4-5 lists other examples.

> Rao NA. Mechanisms of inflammatory response in sympathetic ophthalmia and VKH syndrome. *Eye.* 1997;11:213–216.

Table 4-5 Ocular Inflammatory Diseases Thought to Require a Major Contribution of Th1-Mediated DH Effector Mechanisms

Site	Disease	Presumed Antigen
Conjunctiva	Contact hypersensitivity to contact lens solutions	Thimerosal or other chemicals
	Giant papillary conjunctivitis	Unknown
	Phlyctenulosis	Bacterial antigens
Cornea and sclera	Chronic allograft rejection	Histocompatibility antigens
	Marginal infiltrates of blepharitis	Bacterial antigens
	Disciform keratitis after viral infection	Viral antigens
Anterior uvea	Acute anterior uveitis	Uveal autoantigens, bacterial antigens
	Sarcoid-associated uveitis	Unknown
	Intermediate uveitis	Unknown
Retina and choroid	Sympathetic ophthalmia	Retinal or uveal autoantigens
	Vogt-Koyanagi-Harada syndrome	Retinal or uveal autoantigens
	Birdshot choroiditis	Unknown
Orbit	Acute thyroid orbitopathy	Unknown
	Giant cell arteritis	Unknown

cells. CTLs can also mediate graft rejection and some cases of autoimmunity. In most cases, the ideal antigen for CTLs is an intracellular protein that either occurs naturally or is produced as a result of viral infection. CTLs appear to require help from CD4 helper T-cell signals to fully differentiate. Primed *precursor* CTLs leave the lymph node and migrate to the target tissue, where they are restimulated by the interaction of the CTL antigen receptor and foreign antigens within the antigen pocket of class I molecules (HLA-A, -B, or -C) on the target cell. Additional CD4 T cells help at the site, and expression of other accessory costimulatory molecules on the target is often required to obtain maximal killing.

CTLs kill cells in one of two ways: assassination or suicide induction (Fig 4-7). *Assassination* refers to CTL-mediated *lysis* of targets, using a specialized pore-forming protein called *perforin,* which puts pores, or holes, into cell membranes, causing osmotic lysis of the cell. *Suicide induction* refers to the capability of CTLs to stimulate *programmed cell death* of target cells, called *apoptosis,* using the CD95 ligand, the *FasL,* to activate its receptor on targets. Alternatively, CTLs can release cytotoxic cytokines like TNF to induce apoptosis. Activation of the apoptosis pathway induces the release of target cell enzymes and nucleases that cause fragmentation of chromosomal DNA and blebbing of the cell membrane,

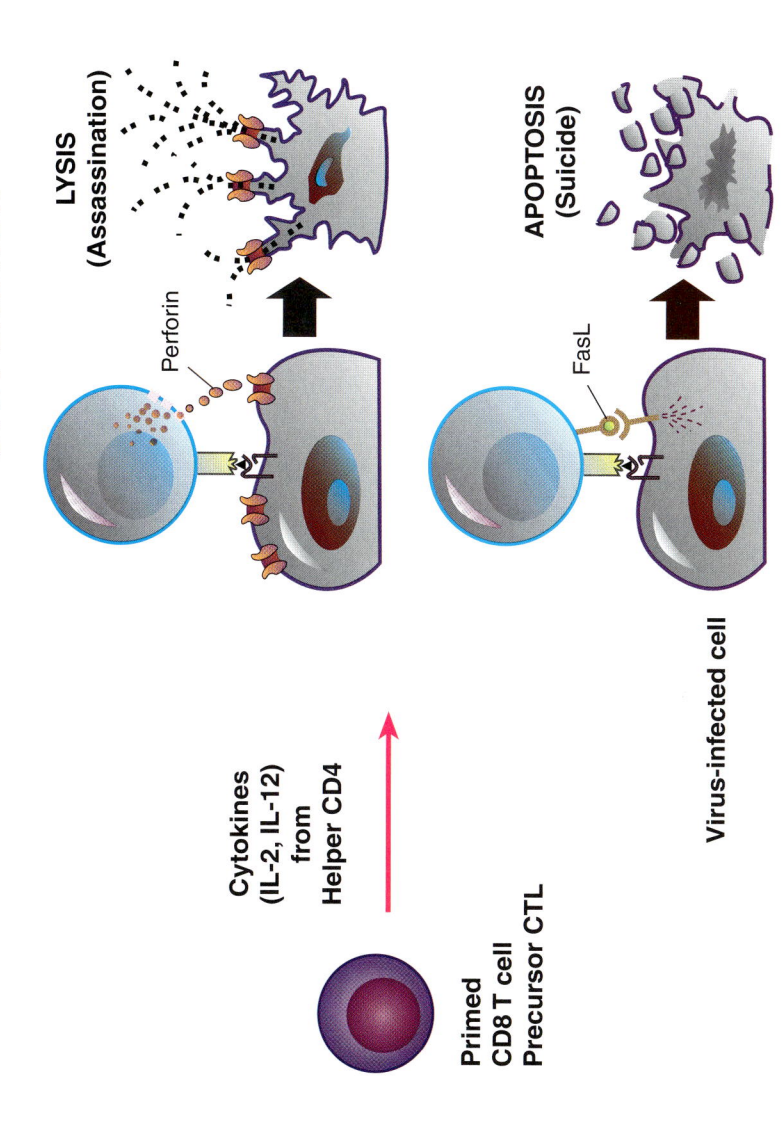

Figure 4-7 Schematic representation of the two major mechanisms of CD8 T-cell cytotoxicity. CD8 T cells, having undergone initial priming in the lymph node, enter the tissue site, where they again encounter antigen in the form of infected target cells. Upon restimulation, usually requiring CD4 helper T-cell factors, they become activated into fully cytolytic T cells. CD8 T cells can kill by lysing the infected cell, using a pore-forming protein called *perforin*. Or cytotoxic lymphocytes (CTLs) can kill by inducing *programmed cell death*, or *apoptosis*, using either FasL or cytokine-mediated mechanisms. *(Illustration by Barb Cousins, modified by Joyce Zavarro.)*

ultimately killing the cell. CTLs produce low-grade lymphocytic infiltrate within tumors or infected tissues and usually kill without causing significant inflammation.

Natural killer (NK) cells. NK cells—a subset of non-T, non-B lymphocytes—were originally called *null cells,* or large granular lymphocytes. They also kill tumor cells and virally infected cells but, unlike CTLs, NK cells do not have a specific antigen receptor. Instead, they are triggered by a less well characterized NK cell receptor. Once triggered, however, NK cells kill target cells using the same molecular mechanisms as CTLs. Since NK cells are not antigen-specific, they theoretically have the advantage of not requiring the time delay caused by induction of the adaptive, antigen-specific CTL immune response. However, NK cells do seem to require some of the same effector activational signals at the tissue site, especially cytokine stimulation. Thus, NK cells are probably most effective in combination with adaptive effector responses.

In some ways NK cells and CTLs are complementary in that they are inversely regulated—that is, cell processes such as diminished class I molecule expression that inhibit CTL function often enhance activation of NK cells, and vice versa. NK cells thereby provide another layer of protection against pathogens that interfere with class I expression, as do many viruses, especially cytomegalovirus. Experimental evidence suggests that NK cells may contribute to antiviral protection in cytomegalovirus and herpes simplex virus infections of the eye.

Lymphokine-activated killer (LAK) cells. LAK cells are T cells that have become nonspecifically activated by iatrogenic administration of immune cytokines such as IL-2 and others. LAK cells kill by various mechanisms, including those described above. Once it was learned that T cells are produced and become activated upon exposure to immune cytokines, or *lymphokines,* clinicians began to evaluate the clinical efficacy of treatment with cytokine immunotherapy. Originally, it was discovered that patients with certain tumors, especially metastatic malignant melanoma, who were treated with large doses of intravenous IL-2, sometimes responded with immune-mediated rejection of the tumor. Efficacy was subsequently improved when CTLs were removed from the blood or even from within metastatic tumor foci (ie, tumor-infiltrating lymphocytes) and treated with cytokines extracorporeally, then reinfused. Currently, numerous biotechnological approaches are being developed to enhance immunotherapy of LAK function for treatment of tumors and viral infections.

Combined Antibody and Cellular Effector Mechanisms

Antibody-dependent cellular cytotoxicity (ADCC)

Antibody can combine with a cell-associated antigen such as a tumor or viral antigen, but if the antibody is not a subclass that activates complement, it may not induce any apparent cytotoxicity. However, because the Fc tail of the antibody is externally exposed, various leukocytes can recognize the Fc domain of the antibody molecule and be directed to the cell through the antibody. When this happens, binding to the antibody activates various leukocyte cytotoxic mechanisms, including degranulation and cytokine production.

Since human leukocytes can express various types of Fc receptors—IgG subclasses have three different Fcg receptors, IgE has two different Fce receptors, and so on—

CLINICAL EXAMPLE

Antiviral immunity in cytomegalovirus (CMV) retinitis CMV retinitis is the most frequent opportunistic ocular infection in patients with AIDS. The majority of most populations have serologic evidence of prior CMV infection, which is typically thought to occur during chldhood or after contact with infected children. The pathophysiology of CMV infection is not entirely understood, but it can be inferred from analysis of animal experiments and human epidemiological studies. The primary afferent phase is usually initiated after upper respiratory tract infection, not uncommonly associated with viremia. The site of processing is unknown. Innate effectors, such as macrophages, natural killer cells, and neutrophils, provide some antiviral activity. However, most investigators think that virus-specific CD8 T cells are the best antiviral effector for controlling active infection. Some evidence also suggests a role for DH T cells. Antibodies are also generated, but they do not seem to play a major role in controlling virus infection, spread, or clearance. Antibodies may limit reinfection, however.

During the primary infection, virus is not completely cleared from the infected host but remains in a chronic state. It was originally thought that virus disseminated to various target tissues such as eye, gut, or kidney and became latent. More recent research suggests that the virus chronically infects the bone marrow and lung, probably persisting in certain macrophage precursor cells. Alternatively, CMV might infect the salivary gland, where it remains in epithelial cells. CMV appears to persist in these sites in a chronic but nonproductive state, and the existence of true latency is debated. However, as long as the host immune response is intact, the virus does not replicate effectively to infect the eye or other target organs.

Immunosuppression allows the virus to reactivate into a productive infection. Virus infects neutrophils, macrophages, and other leukocytes and spreads through the blood to susceptible target sites such as the retina. Alternatively, viremia during a primary CMV infection that occurs in previously uninfected immunosuppressed persons, especially after organ transplantation, can spread virus by a similar mechanism. It is thought that virus-specific CD8 T cells are the most important effector cell in preventing spread, but natural killer cells might also be effective. CD4 T cells play a role primarily by providing helper cytokines to fully activate CD8 T cells. Thus, in AIDS, CMV retinitis presumably occurs late in the disease because CD8 effectors become diminished later in the course of infection than do CD4 T cells. Transfusion of virus-specific CD8 T cells in organ transplant patients and replacement of helper cytokines to activate CD8 T cells in a mouse model of AIDS have both been shown to prevent CMV. Highly active antiretroviral therapy to suppress the HIV viral load has dramatically decreased the incidence of new cases of CMV retinitis in AIDS. The role of intravenous immune globulins, polyclonal antibodies enriched from human sera, in prophylaxis or treatment is controversial, but they may help prevent CMV disease after organ transplantation.

Riddell SR. Pathogenesis of cytomegalovirus pneumonia in immunocompromised hosts. *Semin Respir Infect*. 1995;10:199–208.

> **CLINICAL EXAMPLE**
>
> **Immune responses to malignant melanoma** Several investigators have evaluated the immune response to human uveal melanomas. Although controversial, data suggest that most primary or metastatic uveal melanomas demonstrate *melanoma antigen genes (MAGE)* and that these growing tumors express at least one family of tumor-associated antigens that should be recognized by CD8 cytolytic adaptive immune responses. Tumor-infiltrating lymphocytes were isolated from eyes undergoing enucleation because of large, growing melanomas. Numerous CD8 T cells could be isolated from all tumors, including tumor-specific T cells (indicating that afferent and processing phases had been initiated).
>
> In cell culture, the cytolytic T cells failed to effectively kill melanoma cells. After treatment with the cytokine (or lymphokine) IL-2, however, the CD8 T cells became fully cytolytic and did effectively kill the melanoma cells. The investigators conclude that uveal melanomas might create an immunologic microenvironment that prevents activation of the antitumor effector responses even though sensitized CTLs may be present in the tumor. Lymphokine activation may be a method to overcome this suppressive microenvironment and to upregulate the host's antitumor response to melanoma in order to prevent or control metastases.
>
> Chen PW, Murray TG, Uno T, et al. Expression of MAGE genes in ocular melanoma during progression from primary to metastatic disease. *Clin Exp Metastasis*. 1997;15:509–518.
>
> Niederkorn JY. Immunoregulation of intraocular tumours. *Eye*. 1997; 11:249–254.

leukocyte subsets differ in their capacity to recognize and bind different antibody isotypes. Classically, ADCC was observed to be mediated by a special subset of large granular (non-T, non-B) lymphocytes, called *killer cells*, that induce cell death in a manner similar to CTL. The killer cell itself is nonspecific but gains antigen specificity through interaction with specific antibody. Macrophages, NK cells, certain T cells, and neutrophils can also participate in ADCC using other Fc receptor types. An IgE-dependent form of ADCC might also exist for eosinophils.

ADCC is presumed to be important in tumor surveillance, antimicrobial host protection, graft rejection, and certain autoimmune diseases such as cutaneous systemic lupus erythematosus. Nevertheless, this effector mechanism probably does not play an important role in uveitis, although it might contribute to corneal graft rejection and antiparasitic immunity.

Acute IgE-mediated mast cell degranulation

Mast cells can bind IgE antibodies to their surface through a high-affinity Fc receptor specific for IgE molecules, positioning the antigen-combining site of the bound IgE externally (Fig 4-8). Combination of the antibody with a specific allergen (see the Clinical Example: Allergic conjunctivitis in this chapter) causes degranulation of the mast cell and release of mediators within minutes, producing an acute inflammatory reaction

MAST CELL

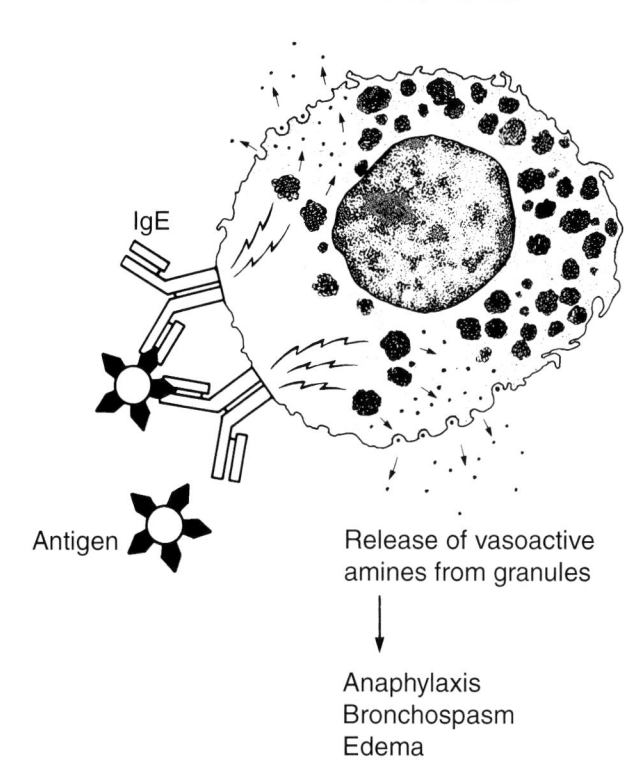

Figure 4-8 Schematic representation of IgE-mediated mast cell degranulation.

IgE

Antigen

Release of vasoactive amines from granules

↓

Anaphylaxis
Bronchospasm
Edema

called *immediate hypersensitivity* (Coombs and Gell Type I), which is characterized by local plasma leakage and itching. When severe, this response can produce a systemic reaction called *anaphylaxis,* which ranges in severity from generalized skin lesions such as erythema, urticaria, or angioedema to severe altered vascular permeability with plasma leakage into tissues that causes airway obstruction or hypotensive shock. Mast cells and vasoactive amines are discussed in greater detail below.

Chronic mast cell degranulation plus Th2 DH

Recent research has suggested that mast cells, B lymphocytes, and T lymphocytes can cooperate in atopic diseases to mediate chronic inflammatory reactions with a pattern that represents a mixture of acute allergy and delayed hypersensitivity. As discussed above, a Th2 subset of $CD4^+$ DH cells not only releases inflammatory mediators but also secretes certain cytokines (IL-4) that induce B cells to synthesize IgE and to recruit and activate eosinophils within a site (IL-5). Since mast cells can degranulate in response to stimuli other than IgE, the precise contributions of IgE-mediated mast cell degranulation in these chronic reactions have not been clarified. This pathogenic mechanism is thought to be especially important in the skin and at mucosal sites.

> **CLINICAL EXAMPLES**
>
> **Allergic conjunctivitis** Allergic conjunctivitis represents a secondary adaptive immune response to a family of antigens called *allergens* that induce predominately an acute IgE–mast cell effector response. The primary response presumably has occurred during a prior exposure to the allergen, often within the nasopharynx, in which afferent and processing phases were initiated. During this primary response, allergen-specific B cells were distributed to specialized areas in various MALT sites. At these sites, the B cells, with T-cell help, switch from IgM-antiallergen production to IgE-antiallergen production. IgE released at the site then combines with Fc receptors of surrounding mast cells, thereby arming the mast cells with a specific allergen receptor (ie, the antigen-recognizing Fab portion of the immunoglobulin). Thus, one mast cell may have bound antibodies specific for numerous different allergens.
>
> When reexposure to allergen occurs in a secondary response at a different site from the initial encounter, allergen must permeate beyond the superficial conjunctival epithelium to the subepithelial region, where the antigen binds allergen-specific IgE on the surface of mast cells. Degranulation occurs within 60 minutes, leading to the release of mediators, causing chemosis and itching. A late response, within 4–24 hours, is characterized by the recruitment of lymphocytes, eosinophils, and neutrophils. The role of Th2 DH or helper T cells in the effector response has not been confirmed for allergic conjunctivitis, but presumably both play a role, especially in B-cell differentiation, since the IgE is thought to be produced locally within the conjunctiva.
>
> **Atopic keratoconjunctivitis** Atopic keratoconjunctivitis is a chronic inflammatory condition of the palpebral and bulbar conjunctiva with features of allergic and cell-mediated inflammation (see BCSC Section 8, *External Disease and Cornea*). Analysis of biopsy specimens reveals the inflammatory infiltration to consist of mast cells and eosinophils, as well as activated CD4 T cells and B cells. Although immunopathogenesis is not clearly defined, a mechanism similar to that of atopic dermatitis can be inferred, combining poorly understood genetic mechanisms, chronic mast cell degranulation, and features of Th2-type delayed hypersensitivity. Immunopathogenesis of vernal conjunctivitis and giant papillary conjunctivitis is probably also similar.

Mediator Systems That Amplify Innate and Adaptive Immune Responses

Although innate or adaptive effector responses may directly induce inflammation, in most cases these effectors instead initiate a process that must be amplified to produce overt clinical manifestations. Molecules generated within the host that induce and amplify inflammation are termed *inflammatory mediators*, and mediator systems include several categories of these molecules (Table 4-6). Most act on target cells through receptor-mediated processes, although some act in enzymatic cascades that interact in a complex fashion.

Plasma-Derived Enzyme Systems

Complement factors

Complement is an important inflammatory mediator in the eye. Components and fragments of the complement cascade, which account for approximately 5% of plasma protein and more than 20 different proteins, represent important endogenous amplifiers of innate and adaptive immunity as well as mediators of inflammatory responses. Both adaptive and innate immune responses can initiate complement activation pathways, which generate products that contribute to the inflammatory process (Fig 4-9). Adaptive immunity typically activates complement by the classic pathway with antigen–antibody (immune) complexes, especially those formed by IgM, IgG1, and IgG3. Innate immunity typically activates complement by the alternative pathway using certain carbohydrate moieties or LPS on the cell wall of microorganisms.

Complement serves the following three basic functions during inflammation:

- Coating of antigenic or pathogenic surfaces by C3b to enhance phagocytosis
- Promotion of lysis of cell membranes through pore formation by membrane attack complexes
- Recruitment of PMNs and induction of inflammation through generation of the anaphylatoxins C3a, C4a, and C5a

The anaphylatoxins, so named because they cause anaphylaxis upon systemic administration into animals, are the principal complement-derived mediators. The effects of these anaphylatoxins include chemotaxis and changes in cell adhesiveness, mediated principally by C5a, and degranulation and release of mediators from mast cells and platelets, mediated by all three (these effects are described below in discussions of vasoactive amines, arachidonic acid (AA) metabolites, and PAFs). The proinflammatory complement mediator C5a also stimulates oxidative metabolism and the production and release of toxic oxygen radicals from leukocytes, as well as the extracellular discharge of leukocyte granule contents.

Walport MT. Advances in immunology: complement—first of two parts. *N Engl J Med.* 2001;344:1058–1060.

Table 4-6 Mediator Systems That Amplify Innate and Adaptive Immune Responses

Plasma-derived enzyme systems: complement, kinins, and fibrin
Vasoactive amines: serotonin and histamine
Lipid mediators: eicosanoids and platelet-activating factors
Cytokines
Reactive oxygen intermediates
Reactive nitrogen products
Neutrophil-derived granules and products

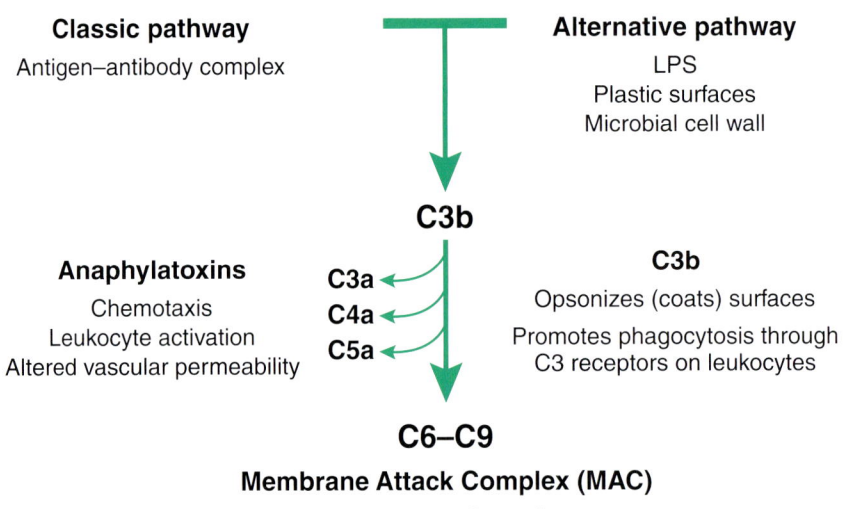

Classic pathway
Antigen–antibody complex

Alternative pathway
LPS
Plastic surfaces
Microbial cell wall

C3b

Anaphylatoxins
Chemotaxis
Leukocyte activation
Altered vascular permeability

C3a
C4a
C5a

C3b
Opsonizes (coats) surfaces
Promotes phagocytosis through C3 receptors on leukocytes

C6–C9
Membrane Attack Complex (MAC)
Forms pores in cell membranes
Osmotic lysis

Figure 4-9 Overview of the essential intermediates of the complement pathway.

Walport MT. Advances in immunology: complement—second of two parts. *N Engl J Med*. 2001;344:1140–1144.

Kinin-forming system

Kinins are low-molecular-weight polypeptides derived from precursors, or *kininogens*, in plasma and tissue fluids. They mediate numerous inflammatory effects, including vasodilation, pain, constriction of smooth muscle, increased vascular permeability, and stimulation of AA metabolism. The generation of kinins proceeds in the multiple steps typical of cascade reactions, and more than one pathway is known. In one pathway, innate triggers such as LPS activate Hageman factor, which in turn converts inactive proenzymes (prekallikrein) into active forms, or *kallikrein*. Substrates for the kallikrein enzymes are kininogens that are converted into kinins. The best-known kinin product of the Hageman factor–dependent pathway is *bradykinin*. Interestingly, the four cascade systems that play major or minor roles during inflammation (kinin, fibrinolytic, clotting, and complement) may all interact with Hageman factor, a plasma protein that can be activated by numerous stimuli, including negatively charged surfaces, collagen, trypsin, plasmin, kallikrein, coagulation factor XI, and LPS.

Fibrin and other plasma factors

Fibrin is the final deposition prouduct of another important plasma-derived enzyme system, and its deposition during inflammation promotes hemostasis, fibrosis, angiogenesis, and leukocyte adhesion. Fibrin is released from its circulating zymogen precursor, *fibrinogen,* upon cleavage by thrombin, also a zymogen, or proenzyme. In situ polymerization of smaller units gives rise to the characteristic fibrin plugs or clots. Fibrin dissolution is mediated by plasmin, which is activated from its zymogen precursor, plasminogen, by plasminogen activators such as tissue plasminogen activator. Thrombin, which is derived principally from platelet granules, is released after any vascular injury that causes platelet aggregation and release.

Fibrin deposition has long been considered a clinical sign of DH, since fibrin deposits in skin lesions of DH reactions give the skin a hardened or indurated feeling upon palpation, and extracellular fibrin deposits are histologically visible. However, significant fibrin deposits occur in forms of inflammation triggered by innate mechanisms as well. The role of fibrin deposition in the eye during uveitis is unknown, but it is thought to promote complications such as synechiae, cyclitic membranes, and tractional retinal detachment.

Vasoactive Amines

Serotonin and *histamine* are small preformed molecules released early during inflammatory responses that cause smooth muscle contraction and strongly influence vascular permeability and blood flow. In addition, histamine can influence cytokine production and receptor expression by leukocytes. Both of these amines subserve other functions as well. For example, serotonin also acts as a neurotransmitter. Vasoactive amines are important mediators for certain types of ocular inflammation, especially allergic reactions on the ocular surface such as vernal conjunctivitis.

Serotonin

Platelets probably provide the principal source of serotonin, which, like histamine, participates in regulating the initial increased blood flow and vascular permeability responses of inflammation. Platelets release serotonin from the granules following activation or aggregation. Since platelet plasma membranes are easily activated and respond rapidly to a wide variety of injuries and inflammatory stimuli, serotonin probably acts synergistically with other platelet-derived inflammatory mediators such as PAFs and thromboxanes. Further platelet aggregation and activation then ensues (see below).

Histamine

Histamine is present in the granules of mast cells and basophils, and it is actively secreted from this source following exposure of cells to a wide range of stimuli. Histamine acts by binding to one of at least three known types of receptors present differentially on target cells. The best-studied pathway for degranulation is antigen cross-linking of IgE bound to mast-cell Fc IgE receptors, but many other inflammatory stimuli can stimulate secretion, including complement, direct membrane injury, and certain drugs. Classically, histamine release has been associated with allergy. The contribution of histamine to intraocular inflammation remains equivocal.

Lipid Mediators

Two groups of lipid molecules synthesized by stimulated cells act as powerful mediators and regulators of inflammatory responses: the acetylated triglycerides, usually called *platelet-activating factors (PAFs),* and the AA metabolites, or *eicosanoids.* Both groups of molecules may be rapidly generated from the same lysophospholipid precursors by the enzymatic action of cellular phospholipases such as phospholipase A$_2$ (Fig 4-10).

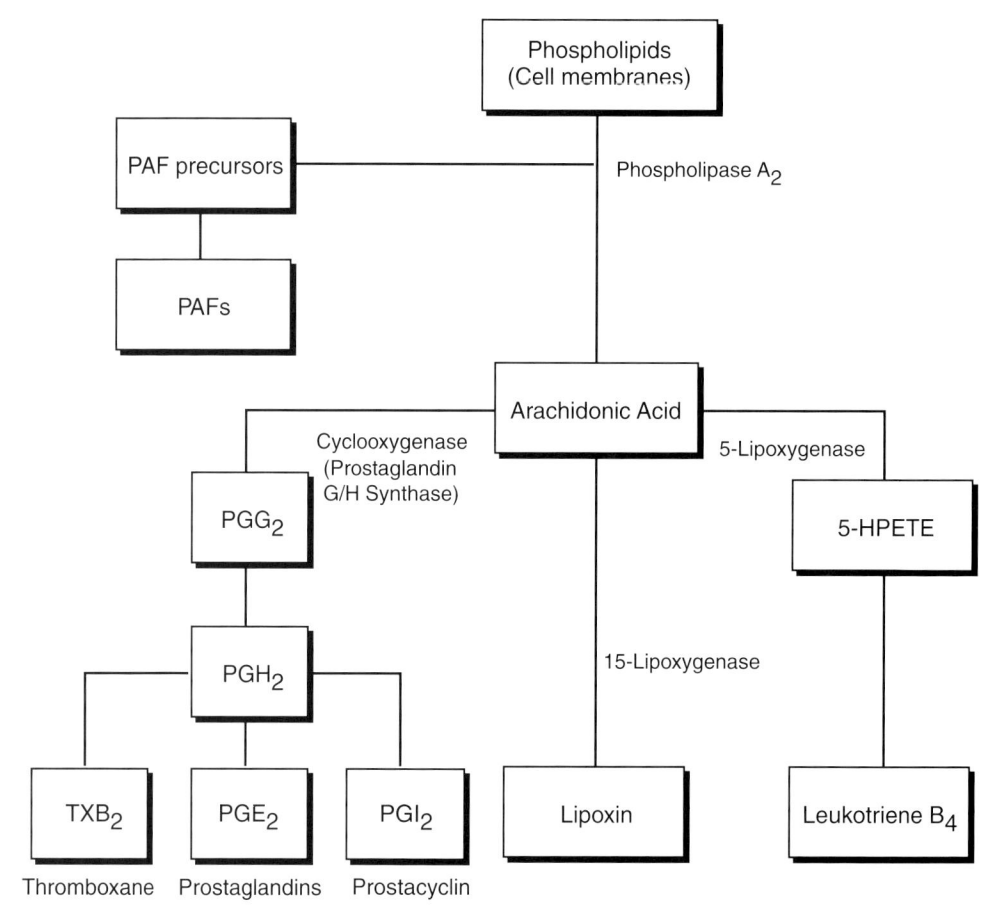

Figure 4-10 Overview of the essential intermediates of the eicosanoid and platelet-activating factor (PAF) pathways. *(Modified with permission from Pepose JS, Holland GN, Wilhelmus KR, eds.* Ocular Infection and Immunity. *St Louis: Mosby; 1996.)*

Eicosanoids

All eicosanoids are derived from AA. AA is liberated from membrane phospholipids by phospholipase A_2, which is activated by various agonists. AA is oxidized by two major pathways to generate the various mediators:

- The cyclooxygenase (COX) pathway, which produces prostaglandins (PGs), thromboxanes, and prostacyclins; COX is also known as prostaglandin G/H synthase (PG/H synthase)
- The 5-lipoxygenase pathway, which produces hydroxyeicosatetraenoic acid, lipoxins, and leukotrienes

Many other important enzymes also function in eicosanoid metabolism.

The COX-derived mediators are evanescent compounds induced in virtually all cells by a variety of stimuli. In general, they act in the immediate environment of their release to directly mediate many inflammatory activities, including effects on vascular permeability, cell recruitment, platelet function, and smooth muscle contraction. Perhaps of even greater importance, COX-derived products act on cells to regulate other functions, and they have very complicated effects on immune responses. Depending on conditions, COX-derived products can either upregulate or downregulate the production of cytokines, enzyme systems, and oxygen metabolites. Two forms of COX exist: COX-1 and COX-2. COX-1 is thought to be constitutively expressed in many cells, especially in cells that use PG for basal metabolic functions, such as the gastric mucosa or the renal tubular epithelium. COX-2 is inducible by many proinflammatory stimuli, including other inflammatory mediators (eg, PAF and some cytokines) and innate stimuli (eg, LPS).

Of the COX-derived mediators, PGs probably play the most important role in ocular inflammation. PGs have long been associated with regulation of vascular permeability in the eye, although their part in mediating cellular infiltration is not completely clear. Among the best characterized PGs are PGE_1 and PGE_2, but their ultimate role in the eye, whether harmful or protective, is unclear. For instance, increased levels of PGE_2 have been associated with uveitis, yet this PG can suppress effector cell function in vitro. The role of PGs in miosis of the pupil during inflammation has generated great interest, yet most PGs have minimal or no significant miotic activity on nonhuman primates or in human eyes. Some PGs have been hypothesized to cause corneal neovascularization.

Finally, PGs may be the cause of cystoid macular edema in association with anterior segment surgery or inflammation. Posterior diffusion of one or more of the eicosanoids through the vitreous is assumed to alter capillary permeability of the perifoveal network, leading to the characteristic pattern of intraretinal fluid accumulation and cyst formation. Clinical trials in humans have indicated that topical treatment with COX inhibitors does diminish the onset of mild cystoid macular edema after cataract surgery and might be efficacious in the treatment of severe persistent cystoid macular edema.

Prostaglandins and other eicosanoids indisputably play a major role in the physiology of the eye, reaching far beyond their putative participation as mediators of inflammation. For example, PGE_1 regulates the alternative (uveoscleral) outflow pathway for aqueous humor, perhaps explaining why IOP is diminished in some inflamed eyes. Latanoprost, a $PGF_{2\alpha}$ analogue, may act with a similar mechanism.

The products of the other major pathway of AA metabolism, the 5-lipoxygenase pathway, are also numerous, and some of them are extremely potent mediators of the inflammatory response. Derivatives of 5-lipoxygenase, an enzyme found mainly in granulocytes and some mast cells, have been also detected in the brain and retina. In contrast with prostaglandins, *leukotrienes* probably contribute significantly to inflammatory infiltration. One of the best characterized is leukotriene B_4, a potent chemotactic factor that also causes lysosomal enzyme release and reactive oxygen radical production by granulocytes. Some leukotrienes may have 1000 times the effect of histamine on vascular permeability. Another lipoxygenase product, lipoxin, is a potent stimulator of superoxide anion.

Platelet-activating factors

PAFs are a family of phospholipid-derived mediators that appear to be important stimuli in the early stage of inflammation. PAFs also serve physiological functions unrelated to inflammation, especially in reproductive biology, physiology of secretory epithelium, and neurobiology. In these physiological roles of PAFs, a de novo biosynthetic pathway has been identified. However, the *remodeling pathway* is the one implicated in PAF inflammatory actions.

Phospholipase A$_2$ metabolizes phosphocholine precursors in cell membranes, releasing AA and PAF precursors, which are then acetylated into multiple species of PAF. PAF release can be stimulated by various innate triggers such as bacterial toxins or trauma and cytokines. PAFs not only activate platelets but also activate most leukocytes as well, which in turn produce and release additional PAFs. The PAFs function by binding to one or more guanosine triphosphate protein–associated receptors on target cells.

In vitro, PAFs induce an impressive repertoire of responses including phagocytosis, exocytosis, superoxide production, chemotaxis, aggregation, proliferation, adhesion, eicosanoid generation, degranulation, and calcium mobilization as well as diverse morphological changes. PAFs seem to be a major regulator of cell adhesion and vascular permeability in many forms of acute inflammation, trauma, shock, and ischemia. PAF antagonists are being developed and tested in clinical trials. Synergistic interactions probably exist among PAFs, nitric oxide, eicosanoids, and cytokines. PAFs have been associated with ocular inflammation, but their precise role is under investigation.

Cytokines

Cytokine is a generic term for any soluble polypeptide mediator that is synthesized and released by cells for the purposes of intercellular signaling and communication. Table 4-7 lists some examples of cytokines that are most likely to be associated with ocular inflammation. Cytokines can be released to signal neighboring cells at the site *(paracrine action),* to stimulate a receptor on its own surface *(autocrine action),* or in some cases to act on a distant site through being released into the blood *(hormonal action).* Traditionally, investigators have subdivided cytokines into families with related activities, sources, and targets, using terms such as *growth factors, interleukins, lymphokines, interferons, monokines,* and *chemokines.* Thus, growth factor traditionally refers to cytokines mediating cell proliferation and differentiation. *Interleukin* or *lymphokine* identifies cytokines thought to mediate intercellular communication among lymphocytes or other leukocytes. *Interferons* are cytokines that limit or interfere with virus infection of a cell. *Chemokines,* originally called *intercrines,* are chemotactic cytokines. However, research has demonstrated that although some cytokines are specific for particular cell types, most cytokines have such multiplicity and redundancy of source, function, and target that this focus on specific terminology is not particularly useful for the clinician. For example, activated macrophages in an inflammatory site synthesize growth factors, interleukins, interferons, and chemokines.

Both innate and adaptive responses result in the production of cytokines. T lymphocytes are the classic cytokine-producing cell of adaptive immunity, but macrophages, mast cells, and even PMNs can also synthesize a wide range of cytokines upon stimulation. Nevertheless, the exact role of individual molecules during the inflammatory response is not clear. Cytokine interactions can be additive, combinatorial (two factors combining for greater effect than the sum of their individual activities), or synergistic (two factors enabling a new activity not manifested by either alone). Further complicating the issue, cytokines usually have multiple functions that overlap and counteract; as a

Table 4-7 Cytokines of Relevance to Ocular Immunology

Family	Example	Major Cell Source	Major Target Cells	Major General Actions	Specific Ocular Actions
Interleukins	IL-1α	Macrophages Many others	Most leukocytes Various ocular cells	Many actions on T and B cells Systemic toxicity (fever, shock)	Altered vascular permeability PMN and macrophage infiltration Langerhans migration to central cornea
	IL-6	Macrophages T cells Mast cells Most ocular epithelium	Most leukocytes Various ocular cells	Many actions on B cells Systemic toxicity (fever, shock)	Altered vascular permeability PMN infiltration High levels in many forms of uveitis and nonuveitic diseases
	IL-2	Th0 or Th1 CD4 T cells	T cells B cells NK cells	Activates CD4 and CD8 T cells Induces Th1	Detectable levels in some forms of uveitis
	IL-4	Th2 CD4 T cells Basophils, mast cells	T cells B cells	Induces Th2, blocks Th1 Induces B cells to make IgE	? Role in atopic and vernal conjunctivitis
	IL-5	Th2 CD4 T cells		Recruits eosinophils	? Role in atopic and vernal conjunctivitis
Alpha chemokines	IL-8	Many cell types	Endothelial cells PMN Many others	Recruits and activates PMN Upregulates CAM on endothelium	Altered vascular permeability PMN infiltration
Beta chemokines	Macrophage chemotactic protein-1 (MCP-1)	Macrophages Endothelium RPE	Endothelial cells Macrophages T cells	Recruits and activates macrophages, some T cells	Recruits macrophages and T cells to eye
Tumor necrosis factors	TNF-α or -β	Macrophages (TNF-α) T cells (TNF-β)		Tumor apoptosis Macrophage and PMN activation Cell adhesion and chemotaxis Fibrin deposition and vascular injury Systemic toxicity (fever, shock)	Altered vascular permeability Mononuclear cell infiltration

(Continues)

Table 4-7 Cytokines of Relevance to Ocular Immunology (Continued)

Family	Example	Major Cell Source	Major Target Cells	Major General Actions	Specific Ocular Actions
Interferons	Interferon gamma (IFN-γ)	Th1 T cells NK cells		Activates macrophages	PMN and macrophage infiltration
	IFN-α	Most leukocytes	Most parenchymal cells	Prevents viral infection of many cells Inhibits hemangioma, conjunctival intraepithelial neoplasia, and other tumors	Innate protection of ocular surface from viral infection, treatment of ocular surface neoplasms
Growth Factors	Transforming growth factor–β (TGF-β)	Many cells Leukocytes, T cells RPE and NPE of ciliary body Pericytes Fibroblasts	Macrophages T cells RPE Glia Fibroblasts	Suppresses T-cell and macrophage inflammatory functions Fibrosis of wounds	Regulator of immune privilege and ACAID
	Platelet-derived growth factors (PDGF)	Platelets Macrophages RPE	Fibroblasts Glia Many others	Fibroblast proliferation	Role in inflammatory membranes, subretinal fibrosis
Neuropeptides	Substance P	Ocular nerves Mast cells	Leukocytes Others	Pain Altered vascular permeability	Altered vascular permeability Leukocyte infiltration, photophobia
	Vasoactive intestinal peptide	Ocular nerves	Leukocytes Others	Suppresses macrophage and T-cell inflammatory function	Role in ACAID and immune privilege

consequence, elimination of the action of a single molecule may have an unpredictable outcome. Moreover, the function of various cytokines might change during the course of an inflammatory response. Finally, not only do innate and adaptive immune responses use cytokines as mediators and amplifiers of inflammation, but cytokines also modulate the initiation of immune responses; the function of most leukocytes is altered by pre-exposure to various cytokines. Thus, for many cytokines, their regulatory role may be as important as their actions as mediators of inflammation.

Reactive Oxygen Intermediates

Under certain conditions, oxygen can undergo chemical modification to transform into highly reactive substances with the potential to damage cellular molecules and inhibit functional properties in pathogens or host cells. BCSC Section 2, *Fundamentals and Principles of Ophthalmology,* discusses the processes involved in greater detail in Part IV, Biochemistry and Metabolism. See especially Chapter 18, Free Radicals and Antioxidants.

Three of the most important oxygen intermediates are superoxide anion, hydrogen peroxide, and the hydroxyl radical:

$$O_2 + e^- \rightarrow O_2^-$$ superoxide anion

$$O_2^- + O_2^- + 2H^+ \rightarrow O_2 + H_2O_2$$ superoxide dismutase catalyzes anions to form hydrogen peroxide

$$H_2O_2 + e^- \rightarrow OH^- + OH^\bullet$$ hydroxyl anion and hydroxyl radical

Oxygen metabolites that are generated by leukocytes, especially PMNs and macrophages, and triggered by immune responses are the most important source during inflammation. A wide variety of stimuli can trigger leukocyte oxygen metabolism, including

- Innate triggers such as LPS or formyl methionine-leucine-proline
- Adaptive effectors such as complement-fixing antibodies or certain cytokines produced by DH T cells
- Other chemical mediator systems such as C5a, PAF, or leukotrienes

Reactive oxygen intermediates can also be generated as part of noninflammatory cellular biochemical processes, especially by electron transport in the mitochondria, detoxification of certain chemicals, or interactions with environmental light or radiation.

The principal mechanism by which oxygen metabolites are activated during inflammation is by the induction of various oxidases in PMNs or macrophage cell membranes, especially NADPH oxidase, but also NADH oxidase, xanthine oxidase, and aldehyde oxidase. NADPH oxidase catalyzes the transfer of electrons from NADPH, the reduced form of nicotinamide-adenine dinucleotide phosphate, or from NADH, the reduced form of nicotinamide-adenine dinucleotide, to oxygen or hydrogen peroxide (H_2O_2) to form intermediates such as the reactive oxygen radical superoxide anion. As shown in the formulas above, the transfer of a single electron to oxygen forms superoxide anion, an unstable radical that may dismutate spontaneously; that is, one of the molecules gains an electron and the other loses one. Otherwise, the reaction can be catalyzed by the enzyme superoxide dismutase to form H_2O_2 and oxygen.

Alternatively, two electrons can be transferred to molecular oxygen, a process that normally occurs in the peroxisomes. This process also results in formation of H_2O_2, a molecule that by itself has feeble inflammatory and microbicidal activity. Moreover, H_2O_2 can be readily neutralized into water and oxygen by enzymes such as catalase in peroxisomes and glutathione peroxidase in the cytosol, as shown in Figure 4-11.

H_2O_2, however, can be converted into molecules with potential inflammatory and antimicrobial activity by at least three chemical processes:

- The Fenton or Haber-Weiss reactions can add one electron to form the hydroxyl anion (OH^-) along with the highly reactive hydroxyl radical ($OH^\bullet$). However, the existence of this pathway in vivo has been disputed.
- In a second, recently discovered, process, H_2O_2 may be catalyzed by myeloperoxidase, an abundant protein found in PMNs, to react with halide or pseudohalide (thiocyanate) substrates to form extremely toxic products that are highly damaging to bacteria and tissues. These include hypohalous acids, halogens, chloramines, and hydroxyl radicals. Hydroxyl radicals interact with several potential cellular targets to cause enzyme and protein damage as a result of cross-linking of sulfhydryl groups; cell membrane injury caused by lipid peroxidation of the lipid bilayers; loss of energization and cellular stores of adenosine triphosphate as a result of loss of integrity of the inner membrane of the mitochondria; and breaks or cross-links in DNA from chemical alterations of nucleotides.

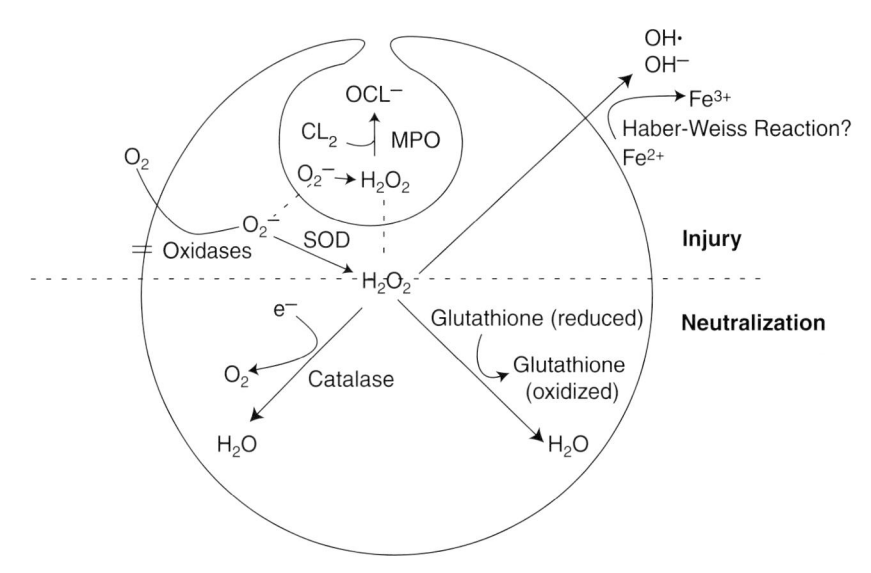

Figure 4-11 Overview of the essential intracellular and extracellular pathways in the generation of reactive oxygen intermediates. Activation of oxidases catalyzes the production of superoxide anion (O_2^-), which can be converted into H_2O_2 by superoxide dismutase (SOD). Catalase (in the peroxisome) and glutathione can neutralize H_2O_2. However, H_2O_2 can be converted into hydroxyl ion (OH^+) or hydroxyl radical ($OH^\bullet$) by the Haber-Weiss reaction. Alternatively, H_2O_2 can be catalyzed by myeloperoxidase (MPO) into hypochlorous anion and other reactive intermediates. *(Reprinted with permission from Pepose JS, Holland GN, Wilhelmus KR, eds.* Ocular Infection and Immunity. *St Louis: Mosby; 1996.)*

- A third inflammatory process involves the formation of peroxynitrite after chemical interaction between superoxide and nitric oxide (see below).

Reactive Nitrogen Products

Another important pathway of host defenses and inflammation involves the toxic products of nitrogen, especially *nitric oxide (NO)*. NO is a highly reactive chemical species that, like reactive oxygen intermediates, can react with various important biochemical functions in microorganisms and host cells. This pathway was first observed in patients with a deficiency of the respiratory burst enzymes. Because of this deficiency, their PMNs and macrophages were unable to generate reactive oxygen intermediates, but they were still able to mount effective antimicrobial function through a toxic nitrogen product, NO.

The formation of NO depends on the enzyme nitric oxide synthetase (NOS), which is located in the cytosol and is NADPH-dependent. NO is formed from the terminal guanidino-nitrogen atoms of L-arginine. Several forms of NO synthetase are known, including several constitutive forms of NOS (cNOS) and an inducible NOS (iNOS). Many normal cells produce basal levels of NO, which is considered secondary to the calcium-dependent, constitutive form of the enzyme. Activation *induces* enhanced production of NO in certain cells, especially macrophages. This enhanced production appears to be secondary to the induced synthesis of a second, calcium-independent form of NO synthetase (iNOS). Many innate and adaptive stimuli modulate induction of iNOS, especially cytokines and bacterial toxins.

How NO functions to kill microorganisms is uncertain. Likely possibilities include interaction with the Fe-S groups of aconitase, an enzyme important for the control of DNA synthesis and RNA production, or complex I and complex II of the mitochondrial electron transport system. During inflammation, NO may also interact with O_2 to form the toxic hydroxyl radical and peroxynitrite ($ONOO^-$). Peroxynitrite displays high chemical reactivity, including great capacity to peroxidate lipids in cell membranes, modify

CLINICAL EXAMPLE

Role of oxygen-mediated damage in experimental uveitis Reactive oxygen intermediates are likely mediators in many forms of ocular inflammation, especially those forms involving the retina. In a series of studies examining a model of autoimmune uveoretinitis, investigators demonstrated that the generation of toxic oxygen intermediates was associated with PMNs and monocyte infiltration. The formation of superoxide anion and hydroxyl radicals was an early event, and peroxidation of photoreceptor membranes, especially the depletion of polyunsaturated fatty acids, occurred simultaneously with the onset of free radical formation and electrophysiological loss of photoreceptor function. Interestingly, the peroxidation products were chemotactic for PMNs, thereby providing a possible mechanism for amplifying the cycle of inflammatory tissue destruction. Some antioxidants were partially protective.

Rao NA. Role of oxygen free radicals in retinal damage associated with experimental uveitis. *Trans Am Ophthalmol Soc.* 1990;88:797–850.

cellular proteins, and damage DNA. NO biology in the eye during uveitis is under active investigation.

Neutrophil-Derived Granule Products

PMNs are also a source of specialized products that can amplify innate or adaptive immune responses. A large number of biochemically defined antimicrobial polypeptides are present in many types of granules found in PMNs. The principal well-characterized antimicrobial polypeptides found in human PMN granules are bactericidal/permeability-increasing protein, defensins, lysozyme, lactoferrin, and the serine proteases (or their homologues).

In addition to antimicrobial polypeptides, the PMNs contain numerous other molecules that may contribute to inflammation. These include hydrolytic enzymes, elastase, metalloproteinases, gelatinase, myeloperoxidase, vitamin B_{12}–binding protein, cytochrome b_{558}, and others. Granule contents are considered to remain inert and membrane-bound when the granules are intact, but they become active and soluble when granules fuse to the phagocytic vesicles or plasma membrane.

Exactly how the various granulocyte products enhance inflammation is not clear. Originally, it was thought that the release of proteases and other enzymes directly degraded the extracellular matrix of inflamed sites, thereby enabling the recruitment of additional leukocytes, damaging the integrity of microvessels, and injuring the attachment substrate of the parenchymal cells. However, recent evidence suggests that hypochlorous acid, derived from reactive oxygen by-products, must interact with proteases and protease inhibitors in a complex fashion to enhance the tissue-destructive effects of PMN granule products. The role of PMN-derived proteases in ocular inflammation remains unclear. Collagenases are thought to contribute to corneal injury and liquefaction during bacterial keratitis and scleritis, especially in *Pseudomonas* infections. Collagenases also contribute to peripheral corneal melting syndromes secondary to rheumatoid arthritis–associated peripheral keratitis.

CHAPTER 5

Special Topics in Ocular Immunology

Immunoregulation of the Adaptive Immune Response

T- and B-cell Antigen Receptor Repertoire

The biology of T-cell and B-cell antigen receptors has become a major area of research. The specificities of T-cell antigen receptors and of B-cell antigen receptors such as surface IgM and IgD must account for tens of thousands (if not millions) of possible antigens in nature. Since antigen receptor specificities are originally generated randomly, before the initial encounter with antigen, this wide range of potential specificities requires that the adaptive immune system generate a huge number of different antibody and T-cell receptor molecules from relatively few associated genes. This diversity requires a very elegant form of molecular *recombination*, or the mixing and matching of genetic segments of immunoglobulin or T-cell receptor germline genes during maturation of T cells and B cells. For B cells, additional recombination and mutation of the receptor genes take place during the immune response. These genetic manipulations do not occur for other types of receptors. Nevertheless, the random formation of antigen receptors implies that the generation of many receptors that recognize self-antigens is possible, leading to the potential for autoimmunity. BCSC Section 2, *Fundamentals and Principles of Ophthalmology*, discusses recombination in Part III, Genetics.

Tolerance and Immunoregulation

A central theme in immunology is the ability of the adaptive immune response to differentiate between *self* and *nonself*, or foreign. The paradox involved was eloquently recognized by Erlich, who coined the term *horror autotoxicus*, or fear of self-poisoning, to convey the idea that a sophisticated mechanism must exist to prevent the immune system from attacking normal tissues. Medawar subsequently enunciated the formal concept of self-tolerance.

In modern immunology, *tolerance* is usually defined as the sum total of the mechanisms by which the immune system differentiates self from foreign to prevent *inflammation-triggering* immune responses against self-antigens. Recent advances in immunology have clarified various mechanisms of immunologic tolerance that prevent widespread autoimmune inflammation. Although a detailed description of these mechanisms is beyond the scope of this book, a brief overview is included below. See also Chapter 2 for a discussion of *T-cell cross-regulation*, the concept that Th1 cells can regulate Th2 activation, and vice versa.

Davidson A, Diamond B. Autoimmune diseases. *N Engl J Med.* 2001;345:340–350.

Clonal deletion

The thymus has the ability to destroy self-reactive T cells during T-cell maturation, resulting in clonal deletion. Perhaps 99% of all T cells that enter the thymus are deleted from the host by this mechanism, suggesting that at least some of the deleted T cells were autoreactive. Thus, clonal deletion provides a mechanism for immunologic unresponsiveness that creates a gap in the repertoire of potential antigens, presumably self-antigens, against which the immune response can mobilize. In mice, clonal deletion has been demonstrated in principle through several different experimental approaches.

The precise role of clonal deletion in immunologic tolerance to ocular autoantigens remains uncertain. Intriguingly, a crystallin protein and S antigen have been detected within the thymus, suggesting the possibility of crystallin-specific and S antigen–specific deletion of T cells. However, actual clonal deletion of autoreactive T cells has not yet been demonstrated for ocular autoantigens. If clonal deletion were complete, lens- or retinal-responsive T cells would be absent during uveitis. Because such T cells can indeed be demonstrated under certain experimental conditions, clonal deletion, if present, must be incomplete.

Anergy

Anergy and *clonal inactivation* are terms that have been used to describe the situation in which antigen-specific T cells or B cells are rendered incapable of mounting a normal inflammation-triggering response to that antigen. For example, when B cells of mice are exposed to antigen early in the developmental process, they are rendered unresponsive to that antigen after maturation. Similarly, several different mechanisms that "tolerize" T cells have been demonstrated. When T cells are presented antigen by nonprofessional antigen-presenting cells (APCs) such as corneal endothelium or Müller cells, they become inactivated from further differentiation into inflammatory effector cells. Although these T cells survive, they are incapable of initiating inflammatory immune responses. Anergy therefore provides an additional mechanism for immunologic unresponsiveness.

Suppression

Suppression, the third classic mechanism for tolerance, postulates that a population of *downregulatory T cells* exists to balance the population of helper and inflammation-enhancing T cells. These downregulatory T cells modulate and diminish the level of activation by the effector or helper T cells. Whereas clonal deletion or anergy supports immunologic unresponsiveness, suppression indicates an active but tolerizing immune response to a specific antigen. The best-characterized mechanism involves the release of immunosuppressive cytokines such as transforming growth factor–β by CD8 suppressor T cells, but several other mechanisms have also been supported by experimental data. Although the physiological importance and mechanism(s) by which suppression is induced and regulated have been challenged, suppression is clearly an important regulatory mechanism for the immune system in general and for ocular immune responses in particular. See Chapter 3 for a discussion of suppression induced during anterior chamber–associated immune deviation.

Potential role of antibody isotype

An interesting paradox can be demonstrated in many healthy people: antiself-antibodies to many major autoantigens can be demonstrated in sera, but these autoantibodies do not seem to cause inflammation. One explanation may be related to the different effector functions of various antibody isotypes (see Table 4-4). The major inflammation-inducing mechanism of antibody is brought about by complement activation, which in turn is a function of the isotype of the antibody molecule itself. As discussed in Chapter 4, isotypes vary in their capacity to activate complement. Preferential activation of B cells that produce complement-fixing antibodies results in inflammation-inducing immunity, since complement activation is initiated following immune complex formation. Conversely, preferential activation of non–complement-fixing antibodies results in high antibody titers but not severe inflammation. Immune complexes opsonize or agglutinate the antigen, but complement is not activated. Therefore, one key to B-cell effector function is determined by the regulation of the class switch from an IgM-synthesizing B cell to one producing an antibody of the other isotypes. This switch is controlled by different T-cell–derived cytokines. By inference, the regulation of this form of B-cell tolerance is passive and under the control of helper T-cell signals.

Male DK, Cooke A, Owen M, et al. *Advanced Immunology.* 3rd ed. St Louis: Mosby; 1996.
Roitt IM, Delves PJ. *Roitt's Essential Immunology.* 10th ed. Malden, MA: Blackwell Science; 2001.

Molecular Mimicry

Autoimmunity may play an important role in the pathogenesis of inflammatory ocular diseases, and one mechanism through which autoimmunity to self-antigens in the eye may be triggered is *molecular mimicry,* the immunologic cross-reaction between epitopes of an unrelated foreign antigen and self-epitopes with similar structures. Theoretically, these epitopes would be similar enough to stimulate an immune response, yet different enough to cause a breakdown of immunologic tolerance.

For example, a foreign antigen such as those present within yeast, viruses, or bacteria can induce an appropriate afferent, processing, and effector immune response. A self-antigen with similar epitopes may induce antimicrobial antibodies or effector lymphocytes to inappropriately cross-react. A dynamic process would then be initiated, causing tissue injury by an autoimmune response that would induce additional lymphocyte responses directed at other self-antigens. Thus, the process would not require the ongoing replication of a pathogen or the continuous presence of the inciting antigen.

> **CLINICAL EXAMPLE**
>
> **Tolerance to lens crystallins** Why does violation of the lens capsule and release of lens proteins during cataract surgery almost always produce only minimal immunologic sequelae? Intuitively, cataract surgery or any type of lens injury and the ensuing release of lens protein would seem likely to initiate an autoimmune attack. Yet even though serum titers of antilens antibodies often rise in patients after cataract surgery, effector T cells, pathogenic antibodies, and true autoimmune uveitis rarely develop. Most investigators think that the protection of the lens is caused by the presence of active immunologic tolerance and that the lens is *not* sequestered from the immune system. Thus, the relative rarity of true autoimmune uveitis directed against the lens indicates the power of protective tolerance to self.
>
> The nature of the T-cell tolerance to the lens, and whether it involves clonal deletion, anergy, suppression, cross-regulation, or a combination thereof is not known. Clonal deletion of antilens T cells is suggested by the detection of a crystallin protein and mRNA within the thymus. Anergy is also suggested by some other animal experiments. Ocular immune privilege (ACAID) may provide an additional mechanism for tolerance by the generation of suppressor T cells. However, tolerance is not complete because responses of antilens helper T cells can be demonstrated under certain experimental conditions, although DH effector cells rarely develop.
>
> B-cell tolerance to lens protein is probably indirect, controlled at the level of the helper T cell. Thus, functional lens-specific B cells certainly exist, since antilens antibody can be identified in the serum of many normal persons and in most patients after cataract surgery. In addition, antibody titers can be stimulated in all animals by cutaneous immunization. An increase in the titer of antilens antibody after immunization or surgery, however, does not necessarily indicate loss of tolerance as long as the antibody titers are predominated by non–complement-fixing isotypes.
>
> Pepose JS, Holland GN, Wilhelmus KR, eds. *Ocular Infection and Immunity.* St Louis: Mosby; 1996.

HLA Associations and Disease

Normal Function of HLA Molecules

All animals with white blood cells express a family of cell surface glycoproteins called *major histocompatibility complex (MHC)* proteins. In humans, the MHC proteins are called *human leukocyte antigen (HLA)* molecules. As discussed in Chapter 2, six different families of HLA molecules have been identified:

- Three class I MHC: HLA-A, -B, -C
- Three class II MHC: HLA-DR, -DP, -DQ

> **CLINICAL EXAMPLE**
>
> **Molecular mimicry and autoimmune uveitis** Molecular mimicry has been suggested as a mechanism for uveitis after finding that the primary amino acid sequence of a variety of foreign antigens (including those of baker's yeast histone, *E coli*, hepatitis B virus, and certain murine and primate retroviruses) showed sequence homology to a pathogenic epitope of the ocular autoantigen S antigen. Immunization of rats with crude extracts prepared from these organisms or synthetic peptides corresponding to the homologous epitopes induced retinal inflammation. In addition, T cells isolated from rats immunized with foreign substances cross-reacted with retinal autoantigens, providing evidence of molecular mimicry between self and nonself proteins. Currently, no definitive clinical evidence suggests that molecular mimicry contributes to autoimmune diseases of the human eye.

A seventh category, HLA-D, does not exist as a specific molecule but instead represents a functional classification as determined by an in vitro assay. Class III MHC molecules and minor MHC antigens have also been identified, but they are not discussed here.

The important role MHC molecules play in immunologic function is discussed in Chapter 2, and Table 5-1 gives a historical perspective, linking MHC molecules and transplantation biology with immune response genes. HLAs are also considered to be human immune response genes, since the HLA type determines the capacity of the APC to bind peptide fragments and thus determines T-cell immune responsiveness.

Allelic Variation

Many different alleles or polymorphic variants of each of the six HLA types exist within the population: more than 25 alleles for HLA-A, 50 for -B, 10 for -C, 100 for -DR, and so on. Since there are six major HLA types and each individual has a pair of each HLA type, or one *haplotype,* from each parent, an APC expresses six pairs of MHC molecules. Thus, with the exception of identical twins, it is rare that two individuals will match all 12 potential haplotypes. Alleles and genetic variations are discussed in greater detail in BCSC Section 2, *Fundamentals and Principles of Ophthalmology,* Part III, Genetics.

Allelic diversity may be designed to provide protection through *population-wide immunity.* Each HLA haplotype theoretically covers a set of antigens to which a particular individual can respond adaptively. Thus, in theory, the presence of many different HLA alleles within a population should ensure that the adaptive immune system in at least some individuals in the whole group will be able to respond to a wide range of potential pathogens. The converse also holds true: Some individuals may be at increased risk for immunologic diseases.

Clinical detection and classification of different alleles

Traditionally, the different alleles of HLA-A, -B, -C, -DR, and -DQ have been detected by reacting lymphocytes with special antisera standardized by international HLA Workshops sponsored by the World Health Organization (WHO). HLA-DP and HLA-D typing requires performance of specialized T-cell culture assays. Traditionally, provisional

Table 5-1 The Major Histocompatibility Complex Locus and the HLA System: A Short History

1940s	Skin autografts succeed, but allografts are rejected unless from a twin
1950s	Transfusion reactions noted against white blood cells among patients matched to RBC antigens, called *human leukocyte antigens (HLA)*
	Antibodies to disparate fetal HLA types noted among multiparous mothers
1960s	Immune response genes in mice control ability to respond to one antigen but not another
	Immune response genes probably code for mouse equivalent of HLA (immune antigen, or Ia)
	Allograft rejection is genetically determined by the major histocompatibility complex (MHC) locus
1970s	Ia in mice and HLA types in humans correlate with transplant rejection, giving rise to the concept that immune response genes are part of the MHC
	Prediction that Ia type in mice and HLA type in humans will correlate with propensity to autoimmunity on basis of immune responsiveness to environmental pathogens
	First HLA association with inflammatory disease (HLA-B27 and ankylosing spondylitis)
1980s	Mechanism of MHC function: HLA required on antigen-presenting cells to activate T cells—class I molecules present to CD8 T cells; class II molecules present to CD4 T cells
	T cells and B cells see antigen differently; B cells see the whole, natural antigen; T cells "see" antigens after they are chopped up into peptides
	Function of class I and II molecules confirmed—antigen fragments are placed within a groove formed by the tertiary structure of the molecule to allow presentation to the T-cell receptor
	Different HLA molecules have different capacity to bind different fragments, explaining role as immune response gene
	Mutations in the binding site within the groove of class I and II molecules may allow some individuals to bind and present certain environmental or self-peptides, thereby predisposing to autoimmunity
1990s	Molecular typing of HLA becoming more available and better than serotyping
	Molecular mechanism of antigen processing well characterized

serotypes pending official recognition were often designated *workshop* (ie, DRw53). More recently, molecular techniques have been developed to characterize the nucleic acid sequence of various MHC alleles. HLA molecules are composed of two chains: α and β chains for class II, an α chain and the $β_2$-microglobulin chain for class I. Since subtle differences in molecular structure can be easily missed during antisera, molecular genotyping is a more precise method to determine MHC types. Thus, the genotype specifies the chain, the major genetic type, and the specific minor molecular variant subtype. For example, genotype DRB1 *0408 refers to the HLA-DR4 molecule β chain with the "—08" minor variant subtype.

New serotypes now must correspond to a specific genotype, and the provisional "w" label is rarely used. Nonetheless, haplotypes currently recognized as a single group will continue to be subdivided into new categories or new subtypes. For example, at least two different A29 subtypes and eight different HLA-B27 subtypes have been recognized. Finally, some investigators have proposed that HLA classification based on similarities of

> **CLINICAL EXAMPLE**
>
> **HLA-B27–associated acute anterior uveitis** Approximately 50% of patients with acute anterior uveitis (AAU) express the HLA-B27 haplotype, and many of these patients also experience other immunologic disorders such as Reiter syndrome, ankylosing spondylitis, inflammatory bowel disease, and psoriatic arthritis (see Chapter 7). Although the immunopathogenesis remains unknown, various animal models permit some informed speculation. Many cases of uveitis or Reiter syndrome follow gram-negative bacillary dysentery or chlamydial infection. The possible role of bacterial lipopolysaccharide and innate mechanisms was discussed in Chapter 4. Experiments in rats and mice genetically altered to express human HLA-B27 molecules seem to suggest that bacterial infection of the gut predisposes rats to arthritis and a Reiter-like syndrome, although uveitis is uncommon.
>
> It has been suggested that chronic intracellular chlamydial infection of a joint, and presumably the eye, might stimulate an adaptive immune response using the endogenous (class I) antigen-processing pathway of the B27 molecule, invoking a CD8 T-cell effector mechanism activated to kill the infection but indirectly injuring the eye. Others have suggested that B27 haplotype might present *Klebsiella* peptide antigens to CD8 T cells, but how a presumed exogenous bacterial antigen would be presented through the class I pathway is unknown. Another hypothesis posits that molecular mimicry may exist between bacterial antigens and an epitope of HLA-B27. Analysis of human AAU fluids and various animal models of AAU and arthritis suggests that anterior uveitis might be a CD4 Th1–mediated DH response, possibly in response to bacteria-derived antigens such as bacterial cell wall antigens or heat shock proteins trapped in the uvea or to endogenous autoantigens of the anterior uvea, possibly melanin-associated antigens, type II collagen, or myelin-associated proteins. How a CD4-predominant mechanism would relate to a class I immunogenetic association is unclear.

peptide binding, rather than on serotyping or genetic typing, may reveal other disease associations.

MHC and Transplantation

As indicated in Table 5-1, failure of *allogeneic* transplanted tissue, from a genetically nonidentical donor, to remain viable was first recognized as an adaptive immune response in the 1940s. The association between transplantation antigens (ie, MHC antigens) and immune response genes was not recognized until decades later. How the immune system recognizes HLA haplotype differences as foreign antigens is not entirely clear. Intuitively, it seems that T cells from the recipient individual should simply ignore APCs from a donor individual bearing a different HLA haplotype. Short-term cell culture experiments (ie, 1–3 days) accordingly show that the recipient's T cells do fail to recognize exogenous foreign antigens presented by the donor APCs, even if the T cells had been previously sensitized. However, if the T-cell cultures and donor APCs are left to react over a longer term (ie, 5–7 days), a significant fraction of the recipient T cells unexpectedly become activated in response to the donor APC HLA molecules, especially class II differences. What remains unknown is whether this *mixed lymphocyte reaction*–induced activation process represents a direct interaction between the foreign HLA and the recipient's T-cell receptor, or if the foreign HLA molecule is processed as a foreign protein and presented by host APCs to host T cells. Both DH and cytotoxic T lymphocyte effector responses are activated by this process, and both appear crucial in transplant rejection, including corneal allograft rejection.

Although antibodies to class I transplantation antigens can also occur in some cases of hyperacute rejection, this mechanism does not appear to be important in corneal graft rejection. In general, HLA matching, especially at DR loci, followed by A and B loci, greatly reduces rejection for many types of organ allografts. Similar observations have not been confirmed for high-risk corneal allograft rejection.

Disease Associations

In 1973, the first association between HLA haplotype and ankylosing spondylitis was identified. Since then, more than 100 other disease associations have been made, including several for ocular inflammatory diseases (Table 5-2). In general, an HLA disease association is defined as the statistically increased frequency of an HLA haplotype in persons with that disease as compared to the frequency in a disease-free population. The ratio of these two frequencies is called *relative risk*, which is the simplest method for expressing the magnitude of an HLA disease association. Nevertheless, several caveats must be kept in mind:

Table 5-2 HLA Associations and Ocular Inflammatory Disease

Disease	HLA Association	Specific Relative Risk (RR) for Associated Subgroup
Acute anterior uveitis	HLA-B27	RR = 8
Reiter syndrome	HLA-B27	RR = 60
Juvenile rheumatoid arthritis	HLA-DR4, -Dw2	Acute systemic disease
Behçet syndrome	HLA-B51	Japanese and Middle Eastern descent RR = 4–6
Birdshot chorioretinitis	HLA-A29, -A29.2	RR = 80–100, for North Americans and Europeans
Intermediate uveitis	HLA-B8, -B51, -DR2 HLA-DR15	RR = 6, possibly the DRB1*1501 genotype
Sympathetic ophthalmia	HLA-DR4	
VKH syndrome	HLA-DR4	Japanese and North Americans
Sarcoidosis	HLA-B8	Acute systemic disease
	HLA-B13	Chronic systemic disease but not for eye
Multiple sclerosis	HLA-B7, -DR2	
Ocular histoplasmosis syndrome (OHS)	HLA-B7, -DR2	RR = 12
Retinal vasculitis	HLA-B44	Britons

- The association is only as strong as the clinical diagnosis. Diseases that are difficult to diagnose on clinical features may obscure real associations.
- The association depends on the validity of the haplotyping. Older literature often reflects associations based on HLA classifications (some provisional) that might have changed.
- The HLA association identifies persons at risk and is not a diagnostic marker. The associated haplotype is not necessarily present in all persons affected with the specific disease, and its presence in a person does not ensure the correct diagnosis.
- The concept of linkage disequilibrium proposes that if two genes are physically near on the chromosome, they may be inherited together rather than undergo genetic randomization in a population. Thus, HLA may be coinherited with an unrelated disease gene, and sometimes two HLA haplotypes can occur together more frequently than predicted by their independent frequencies in the population.

At least four theoretical explanations have been offered for HLA disease associations. The most direct theory postulates that HLA molecules act as peptide-binding molecules for etiologic antigens or infectious agents. Thus, persons bearing a specific HLA molecule might be predisposed to processing certain antigens, such as an infectious agent that cross-reacts with a self-antigen, and other persons lacking that haplotype would not be so predisposed. Specific variations or mutations in the peptide-binding region would greatly influence this mechanism, and these variations can be detected only by molecular typing. Preliminary data in support of this theory have been provided for type 1 diabetes.

A second theory proposes molecular mimicry between bacterial antigens and an epitope of an HLA molecule (ie, an antigenic site on the molecule itself). An appropriate antibacterial effector response might inappropriately initiate a cross-react effector response with an epitope of the HLA molecule. The third theory suggests that the T-cell antigen receptor (gene) is really the true susceptibility factor. Since a specific T-cell receptor uses a specific HLA haplotype, a strong correlation would exist between an HLA and the T-cell antigen receptor repertoire. A fourth theory implicates an innate cause unrelated to the role of HLAs in adaptive immunity. For example, transgenic mice genetically altered to express the HLA-B51 molecule, which is associated with Behçet syndrome, develop polymorphonuclear neutrophils with enhanced activation and perhaps exaggerated innate effector function.

Immunotherapeutics

BCSC Section 2, *Fundamentals and Principles of Ophthalmology,* includes chapters on pharmacologic principles and ocular pharmacotherapeutics in Part V, Ocular Pharmacology. See also Chapter 6 of this volume, under "Medical Management of Uveitis."

> Jabs DA, Rosenbaum JT, Foster CS, et al. Guidelines for the use of immunosuppressive drugs in patients with ocular inflammatory disorders: recommendations of an expert panel. *Am J Ophthalmol.* 2000;130:492–513.
>
> Solomon SD, Cunningham ET Jr. Use of corticosteroids and noncorticosteroid immunosuppressive agents in patients with uveitis. *Comprehensive Ophthalmology Update.* 2001; 165:273–286.

Nonsteroidal Anti-Inflammatory Drugs (NSAIDs)

NSAIDs are a family of aspirin-like drugs that inhibit the production of prostaglandins by acting on cyclooxygenase (COX). COX itself has a complex structure that includes a helical channel at the enzymatically active site that oxidizes arachidonic acid. Aspirin and most NSAIDs act by various mechanisms to reversibly or irreversibly inhibit the arachidonic acid–binding site in the channel of both COX-1 and COX-2. COX-2–specified NSAIDs selectively block the inflammation mediated by COX-2 without the adverse effects of stomach lesions and renal toxicity that often arise from COX-1 inhibition. Topical or systemic NSAIDs are moderately effective at inhibiting COX in the eye but appear to have only mild anti-inflammatory efficacy for most types of acute ocular inflammation. Nevertheless, some authorities think that such agents can play an important supplementary role in the treatment of uveitis.

Glucocorticosteroids

The mainstay of uveitis therapy is topical, periocular, or systemic administration of glucocorticosteroids. Corticosteroids bind intracellular receptors that translocate into the nucleus, where the drug acts to alter DNA transcription into mRNA. Systemically administered, corticosteroids can alter the homing pattern of T cells and other effector cells to prevent recruitment into sites of inflammation. Local corticosteroids suppress inflammation through many cellular mechanisms, but the most potent is direct inhibition of most types of inflammatory mediator synthesis or release by effector cells, especially macrophages and neutrophils as well as T cells.

Cytotoxic Chemotherapy

Systemic immunosuppression with cytotoxic chemotherapy includes a wide variety of unrelated compounds often used in treating cancer (see further discussion in Chapter 6):

- Alkylating agents such as cyclophosphamide (Cytoxan) and chlorambucil (Leukeran)
- Antimetabolites such as methotrexate (Rheumatrex), azathioprine (Imuran), and mycophenolate mofetile (Cellcept)

Alkylating agents are presumed to cross-link DNA, thereby preventing cell division. These agents presumably function to prevent the bone marrow from replenishing lymphocytes and other effector subpopulations that mediate inflammation. Methotrexate is a folate analogue that inhibits folate metabolism to block purine ring biosynthesis, ultimately affecting pathways that require nucleotide precursors, such as DNA and mRNA synthesis. Thus, this drug will theoretically inhibit protein synthesis in nondividing effector cells, limit activation and differentiation of T cells within lymphoid tissue, and suppress effector cell expansion within bone marrow. Azathioprine works by a similar mechanism. The ability of any of these drugs to target effector cells within the eye is unknown, but experimental data in animals suggest that local delivery of some cytotoxic agents may be efficacious.

Cyclosporine

Systemic immunosuppression with the T-cell inhibitor cyclosporine is often an effective therapy for severe uveitis. Cyclosporine is a lipid-soluble fungus-derived cyclic polypeptide that binds an intracellular receptor. It acts to block helper T-cell activation and differentiation by various mechanisms, as well as by blocking some functions of APCs. Cyclosporine appears to have limited actions on other effector cell subsets, presumably acting primarily within lymphoid tissue to inhibit immune processing. However, clinical experience with topical cyclosporine and experimental data with a device for intraocular drug delivery of cyclosporine during uveitis indicate that it can also function to inhibit T-cell effector responses locally within the eye.

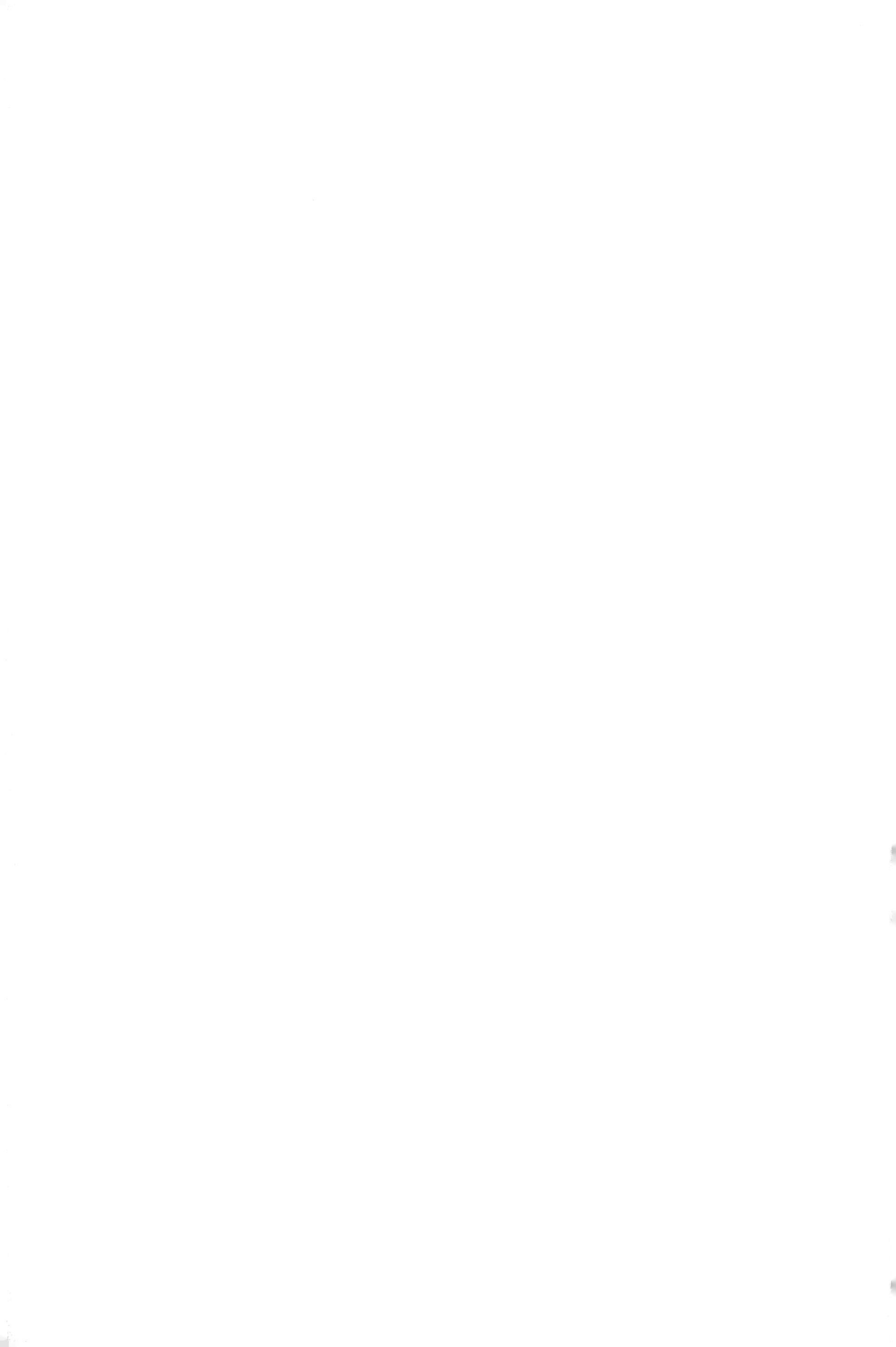

PART II

Intraocular Inflammation and Uveitis

CHAPTER 6

Clinical Approach to Uveitis

The uvea of the eye consists of the iris, ciliary body, and choroid, which is the eye's major blood supply. *Uveitis* is broadly defined as inflammation (ie, *-itis*) of the uvea (from the Latin *uva,* meaning "grape"). The study of uveitis is complicated by the fact that the causes of inflammatory reaction of the inner eye can be infectious, traumatic, neoplastic, or autoimmune. In addition, processes that may only secondarily involve the uvea, such as ocular toxoplasmosis, a disease that primarily affects the retina, may cause a marked inflammatory spillover into the choroid and vitreous.

This chapter uses an anatomical flowchart approach to uveitis diagnosis to untangle the myriad types of inflammation of the inner eye and introduce a systematic classification of these many manifestations. One simple approach is, first, to determine the *symptoms* of uveitis that are causing the patient to seek help and, next, to complete the basic examination evaluating the *signs* pertinent to uveitis. Since uveitis is frequently associated with systemic disease, a careful history and review of systems is an important first step in elucidating the cause of the patient's inflammatory disease. Next, a thorough examination is done to determine the type of inflammation present.

Each patient demonstrates only a portion of the possible symptoms and signs of uveitis. After the physician has used the information obtained from the history and physical examination to determine the *anatomical classification* of uveitis, he or she can use several *associated factors* to further subcategorize, leading in turn to the choice of *laboratory studies* and *therapeutic options.*

> Albert DM, Jakobiec FA, eds. *Principles and Practice of Ophthalmology.* 2nd ed. Philadelphia: Saunders; 1999.
> Foster CS, Vitale AT. *Diagnosis and Treatment of Uveitis.* Philadelphia: WB Saunders; 2002.
> Michelson JB. *A Color Atlas of Uveitis Diagnosis.* 2nd ed. St Louis: Mosby; 1991.
> Nussenblatt RB, Whitcup SM, Palestine AG. *Uveitis: Fundamentals and Clinical Practice.* 2nd ed. St Louis: Mosby; 1996.
> Rao NA, Augsburger JJ, Forster DJ. *The Uvea: Uveitis and Intraocular Neoplasms.* New York: Gower; 1992.

Symptoms of Uveitis

The most common symptoms of uveitis are blurred vision, floaters, pain, photophobia, and redness (Table 6-1). These symptoms vary with the type of inflammation (eg, acute or chronic) as well as with the specific ocular structures involved. Blurred vision may

102 • Intraocular Inflammation and Uveitis

Table 6-1 **Symptoms of Uveitis**

> Redness
> Pain
> Photophobia
> Epiphora
> Visual disturbances
>   Diffuse blur—caused by:
>   Myopic or hyperopic shift
>   Inflammatory cells
>   Cataract
>   Scotoma (central or peripheral)
>   Floaters

result from refractive error such as a myopic or hyperopic shift associated with macular edema, hypotony, or change in lens position. Other possible causes of blurred vision include opacities in the visual axis from inflammatory cells, fibrin, or protein in the anterior chamber; keratic precipitates (KPs); secondary cataract; vitreous debris; macular edema; and retinal atrophy.

The pain of uveitis usually results from acute onset of inflammation in the region of the iris, as in acute iritis, or from secondary glaucoma. The pain associated with ciliary spasm in iritis may be a referred pain that seems to radiate over a larger area served by cranial nerve V *(trigeminal nerve)*. Epiphora and photophobia are usually present when inflammation involves the iris, cornea, or iris–ciliary body. Occasionally, uveitis is discovered on a routine ophthalmic examination in an asymptomatic patient.

Signs of Uveitis

Part I of this volume reviews the basic concepts of immunology, which can be used to understand the symptoms and signs of inflammation in uveitis. An inflammatory response to infectious, traumatic, neoplastic, or autoimmune processes produces the signs of uveitis (Table 6-2). Chemical mediators of the acute stage of inflammation include serotonin, complement, and plasmin. Leukotrienes, kinins, and prostaglandins modify the second phase of the acute response through antagonism of vasoconstrictors. Activated complement is a leukotactic agent. Polymorphonuclear leukocytes, eosinophils, and mast cells may all contribute to signs of inflammation. However, the lymphocyte is, by far, the predominant inflammatory cell in the inner eye in uveitis. These chemical mediators result in vascular dilatation *(ciliary flush)*, increased vascular permeability *(aqueous flare)*, and chemotaxis of inflammatory cells into the eye *(aqueous and vitreous cellular reaction)*.

Anterior Segment

Signs of uveitis in the anterior portion of the eye include

- KPs (Figs 6-1, 6-2)
- Cells
- Flare (Fig 6-3)

Table 6-2 Signs of Uveitis

Eyelid and skin
 Vitiligo
 Nodules

Conjunctiva
 Perilimbal or diffuse injection
 Nodules

Corneal endothelium
 Keratic (cellular) precipitates (diffuse or gravitational)
 Fibrin
 Pigment (nonspecific)

Anterior/posterior chamber
 Inflammatory cells
 Flare (proteinaceous influx)
 Pigment (nonspecific)

Iris
 Nodules
 Posterior synechiae
 Atrophy
 Heterochromia

Angle
 Peripheral anterior synechiae
 Nodules
 Vascularization

Intraocular pressure
 Hypotony
 Secondary glaucoma

Vitreous
 Inflammatory cells (single/clumped)
 Traction bands

Pars plana
 Snowbanking

Retina
 Inflammatory cells
 Inflammatory cuffing of blood vessels
 Edema
 Cystoid macular edema
 RPE: hypertrophy/clumping/loss
 Epiretinal membranes

Choroid
 Inflammatory infiltrate
 Atrophy
 Neovascularization

Optic nerve
 Edema (nonspecific)
 Neovascularization

- Fibrin
- Hypopyon
- Pigment dispersion
- Pupillary miosis
- Iris nodules (Fig 6-4)
- Synechiae, both anterior and posterior (Fig 6-5)
- Band keratopathy (may also be seen in the cornea with long-standing uveitis)

Perilimbal vascular engorgement (ciliary flush) or diffuse injection of the conjunctiva, episclera, or both is typical with acute anterior uveitis. With increased capillary permeability, the anterior chamber reaction can be described as

- Serous (aqueous flare caused by protein influx)
- Purulent (Polymorphonuclear leukocytes and necrotic debris causing hypopyon)
- Fibrinous (plastic, or intense fibrinous exudate)
- Sanguinoid (inflammatory cells with erythrocytes manifested by hypopyon mixed with hyphema)

The intensity of the cellular reaction in the anterior chamber is graded according to the number of inflammatory cells seen in a 1×3-mm high-powered beam at full intensity at a 45°–60° angle:

104 • Intraocular Inflammation and Uveitis

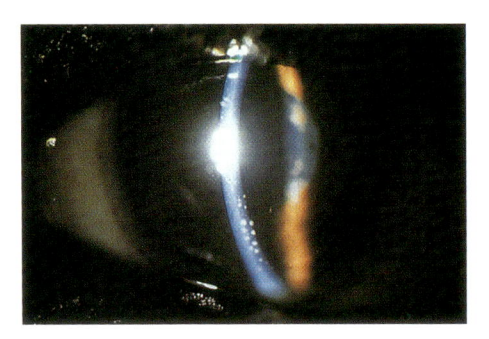

Figure 6-1 Keratic precipitates (medium and small) with broken posterior synechiae. *(Photograph courtesy of H. Jane Blackman, MD.)*

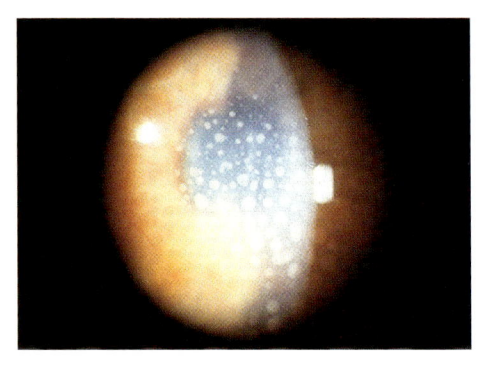

Figure 6-2 Large "mutton fat" keratic precipitates in a patient with sarcoidosis. Large KPs such as these generally indicate a granulomatous disease process. *(Photograph courtesy of David Forster, MD.)*

Figure 6-3 Aqueous flare (4+) in acute iritis.

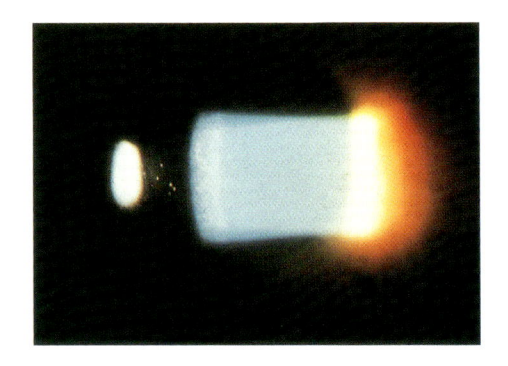

0	no inflammatory cells
trace	<5 cells
1+	5–10 cells
2+	10–20 cells
3+	20–30 cells
4+	cells too numerous to count

KPs are collections of inflammatory cells on the corneal endothelium. When newly formed, they tend to be white and smoothly rounded, but they then become crenated (shrunken), pigmented, or glassy. Large yellowish KPs are described as *mutton-fat KPs;* these are usually associated with granulomatous types of inflammation (see later discussion of the distinction between granulomatous and nongranulomatous inflammation).

Uveitis is sometimes classified as either granulomatous or nongranulomatous. However, this classification system is limited because different experimental doses of the same antigen can produce either appearance; and sarcoidosis, often considered the classic example of granulomatous uveitis, can also present with a nongranulomatous appearance within the eye.

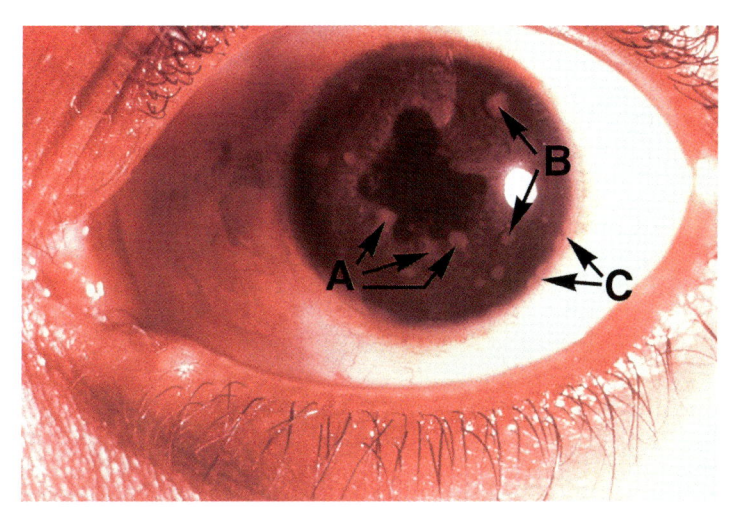

Figure 6-4 Posterior synechiae and iris nodules in a patient with sarcoidosis. Note the three types of iris nodules: **A,** Koeppe nodules (pupillary border); **B,** Busacca nodules (midiris); and **C,** Berlin nodules (iris angle). *(Photograph courtesy of David Forster, MD.)*

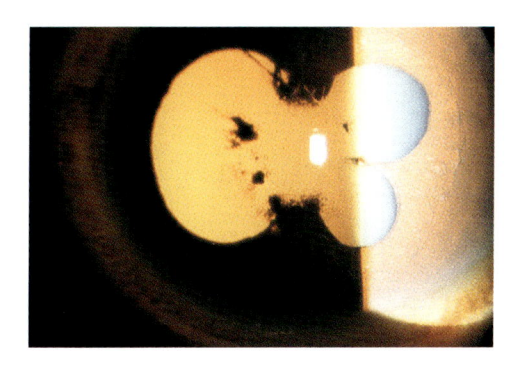

Figure 6-5 Multiple posterior synechiae preventing complete dilation of the pupil. *(Photograph courtesy of David Forster, MD.)*

Iris involvement may manifest as either anterior or posterior synechiae, iris nodules (Koeppe nodules at the pupillary border and Busacca nodules within the iris stroma, and Berlin nodules in the angle), iris granulomas, heterochromia (eg, Fuchs heterochromic iridocyclitis), or stromal atrophy (eg, herpetic uveitis).

With uveitic involvement of the ciliary body and trabecular meshwork, IOP often is low secondary to decreased aqueous production or increased alternative outflow, but IOP may increase precipitously if the meshwork becomes clogged by inflammatory cells or debris, or if the trabecular meshwork itself is the site of inflammation *(trabeculitis)*. Pupillary block with iris bombé and secondary angle closure may also lead to an acute rise in IOP.

Intermediate Segment

Signs in the intermediate anatomical area of the eye include

- Vitreal inflammatory cells, which are graded from 0 to 4+ in density
- *Snowball opacities,* which are common with sarcoidosis or intermediate uveitis

- Exudates over the pars plana *(snowbanking)*
- Vitreal strands

Chronic uveitis may be associated with cyclitic membrane formation with secondary ciliary body detachment and hypotony.

Posterior Segment

Signs in the posterior segment of the eye include

- Retinal or choroidal inflammatory infiltrates
- Inflammatory sheathing of arteries or veins
- Perivascular inflammatory cuffing
- Retinal pigment epithelial hypertrophy or atrophy
- Atrophy or swelling of the retina, choroid, or optic nerve head
- Pre- or subretinal fibrosis
- Exudative, tractional, or rhegmatogenous retinal detachment
- Retinal or choroidal neovascularization

Retinal and choroidal signs may be unifocal, multifocal, or diffuse. The uveitis can be diffuse throughout the eye *(panuveitis)* or appear dispersed with spillover from one area to another, as with toxoplasmosis primarily involving the retina but showing anterior chamber inflammation as well.

Classification of Uveitis

There are several methods of classifying uveitis. The International Uveitis Study Group has proposed an anatomical classification of uveitis divided into four categories with associated specific causes. Discussion in this book follows this basic classification into four groups:

- Anterior uveitis
- Intermediate uveitis
- Posterior uveitis
- Panuveitis (also called *diffuse uveitis*)

> Bloch-Michel E, Nussenblatt RB. International Uveitis Study Group recommendations for the evaluation of intraocular inflammatory disease. *Am J Ophthalmol.* 1987;103:234–235.

Anterior Uveitis

Anterior uveitis can have a range of presentations, from a quiet white eye with low-grade inflammatory reaction apparent only on close examination to a painful red eye with moderate or severe inflammation. Inflammation confined to the anterior chamber is called *iritis;* if it spills over into the retrolental space, it is called *iridocyclitis;* if it involves the cornea, it is called *keratouveitis;* and if the inflammatory reaction involves the sclera and uveal tract, it is called *sclerouveitis.*

By far, most types of anterior uveitis are sterile inflammatory reactions, whereas many of the posterior uveitic syndromes are infectious in origin. In contrast to endophthalmitis from an infectious source, only two noninfectious causes—typically the diseases associated with HLA-B27 and Behçet syndrome—are associated with hypopyon. Many cases of anterior uveitis are isolated instances of unknown cause that often resolve within 6 weeks, such as idiopathic iritis. Glaucomatocyclitic crisis causes a moderately inflamed eye with elevated IOP that subsides quickly over a few weeks. Blunt trauma is a fairly common cause of a generally self-limited uveitis.

The anterior uveitis associated with juvenile rheumatoid arthritis (JRA) can be deceptive, because although the conjunctiva appears quiet externally, the anterior segment may be severely involved in a child without any symptomatic complaints. Another low-grade inflammation of the anterior portion of the eye is seen in Fuchs heterochromic iridocyclitis. Here the damage to the anterior segment is apparently minimal, but the eye needs continued observation because of the commonly occurring secondary complications of cataract and glaucoma. Chapter 7 discusses anterior uveitis in greater detail.

Intermediate Uveitis

Inflammation of the middle portion of the eye manifests primarily as floaters affecting the vision; the eye frequently appears quiet externally. Visual loss is primarily a result of chronic cystoid macular edema or, less commonly, cataract formation. See Chapter 8 of this volume for discussion, as well as Table 6-4 later in this chapter.

Posterior Uveitis

Posterior uveitis may present either with a quiet-appearing eye or with inflammation spilling over to the anterior segment. Inflammation may affect the retina alone *(retinitis)*, the choroid alone *(choroiditis)*, or both layers (*retinochoroiditis*, in which the retina is primarily involved, with secondary involvement of the choroid; and *chorioretinitis*, in which the choroid is primarily affected, with secondary involvement of the retina). The inflammation can be focal, diffuse, or multifocal. Visual symptoms of posterior uveitis may be caused by involvement of the macula or a reduction in peripheral vision. When inflammatory processes involving the retina spill over into the vitreous (ie, retinitis with vitritis), floaters are a common symptom.

Infectious involvement is more common in the retina and choroid than in the anterior segment of the eye. Infections may be viral, bacterial, protozoal, or fungal and have various presentations. Associated systemic findings thus take on particular importance in providing diagnostic clues. Clinical appearance guides the diagnostic workup, with laboratory evaluations frequently required for corroboration. See Chapter 9 for discussion, as well as Table 6-4 later in this chapter.

Panuveitis (Diffuse Uveitis)

Uveitis can affect the entire inner eye. Some patients follow a stormy course, while others have a quiet-appearing eye that nonetheless experiences a slowly debilitating course. Sarcoidosis and syphilis commonly cause a bilateral panuveitis, whereas endophthalmitis generally is a unilateral process. Chapter 10 discusses panuveitis in greater depth, and Chapter 11 covers endophthalmitis.

Review of the Patient's Health and Other Associated Factors

Many factors other than ocular symptoms and signs can aid in the classification or identification of uveitis (Table 6-3). A comprehensive history and review of systems is of paramount importance in helping to elucidate the cause of uveitis. In this regard, a uveitis survey such as that shown at the end of this chapter can be very helpful.

Determining whether the onset was sudden or slow and insidious may help the clinician to narrow the range of diagnostic possibilities. Uveitis may be subcategorized as acute or chronic: *acute* is generally the term used to describe episodes of sudden onset that usually resolve within a few weeks to months, whereas *chronic* uveitis persists for several months to years.

Whether the inflammation is severe or low grade can influence categorization and prognosis. The inflammatory process may occur in one or both eyes, or it may alternate between them. The distribution of ocular involvement—focal, multifocal, or diffuse—is also helpful to note when classifying uveitis. The age, gender, sexual practices, and racial background of the patient are important findings in some uveitic syndromes.

Chronic uveitis can be further characterized histopathologically as being either granulomatous or nongranulomatous. *Nongranulomatous* inflammation typically has a lymphocytic and plasma cell infiltrate, whereas *granulomatous* reactions also include epithelioid and giant cells. Discrete granulomas are characteristic of sarcoidosis; diffuse granulomatous inflammation appears in Vogt-Koyanagi-Harada (VKH) disease and sympathetic ophthalmia. Zonal granulomatous disease can be seen with lens-induced uveitis. However, the physician should be aware that the *clinical* appearance of uveitis as granulomatous or nongranulomatous may not necessarily correlate with the *histopathologic* description and may instead be related to the stage in which the disease is first seen, the amount of presenting antigen, or the host's state of immunocompromise (eg, in a patient being treated with corticosteroids).

Although ocular inflammation may be an isolated process involving only the eye, it can also be associated with a systemic condition. However, the ocular inflammation frequently does not correlate with the inflammatory activity elsewhere in the body, so it is important for the clinician to carefully review systems. In some cases, the uveitis may actually precede the development of inflammation at other body sites. The presence of immunocompromise, use of intravenous drugs, hyperalimentation, and the patient's occupation are just a few risk factors that can direct the investigation of uveitis. Neoplastic disease can masquerade as inflammatory disease. Large cell lymphoma (previously called *reticulum cell sarcoma*), retinoblastoma, leukemia, and malignant melanoma may all be mistaken for uveitis. In addition, juvenile xanthogranuloma, pigment dispersion syndrome, retinal detachment, retinitis pigmentosa, and ischemia all must be considered in the differential diagnosis of uveitis.

The chapters that follow describe discrete uveitis entities. However, many patients do not present with the classic symptoms and signs of a particular disease. Some of these patients require monitoring through follow-up visits, and laboratory tests may need to be repeated at a later date, as the clinical appearance may be unclear or change with time and treatment. The presentation of disease can also be modified by prior therapy or by a delay in seeing the physician.

Table 6-3 **Associated Factors in Diagnosis of Uveitis**

Modifying Factors	Associated Factors Suggesting Systemic Conditions
Time course of disease	Immune system status
Acute	Systemic medications
Relapsing	Trauma history
Chronic	Travel history
Severity	Social history
Severe	Eating habits
Quiescent	Pets
Distribution of uveitis	Sexual practices
Unilateral	Occupation
Bilateral	Drug use
Alternating	
Focal	
Multifocal	
Diffuse	
Patient's sex	
Patient's age	
Patient's race	

Differential Diagnosis and Prevalence of Uveitic Entities

Once a comprehensive history has been taken and a physical examination performed, the most likely causes are ranked in a list based on how well the individual patient's type of uveitis "fits" with the various known uveitic entities. This *naming-meshing system*, described by Smith and Nozik, first names the type of uveitis based on anatomical criteria as well as other associated factors (eg, acute versus chronic, unilateral versus bilateral) and then matches the pattern of uveitis exhibited by the patient with a list of potential uveitic entities that share similar characteristics. One such system for helping to identify a possible cause for a particular patient's uveitis is outlined in Table 6-4.

A knowledge of the prevalence of the various causes seen in uveitis survey populations is also helpful in determining the most probable cause of the uveitis. Numerous studies have been performed to determine the prevalence of various types of uveitis, but the data often vary from one study to another depending on whether the study was performed at a tertiary referral center or was community-based. The location of the study population also produces differing results. For example, the prevalence of cytomegalovirus retinitis would be expected to be much higher in large urban areas with higher rates of AIDS, whereas ocular histoplasmosis would be more prevalent in rural areas in the midwestern United States. Certain types of uveitis also show large, worldwide variations. For example, entities such as Behçet syndrome and VKH disease are much more common in Japan than in Europe or the United States.

Table 6-5 summarizes the data from three surveys, comparing the prevalence of various types of uveitis in both referral-based and community-based populations. In general, the data demonstrate that idiopathic causes are frequently found in anterior uveitis and that infectious causes are more common in posterior uveitis. Also, most

Table 6-4 Flowchart for Evaluation of Uveitis Patients

Type of Inflammation	Associated Factors	Suspected Disease	Laboratory Tests
		Panuveitis	
	See entities described below: sarcoidosis, toxoplasmosis, toxocariasis, endophthalmitis, VKH syndrome, sympathetic ophthalmia, syphilis, cysticercosis		
		Anterior Uveitis	
Acute/sudden onset, severe with or without fibrin membrane or hypopyon	Arthritis, back pain, GI/GU symptoms Aphthous ulcers Postsurgical, posttraumatic None	Seronegative spondyloarthropathies Behçet syndrome Infectious endophthalmitis Idiopathic	HLA-B27, sacroiliac films HLA-B5, -B51 Vitreous culture, vitrectomy Possibly HLA-B27
Moderate severity (red, painful)	Shortness of breath, African descent Posttraumatic Increased IOP Poor response to steroids Post-cataract extraction None	Sarcoidosis Traumatic iritis Glaucomatocyclitic crisis, herpetic iritis Syphilis Low-grade endophthalmitis, IOL-related iritis Idiopathic	Serum ACE, lysozyme; chest x-ray; gallium scan; biopsy RPR, VDRL (screening); FTA-ABS (confirmatory) Consider vitrectomy, culture
Chronic; minimal redness, pain	Child, especially with arthritis Heterochromia, diffuse KP, unilateral Postsurgical None	JRA-related iridocyclitis Fuchs heterochromic iridocyclitis Low-grade endophthalmitis (eg, *P acnes*); IOL-related Idiopathic	ANA, ESR None Consider vitrectomy, capsulectomy with culture
		Intermediate Uveitis	
Mild to moderate	Shortness of breath, African descent Tick exposure, erythema chronicum migrans rash Neurologic symptoms Over age 50 None	Sarcoidosis Lyme disease Multiple sclerosis Intraocular lymphoma Pars planitis	As above ELISA MRI of brain Vitrectomy, cytology

Posterior Uveitis

Chorioretinitis *with vitritis*

Focal	Adjacent scar; raw meat ingestion	Toxoplasmosis	ELISA
	Child; history of geophagia	Toxocariasis	ELISA
	HIV infection	CMV retinitis	As above
Multifocal	Shortness of breath	Sarcoidosis	PPD, chest x-ray
		Tuberculosis	
	Peripheral retinal necrosis	Acute retinal necrosis (ARN)	VZV, HSV titers (ELISA), possibly vitrectomy/retinal biopsy
		Progressive outer retinal necrosis (PORN, if immunocompromised)	
	AIDS	Syphilis, toxoplasmosis	As above
	IV drug use, hyperalimentation, immunosuppression	*Candida, Aspergillus*	Blood, vitreous cultures
	Visible intraocular parasite; from Africa or Central or South America	Cysticercosis	
		Onchocerciasis	
	Over age 50	Intraocular lymphoma	As above
	None	Birdshot choroidopathy	HLA-A29, fluorescein angiography (FA)
		Multifocal choroiditis with panuveitis	Rule out TB, sarcoidosis, syphilis
Diffuse	Dermatologic/CNS symptoms; serius RD	Vogt-Koyanagi-Harada syndrome (VKH)	FA, lumbar puncture to document CSF pleocytosis
	Postsurgical/traumatic, bilateral	Sympathetic ophthalmia	FA
	Postsurgical/traumatic, unilateral	Infectious endophthalmitis	As above
	Child, history of geophagia	Toxocariasis	As above

Chorioretinitis *without vitritis*

Focal	None; history of carcinoma	Neoplastic	Metastatic workup
Multifocal	Ohio/Mississippi Valley	Ocular histoplasmosis	FA if macula involved
	Lesions confined to posterior pole	White dot syndromes (eg, APMPPE, MEWDS, PIC)	FA
	Geographic (maplike) pattern of scars	Serpiginous choroidopathy	FA
Diffuse	From Africa, Central/South America	Onchocerciasis	

Vasculitis

	Aphthous ulcers, hypopyon	Behçet syndrome	As above
	Malar rash, female, arthralgias	Systemic lupus erythematosus (SLE)	ANA

Table 6-5 Most Common Causes or Uveitis

	University/Referral–Based			Community-Based
	Henderly (1987)	Rodriguez (1996)	McCannel (1996)	McCannel (1996)
Anterior	27.8%	51.5%	60.6%	90.6%
Idiopathic	12.1	19.5	30.5	52.1
HLA-B27 +/seronegative spondyloarthropathies	5.8	11.2	10.8	17.4
Juvenile rheumatoid arthritis associated	2.8	5.6	2.3	1.4
Herpes simplex/zoster	2.5	5.0	11.3	7.5
Fuchs heterochromic	1.8	2.6	1.4	0.9
Intraocular lens related	1.0	0.6	0.9	0.9
Sarcoidosis	0	3.0	0.5	0.9
Traumatic	0	0	0	5.2
Intermediate	15.4%	13.0%	12.2%	1.4%
Idiopathic	–	9.1	12.2	0.9
Sarcoidosis	–	2.9	–	–
Multiple sclerosis	–	1.1	–	0.5
Posterior	38.4%	19.4%	14.6%	4.7%
Toxoplasmosis	7.0	4.8	3.5	4.2
Retinal vasculitis	6.8	1.3	1.4	0.5
Idiopathic	3.7	1.3	2.3	0
Ocular histoplasmosis	3.5	0.2	0.5	0
Toxocariasis	2.6	0.5	0.5	0
Cytomegalovirus retinitis	2.5	2.3	*	*
Serpiginous choroidopathy	2.0	0.3	0.5	0
Acute multifocal placoid pigment epitheliopathy	1.8	0.4	0	0
Necrotizing herpetic retinopathy (ARN/PORN)	1.3	1.1	2.8	0
Birdshot choroidopathy	1.2	1.5	0.9	0
Sarcoidosis	0	1.5	0	0
Panuveitis	18.4%	16.0%	9.4%	1.4%
Idiopathic	8.2	3.6	2.5	0.5
Sarcoidosis	3.9	2.3	0.3	0
Vogt-Koyanagi-Harada	3.3	0.9	1.6	0.5
Multifocal choroiditis with panuveitis	–	1.9	0.6	0
Behçet syndrome	1.8	1.9	0.6	0

* Cases of CMV retinitis were excluded from the causes of *general* uveitis in this study. When included in all cases of uveitis, CMV retinitis accounted for 32.6% of university/referral–based patients and 7.0% of community-based patients.

university/referral–based studies probably overestimate the prevalence of intermediate and posterior uveitis compared to cases seen in the community.

> Henderly DE, Genstler AJ, Smith RE, et al. Changing patterns of uveitis. *Am J Ophthalmol.* 1987;103:131–136.
>
> McCannel CA, Holland GN, Helm CJ, et al. Causes of uveitis in the general practice of ophthalmology. UCLA Community-Based Uveitis Study Group. *Am J Ophthalmol.* 1996; 121:35–46.
>
> Rodriguez A, Calonge M, Pedroza-Seres M, et al. Referral patterns of uveitis in a tertiary eye care center. *Arch Ophthalmol.* 1996;114:593–599.

Laboratory and Medical Evaluation

The diagnosis may require laboratory and medical evaluation guided by the history and physical examination. *There is no one standardized battery of tests that needs to be ordered for all patients with uveitis.* Rather, a tailored approach should be taken based on the most likely causes for each patient. Once a list of differential diagnoses is compiled, appropriate laboratory tests can then be ordered, if necessary. Many patients require only one or a few diagnostic tests. When the history and physical examination do not clearly indicate the cause, most uveitis specialists recommend a subset of core tests, including complete blood count, erythrocyte sedimentation rate, angiotensin-converting enzyme, lysozyme, syphilis serologic profile, and chest radiographs. Risk factors may also indicate testing for tuberculosis and Lyme disease. Table 6-4 lists some of the laboratory tests that may be useful for particular presentations of uveitis. These laboratory tests are discussed further in the chapters that follow, covering the various types of uveitis.

In the evaluation of patients with certain types of uveitis, ancillary testing can be extremely helpful:

- *Fluorescein angiography* may show the presence of cystoid macular edema, choroiditis, vascular involvement, serous retinal detachment, and choroidal neovascularization.
- *Ultrasonography* can be useful in demonstrating vitreous opacities, choroidal thickening, retinal detachment, or cyclitic membrane formation, particularly if media opacities preclude a view of the posterior segment.
- *Vitreous biopsy* may be necessary for a diagnostic evaluation in suspected cases of large cell lymphoma (formerly called *reticulum cell sarcoma*) or bacterial or fungal endophthalmitis. Fluid may also be analyzed for the polymerase chain reaction to determine the cause of certain cases.
- *Chorioretinal biopsy* may be useful when the diagnosis cannot be confirmed on the basis of clinical appearance or other laboratory investigations (eg, certain cases of necrotizing retinitis in patients with AIDS or suspected cases of intraocular lymphoma).

Many patients with mild, self-limited uveitis need no referral to a uveitis specialist. However, in uveitis with a chronic or downwardly spiraling course, referring the patient to a uveitis specialist may be helpful not only in eliciting the cause and determining the therapeutic regimen but also in reassuring the patient that all avenues are being explored. Evaluation of vision-threatening uveitis may require coordination with other medical or surgical consultants (eg, in pursuing the diagnosis of HIV-related diseases or in kidney transplant patients on immunosuppressive therapy). Discussion with the patient and other specialists about the prognosis and complications of uveitis helps to determine the appropriate therapy. Therapy for uveitis ranges from simple observation to medical or surgical intervention (Table 6-6).

114 • Intraocular Inflammation and Uveitis

Table 6-6 **Therapy for Uveitis**

Observation
    For development of complications
    For change in the appearance/severity/progression

Medical therapy
Cycloplegics
    To relieve pain
    To break posterior synechiae/pupillary block
Corticosteroids
    Topical drops/ointment
    Sub-Tenon's injection
    Oral or intravenous injection
Immunosuppressives
    Alkylating agents
    Antimetabolites
    T-cell suppressors

Surgical therapy
Diagnostic procedures
    Anterior chamber aspiration
    Vitreous biopsy
Reparative procedures
    Cataract extraction
    Pupillary reconstruction
    Glaucoma surgery
    Epiretinal membrane peeling
    Scleral buckle
    Vitrectomy

Medical Management of Uveitis

Generally, medical therapy includes topical or systemic corticosteroids and may also include topical cycloplegics. Immunosuppressive therapy may be required in patients with severe uveitis unresponsive to corticosteroid therapy or in patients with severe corticosteroid-induced complications. The choice of therapeutic approach depends on the relative risk of complications of uveitis, of which the most common are cataracts, cystoid macular edema, glaucoma, and hypotony. Treatment should be tailored as specifically as possible to the individual patient and adjusted according to response. The physician should consider the patient's systemic involvement and other factors such as age, immune status, and tolerance for side effects. See also the discussion "Immunotherapeutics" in Chapter 5.

Mydriatic and Cycloplegic Agents

Topical mydriatic and cycloplegic agents are beneficial for breaking or preventing the formation of posterior synechiae and for relieving photophobia secondary to ciliary spasm. The stronger the inflammatory reaction, the stronger or more frequent the dosage of cycloplegic. Short-acting drops such as cyclopentolate hydrochloride (Cyclogyl) or long-acting drops such as atropine may be used. Most cases of acute anterior uveitis require only short-acting cycloplegics; these allow the pupil to remain mobile and permit rapid recovery upon discontinuation. Patients with chronic uveitis and moderate flare in the anterior chamber (eg, JRA-associated iritis) may need to be maintained on short-acting agents (eg, tropicamide) on a long-term basis to prevent posterior synechiae.

Corticosteroids

Corticosteroids are the mainstay of uveitis therapy (Table 6-7). Because of their potential side effects, however, they should be reserved for specific indications:

- Treatment of active inflammation in the eye
- Prevention or treatment of complications such as cystoid macular edema
- Reduction of inflammatory infiltration of the retina, choroid, or optic nerve

Complications of corticosteroid therapy are numerous and can be seen with any mode of administration. Therefore, these agents should be used only when the benefits of therapy outweigh the risks of the medications themselves. Corticosteroids are not always

Table 6-7 Corticosteroids Frequently Used in Uveitis Therapy and Their Complications

Route of Administration	Complications
Topical Prednisolone acetate Prednisolone sodium phosphate Fluorometholone Dexamethasone phosphate Rimexalone	Cataract formation Elevation of IOP Worsening of external infection Corneal/scleral thinning or perforation
Periocular *Long-acting* Methylprednisolone acetate (Depo-Medrol) Triamcinolone acetonide (Kenalog) Triamcinolone diacetate (Aristocort) *Short-acting* Hydrocortisone sodium succinate (Solu-Cortef) Betamethasone (Celestone)	Same complications as topical above Ptosis Scarring of conjunctiva/Tenon's capsule Worsening of infectious uveitis Scleral perforation Hemorrhage
Systemic Prednisone Triamcinolone Dexamethasone Methylprednisolone	Same complications as topical above Increased appetite Weight gain Peptic ulcers Sodium and fluid retention Osteoporosis/bone fractures Aseptic necrosis of hip Hypertension Diabetes mellitus Menstrual irregularities Mental status changes Exacerbation of systemic infections Impaired wound healing Acne Others

indicated in patients with chronic flare or in the therapy of specific diseases such as Fuchs heterochromic iridocyclitis, pars planitis without macular edema, or a peripheral lesion of toxoplasmosis (ie, a lesion that does not threaten the papillomacular bundle).

The amount and duration of corticosteroid therapy must be individualized. It is generally preferable to begin therapy with a high dose of corticosteroids (topical or systemic) and taper the dose as the inflammation subsides, rather than beginning with a low dose that may have to be progressively increased to control the inflammation. To minimize complications of therapy, patients should be maintained on the minimal amount of corticosteroid needed to control the inflammation. If steroid therapy is needed for longer than 2–3 weeks, the dosage should be tapered before discontinuation. The dosage may need to be increased when surgical intervention is required to prevent postoperative exacerbation of the uveitis.

Topical administration

Topical corticosteroid drops are effective primarily for anterior uveitis, although they may have beneficial effects on vitritis or macular edema in patients who are pseudophakic or aphakic. Topical corticosteroid drops are given in dosages ranging from once daily to hourly. They can also be given in an ointment form for nighttime use or if preservatives in the eyedrops are not well-tolerated. Of the topical preparations, rimexolone, loteprednol, and fluorometholone have been shown to have less of an ocular hypertensive effect than the other medications and may be particularly useful in patients who are steroid responders. It is unclear whether these agents are as effective as prednisolone in controlling inflammation, however. Also, some generic forms of prednisolone may have less of an anti-inflammatory effect than brand-name products; this should be considered when patients do not respond adequately to topical corticosteroid therapy.

Periocular administration

Periocular corticosteroids are generally given as depot injections when a more posterior effect is needed or when a patient is noncompliant or poorly responsive to topical or systemic administration. They are often preferred for patients with intermediate or posterior uveitis or those with cystoid macular edema, since they deliver a therapeutic dose of medication close to the site of inflammation and have little if any systemic side effects.

Periocular injections can be performed using either a transseptal or a sub-Tenon's approach (Fig 6-6). With a sub-Tenon's injection, a 25-gauge ⅝″ needle is used. If the injection is given in the superotemporal quadrant (the preferred location), the upper eyelid is retracted and the patient is instructed to look down and nasally. After anesthesia is applied with a cotton swab soaked in proparacaine or tetracaine, the needle is placed bevel-down against the sclera and advanced through the conjunctiva and Tenon's capsule using a side-to-side movement, which allows the physician to determine whether the needle has entered the sclera or not. As long as the globe does not torque with the side-to-side movement of the needle, the physician can be reasonably sure that the needle has not penetrated the sclera. Once the needle has been advanced to the hub, the steroid is injected into the sub-Tenon's space.

Periocular injections should not be used in cases of infectious uveitis (eg, toxoplasmosis) and should also be avoided in patients with necrotizing scleritis since scleral

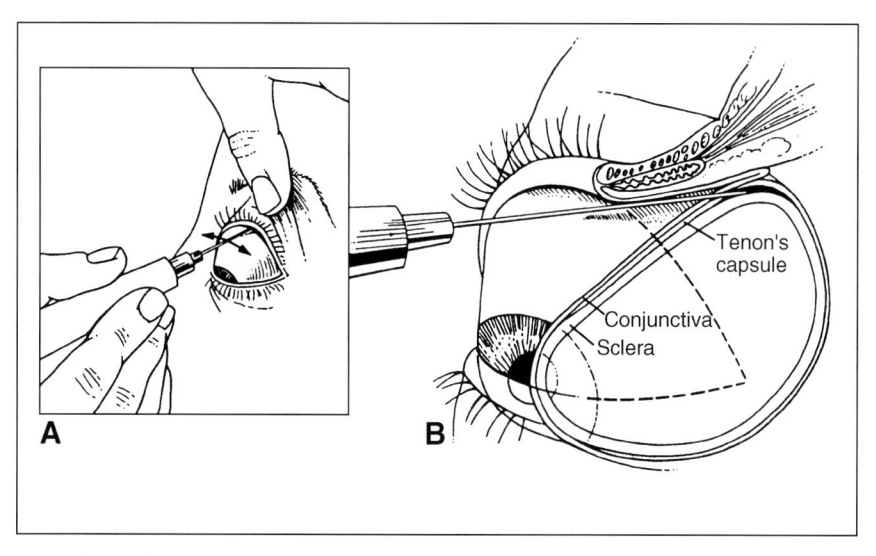

Figure 6-6 Posterior sub-Tenon's injection. **A,** The correct position of the operator's hands and the needle. The *arrows* indicate the direction of the side-to-side circumferential motion (here exaggerated for emphasis). **B,** The positioning of the tip of the needle in its ideal location between Tenon's capsule and the sclera. *(Reproduced with permission from Smith RE, Nozik RA.* Uveitis: A Clinical Approach to Diagnosis and Management. *2nd ed. Baltimore: Williams & Wilkins; 1989.)*

thinning and possible perforation may result. The physician should be aware that periocular corticosteroid injections have the potential to raise the IOP precipitously or for a long time, particularly with the longer-acting agents (triamcinolone or methylprednisolone).

Systemic administration

Oral or *intravenous* therapy may supplement or replace other routes of administration. Systemic corticosteroids are used for vision-threatening chronic uveitis that threatens vision when topical steroids are insufficient or when the systemic disease also requires therapy. The many side effects of both short- and long-term corticosteroids must be discussed with patients, and their general health must be closely monitored, often with the assistance of an internist. Patients maintained on long-term steroid therapy, particularly elderly patients and postmenopausal women, should supplement their diet with calcium and vitamin D to lessen the chances of osteoporosis.

Intravitreal administration

A more recent mode of therapy is the use of intravitreal corticosteroids. These can be administered by injection or by implantation of a sustained-release device and have been shown to be useful in the treatment of chronic uveitis and uveitic cystoid macular edema. The sustained-release device holds particular promise in treating long-standing inflammation, as the devices can release medication for several years after implantation, potentially allowing the reduction or elimination of systemic corticosteroids and immunosuppressive agents. As with other routes of administration for corticosteroids, intraocular pressure must be monitored regularly in these patients.

Antcliff RJ, Spalton DJ, Stanford MR, et al. Intravitreal triamcinolone for uveitic cystoid macular edema: an optical coherence tomography study. *Ophthalmology.* 2001;108:765–772.

Jaffe GJ, Ben-Nun J, Guo H, et al. Fluocinolone acetonide sustained drug delivery device to treat severe uveitis. *Ophthalmology.* 2000;107:2024–2033.

Immunomodulating and Immunosuppressive Agents

Other medications that modulate the immune system are the nonsteroidal anti-inflammatory agents (NSAIDs) and immunosuppressive agents.

NSAIDs

Topical NSAIDs may be useful in the treatment of postoperative inflammation and cystoid macular edema, but their usefulness in treating endogenous anterior uveitis has not been proven. Several studies have shown that systemic NSAIDs benefit patients with chronic iridocyclitis (eg, JRA-associated iridocyclitis); NSAIDs may allow the practitioner to maintain the patient on a lower dose of topical corticosteroids. Potential complications of systemic NSAIDs include gastric ulceration, GI bleeding, nephrotoxicity, and hepatotoxicity.

Immunosuppressive medications

The addition of immunosuppressive medications may greatly benefit patients with severe sight-threatening uveitis or who are resistant to or intolerant of corticosteroids. These agents are thought to work by killing the rapidly dividing clones of lymphocytes that are responsible for the inflammation (see Part I, Immunology). As more evidence accumulates about the complications of long-term systemic corticosteroid use, immunosuppressive agents are being used with increasing frequency as steroid-sparing agents. While early use of immunosuppressive agents is indicated in certain diseases (see below), these drugs should also be considered in patients who require chronic corticosteroid therapy (longer than 6 months) at doses greater than 10 mg/day.

Indications The following indications generally apply to the therapeutic use of immunosuppressive agents in uveitis:

- Vision-threatening intraocular inflammation
- Reversibility of the disease process
- Inadequate response to corticosteroid treatment
- Contraindication of corticosteroid treatment because of systemic problems or intolerable side effects

Corticosteroids are the mainstay of initial therapy, but certain specific uveitis entities also warrant the early use of immunosuppressive agents for treatment of intraocular inflammation, including Behçet syndrome, sympathetic ophthalmia, VKH disease, and necrotizing sclerouveitis. Although these disorders may initially respond well to corticosteroids, the initial treatment of these entities with immunosuppressive agents has been shown to improve the long-term prognosis and to lessen the visual morbidity.

Relative indications for these agents include conditions that are initially treated with corticosteroids but do not respond adequately and patients who develop serious corticosteroid-induced side effects. Examples in this category include intermediate uveitis (pars planitis), retinal vasculitis, panuveitis, and chronic iridocyclitis.

Treatment Before initiating therapy with any immunosuppressive agent, the physician should consider these guidelines:

- Absence of infection
- Absence of hematologic contraindications
- Meticulous follow-up by an ophthalmologist or internist familiar with the use of these medications
- Objective evaluation of the disease process
- Informed consent

Several classes of immunosuppressive medications exist. These include antimetabolites, alkylating agents, and inhibitors of T-cell signaling. These agents are outlined in Table 6-8, along with their mechanisms of action, dosages, and potential complications. It should be noted that no therapeutic response may occur for several weeks after initiation of immunosuppressive therapy; therefore, most patients need to be maintained on corticosteroid therapy until the immunosuppressive agent begins to take effect, at which time the corticosteroid dose may be gradually tapered.

Numerous studies have shown methotrexate to be effective in the treatment of various types of uveitis, including JRA-associated iridocyclitis, sarcoidosis, panuveitis, and scleritis. Treatment with this medication is unique in that it is given as a *weekly* dose, usually starting at 7.5–10.0 mg/week and gradually increasing to a maintenance dose of 15–25 mg/week. It can be administered either orally or subcutaneously and is usually well-tolerated. Azathioprine, cyclophosphamide, and chlorambucil have been found to be beneficial in patients with intermediate uveitis, VKH disease, sympathetic ophthalmia, and Behçet syndrome.

Table 6-8 Immunosuppressive Medications in the Treatment of Uveitis

Medication	Mechanism of Action	Dosage	Potential Complications
Antimetabolites			
Methotrexate (Rheumatrex)	Folate analogue; inhibits dihydrofolate reductase	7.5–25.0 µg/wk PO or SC	GI upset, fatigue, hepatotoxicity, pneumonitis
Azathioprine (Imuran)	Alters purine metabolism	50–150 mg/d	GI upset, hepatotoxicity
Mycophenolate mofetil (CellCept)	Inhibits purine synthesis	1–2 g/d	Diarrhea, nausea, GI ulceration
Alkylating agents			
Cyclophosphamide (Cytoxan)	Cross-links DNA	1–2 mg/d	Hemorrhagic cystitis, sterility, increased risk of malignancy
Chlorambucil (Leukeran)	Cross-links DNA	2–12 mg/d	Sterility, increased risk of malignancy
Inhibitors of T-cell signaling			
Cyclosporine (Neoral, Sandimmune)	Inhibits NF-AT activation	2.5–5.0 mg/kg/d	Nephrotoxicity, hypertension, gingival hyperplasia, GI upset, paresthesias
Tacrolimus (Prograf)	Inhibits NF-AT activation	0.2 mg/kg/d	Nephrotoxicity, hypertension, diabetes mellitus

Cyclosporine likewise has been shown to be effective in the treatment of intermediate uveitis and several types of posterior uveitis, including Behçet syndrome and VKH disease. Our understanding of cyclosporine's exact mechanism of action remains incomplete, but the primary effects appear to be related to inhibition of T-cell activation and recruitment. The most likely mechanism for this inhibition is interference with signaling from the T-cell receptor to genes that code for the various lymphokines and other substances (such as IL-2) that are necessary for T-cell activation. Cyclosporine preferentially inhibits the T helper-inducer and cytotoxic subsets, with minimal effects on T-suppressor cells. The most common complications include renal toxicity and hypertension. The renal impairment is often reversible if the dose is decreased, but irreversible damage to the tubules has occurred in patients on prolonged therapy. Additional side effects include paresthesia, gastrointestinal upset, fatigue, hypertrichosis, and gingival hyperplasia.

Because of the potentially serious complications associated with the use of these medications, patients must be monitored closely by a practitioner who is experienced with these agents. Regular blood monitoring, including complete blood count and liver and renal function tests, should be performed. Serious complications include renal and hepatic toxicity, bone marrow suppression, and increased susceptibility to infection. In addition, the alkylating agents may cause sterility and have been associated with an increased risk of future malignancies such as leukemia or lymphoma. All of these agents are potentially teratogenic, and patients should be advised to refrain from becoming pregnant while on them. The physician should consider obtaining informed consent prior to beginning therapy. In summary, while these agents may be associated with serious life-threatening complications, they can be extremely effective in the treatment of ocular inflammatory disease in patients unresponsive to, or intolerant of, systemic corticosteroids.

Other Immunomodulatory Agents

Cytokine inhibitors such as etanercept and infliximab are being studied for the treatment of uveitis. One study found that infliximab use resulted in a rapid resolution of posterior segment inflammation in patients with Behçet syndrome after a single intravenous infusion. Small studies have shown interferon alfa-2b and intravenous immune globulin to be beneficial in some patients with uveitis.

> Jabs DA, Rosenbaum JT, Foster CS, et al. Guidelines for the use of immunosuppressive drugs in patients with ocular inflammatory disorders: recommendations of an expert panel. *Am J Ophthalmol.* 2000;130:492–513.
>
> Samson CM, Waheed N, Baltatzis S, et al. Methotrexate therapy for chronic noninfectious uveitis: analysis of a case series of 160 patients. *Ophthalmology.* 2001;108:1134–1139.
>
> Sfikakis PP, Theodossiadis PG, Katsiari CG, et al. Effect of infliximab on sight-threatening panuveitis in Behçet's disease. *Lancet.* 2001;358:295.
>
> Solemon SD, Cunningham ET Jr. Use of corticosteroids and non-corticosteroid immunosuppressive agents in patients with uveitis. *Comprehensive Ophthalmology Update.* 2001;1:273–288.
>
> Vitale AT, Rodriguez A, Foster CS. Low-dose cyclosporin A therapy in treating chronic, non-infectious uveitis. *Ophthalmology.* 1996;103:365–378.

Surgery

Surgical therapy may include diagnostic evaluation such as paracentesis or vitreous and/or chorioretinal biopsy to rule out neoplastic or acute infectious processes. Therapeutic vitrectomy may be beneficial in cases of recalcitrant vitritis or cystoid macular edema (or both) that have not responded to medical therapy. As mentioned earlier, implantation of a sustained-release delivery system containing a corticosteroid or other immunomodulating agent may become more commonplace in the years ahead. Other surgical approaches are restorative and address a particular complication, such as cataract extraction or filtering surgery. See Chapter 13, Complications of Uveitis, for further discussion of surgery. See also the volumes of the BCSC that deal with these conditions in detail: Section 10, *Glaucoma;* Section 11, *Lens and Cataract;* and Section 12, *Retina and Vitreous.*

Diagnostic Survey for Uveitis (to be filled in by patient)

FAMILY HISTORY

These questions refer to your grandparents, parents, aunts, uncles, brothers and sisters, children, or grandchildren.

Has anyone in your family ever had any of the following?

Cancer	Yes	No
Diabetes	Yes	No
Allergies	Yes	No
Arthritis or rheumatism	Yes	No
Syphilis	Yes	No
Tuberculosis	Yes	No
Sickle cell disease or trait	Yes	No
Lyme disease	Yes	No
Gout	Yes	No

Has anyone in your family had medical problems in any of the areas listed below?

Eyes	Yes	No
Skin	Yes	No
Kidneys	Yes	No
Lungs	Yes	No
Stomach or bowel	Yes	No
Nervous system or brain	Yes	No

SOCIAL HISTORY

Age (years):   Current job:

Have you ever lived outside of the USA?	Yes	No
If yes, where?		
Have you ever owned a dog?	Yes	No
Have you ever owned a cat?	Yes	No
Have you ever eaten raw meat or uncooked sausage?	Yes	No
Have you ever had unpasteurized milk or cheese?	Yes	No
Have you ever been exposed to sick animals?	Yes	No
Do you drink untreated stream, well, or lake water?	Yes	No
Do you smoke cigarettes?	Yes	No
Have you ever used intravenous drugs?	Yes	No
Have you ever had bisexual or homosexual relationships?	Yes	No
Have you ever taken birth control pills?	Yes	No

PERSONAL MEDICAL HISTORY

Are you allergic to any medications?	Yes	No
If yes, which medications?		

Please list the medications that you are currently taking, including nonprescription drugs such as aspirin, Advil, antihistamines, etc:

Please list all the eye operations you have had (including laser surgery) and the dates of the surgeries:
_____
_____
_____
_____

Please list all operations you have had and the dates of the surgeries:
_____
_____
_____
_____

Have you ever been told that you have the following conditions?

Anemia (low blood count)	Yes	No
Cancer	Yes	No
Diabetes	Yes	No
Hepatitis	Yes	No
High blood pressure	Yes	No
Pleurisy	Yes	No
Pneumonia	Yes	No
Ulcers	Yes	No
Herpes (cold sores)	Yes	No
Chickenpox	Yes	No
Shingles (zoster)	Yes	No
German measles (rubella)	Yes	No
Measles (rubeola)	Yes	No
Mumps	Yes	No
Chlamydia or trachoma	Yes	No
Syphilis	Yes	No
Gonorrhea	Yes	No
Any other sexually transmitted disease	Yes	No
Tuberculosis (TB)	Yes	No
Leprosy	Yes	No
Leptospirosis	Yes	No
Lyme disease	Yes	No
Histoplasmosis	Yes	No
Candida or moniliasis	Yes	No
Coccidioidomycosis	Yes	No
Sporotrichosis	Yes	No
Toxoplasmosis	Yes	No
Toxocariasis	Yes	No
Cysticercosis	Yes	No
Trichinosis	Yes	No
Whipple disease	Yes	No
AIDS	Yes	No
Hay fever	Yes	No
Allergies	Yes	No
Vasculitis	Yes	No
Arthritis	Yes	No
Rheumatoid arthritis	Yes	No

(Continues)

Lupus (systemic lupus erythematosus)	Yes	No
Scleroderma	Yes	No

Have you ever had any of the following illnesses?

Reiter syndrome	Yes	No
Colitis	Yes	No
Crohn disease	Yes	No
Ulcerative colitis	Yes	No
Adamatiades–Behçet disease	Yes	No
Sarcoidosis	Yes	No
Ankylosing spondylitis	Yes	No
Erythema nodosa	Yes	No
Temporal arteritis	Yes	No
Multiple sclerosis	Yes	No
Serpiginous choroiditis	Yes	No
Fuchs heterochromic iridocyclitis	Yes	No
Vogt-Koyanagi-Harada syndrome	Yes	No

Have you ever had any of the following illnesses?

GENERAL HEALTH

Chills	Yes	No
Fever (persistent or recurrent)	Yes	No
Night sweats	Yes	No
Fatigue (tire easily)	Yes	No
Poor appetite	Yes	No
Unexplained weight loss	Yes	No
Do you feel sick?	Yes	No

HEAD

Frequent or severe headaches	Yes	No
Fainting	Yes	No
Numbness or tingling in your body	Yes	No
Paralysis in parts of your body	Yes	No
Seizures or convulsions	Yes	No

EARS

Hard of hearing or deafness	Yes	No
Ringing or noises in your ears	Yes	No
Frequent or severe ear infections	Yes	No
Painful or swollen ear lobes	Yes	No

NOSE AND THROAT

Sore in your nose or mouth	Yes	No
Severe or recurrent nosebleeds	Yes	No
Frequent sneezing	Yes	No
Sinus trouble	Yes	No
Persistent hoarseness	Yes	No
Tooth or gum infections	Yes	No

SKIN

Rashes	Yes	No
Skin sores	Yes	No
Sunburn easily (photosensitivity)	Yes	No
White patches of skin or hair	Yes	No
Loss of hair	Yes	No
Tick or insect bites	Yes	No
Painfully cold fingers	Yes	No
Severe itching	Yes	No

RESPIRATORY

Severe or frequent colds	Yes	No
Constant coughing	Yes	No
Coughing up blood	Yes	No
Recent flu or viral infection	Yes	No
Wheezing or asthma attacks	Yes	No
Difficulty breathing	Yes	No

Have you ever had any of the following symptoms?

CARDIOVASCULAR

Chest pain	Yes	No
Shortness of breath	Yes	No
Swelling of your legs	Yes	No

BLOOD

Frequent or easy bruising	Yes	No
Frequent or easy bleeding	Yes	No
Have you received blood transfusions?	Yes	No

GASTROINTESTINAL

Trouble swallowing	Yes	No
Diarrhea	Yes	No
Bloody stools	Yes	No
Stomach ulcers	Yes	No
Jaundice or yellow skin	Yes	No

BONES AND JOINTS

Stiff joints	Yes	No
Painful or swollen glands	Yes	No
Stiff lower back	Yes	No
Back pain while sleeping or awakening	Yes	No
Muscle aches	Yes	No

(Continues)

GENITOURINARY

Kidney problems	Yes	No
Bladder trouble	Yes	No
Blood in your urine	Yes	No
Urinary discharge	Yes	No
Genital sores or ulcers	Yes	No
Prostatitis	Yes	No
Testicular pain	Yes	No
Are you pregnant?	Yes	No
Do you plan to be pregnant in the future?	Yes	No

(Adapted with permission from Foster CS, Vitale AT. *Diagnosis and Treatment of Uveitis.* Philadelphia: Saunders; 2002.)

CHAPTER 7

Anterior Uveitis

Because uveitis may occur secondarily to inflammation of the cornea and sclera, the physician should evaluate these structures to rule out a primary keratitis or scleritis. Inflammation of the sclera and the cornea is covered in depth in BCSC Section 8, *External Disease and Cornea*, and not in this chapter.

Acute Anterior Nongranulomatous Iritis and Iridocyclitis

The classic presentation of acute anterior uveitis is a triad of pain, redness, and photophobia. Fine keratic precipitates (KPs) and fibrin dust the corneal endothelium in most cases. Endothelial dysfunction may cause the cornea to become acutely edematous. The anterior chamber shows an intense cellular response and variable flare. Severe cases may show a protein coagulum in the aqueous or, less commonly, a hypopyon (Fig 7-1). Occasionally, a fibrin net forms across the pupillary margin (Fig 7-2), potentially producing a seclusion membrane and iris bombé. Iris vessels may be dilated, and rarely, a spontaneous hyphema occurs. Cells may also be present in the anterior vitreous, and in rare cases patients develop severe, diffuse vitritis. Fundus lesions are not characteristic, although cystoid macular edema, disc edema, pars plana exudates, or small areas of peripheral localized choroiditis may be noted. Occasionally, IOP may be elevated because of blockage of the trabecular meshwork by debris and cells or by pupillary block.

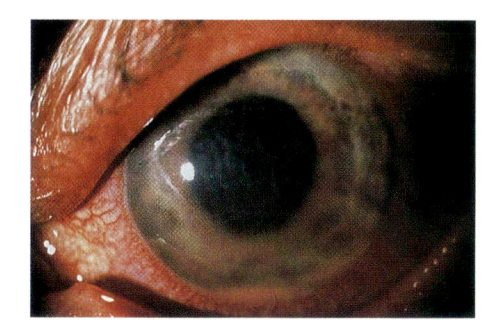

Figure 7-1 Acute HLA-B27–positive anterior uveitis with pain, photophobia, marked injection, fixed pupil, loss of iris detail from corneal edema, and hypopyon. *(Photograph courtesy of David Meisler, MD.)*

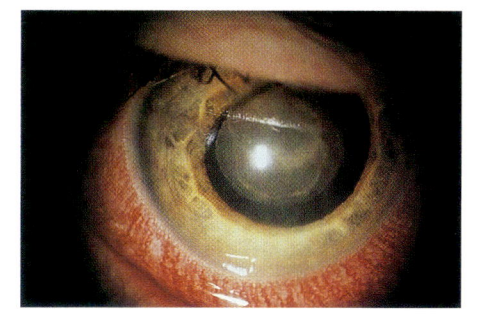

Figure 7-2 Ankylosing spondylitis, acute unilateral iridocyclitis, severe anterior chamber reaction with central fibrinous exudate contracting anterior to the lens capsule and posterior synechiae from 10 o'clock to 12 o'clock. *(Photograph courtesy of David Meisler, MD.)*

The attack of inflammation usually lasts several days to weeks. Typically, an attack is acute and unilateral, with a history of episodes alternating between the two eyes. Recurrences are common. Either eye may be affected, but recurrence is rarely bilateral. If damage to the vascular endothelium can be minimized, no silent, ongoing damage or low-grade inflammation should occur between attacks.

> Cunningham ET Jr. Diagnosis and management of anterior uveitis. In: *Focal Points: Clinical Modules for Ophthalmologists.* San Francisco: American Academy of Ophthalmology; 2002;20:1.
>
> D'Alessandro LP, Forster DJ, Rao NA. Anterior uveitis and hypopyon. *Am J Ophthalmol.* 1991;112:317–321.
>
> Rodriguez A, Akova YA, Pedroza-Seres M, et al. Posterior segment ocular manifestations in patients with HLA-B27–associated uveitis. *Ophthalmology.* 1994;101:1267–1274.

Corticosteroids are the mainstay of treatment to reduce inflammation, prevent cicatrization, and minimize damage to the uveal vasculature. Topical corticosteroids are the first line of treatment, and they often need to be given every 1–2 hours. If necessary, periocular or oral steroids may be used for severe episodes. Initial attacks may require all three routes of treatment, particularly in the severe cases found mostly in younger patients.

Severely damaged vessels may leak continuously, transforming the typical course from acute and intermittent to chronic and recalcitrant. This chronic course must be avoided at all costs by timely diagnosis, aggressive initial therapy, and patient compliance. Maintenance therapy is not indicated once the active inflammation has been controlled.

Cycloplegic/mydriatic agents are used both to relieve pain and to break and prevent synechiae formation. They may be given topically or with conjunctival cotton pledgets soaked in tropicamide (Mydriacyl), cyclopentolate, and phenylephrine hydrochloride (Fig 7-3).

HLA-B27–Related Diseases

HLA-B27 denotes a genotype located on the short arm of chromosome 6. Although it is present in only 1.4%–8.0% of the general population, 50%–60% of patients with acute iritis may be HLA-B27–positive. Racial background and national origin both affect the prevalence of HLA-B27 positivity. The precise trigger for acute iritis in genetically susceptible persons is not clear. The HLA-B27 test should be performed on patients with

Figure 7-3 Acute iridocyclitis after intensive topical steroids and perilimbal subconjunctival dilating agents, leaving an anterior capsular ring of pigment following posterior synechiolysis.
(Photograph courtesy of John D. Sheppard, Jr, MD.)

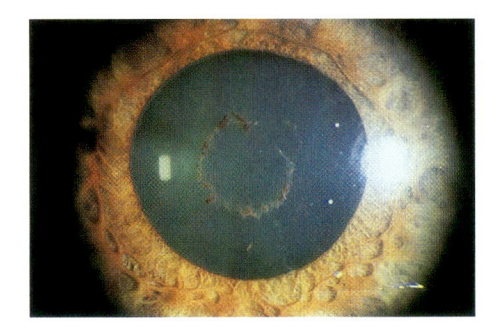

recurrent anterior nongranulomatous uveitis, but the test does not provide an absolute diagnosis.

> Power WJ, Rodriguez A, Pedroza-Seres M, et al. Outcomes in anterior uveitis associated with the HLA-B27 haplotype. *Ophthalmology*. 1998;105:1646–1651.

Several autoimmune diseases known as the *seronegative spondyloarthropathies* are strongly associated with both acute anterior uveitis and HLA-B27 positivity. Patients with these diseases, by definition, do not have a positive rheumatoid factor. The seronegative spondyloarthropathies include

- Ankylosing spondylitis
- Reiter syndrome (reactive arthritis)
- Inflammatory bowel disease
- Psoriatic arthritis
- Postinfectious, or reactive, arthritis

These entities are sometimes clinically indistinguishable, and all may be associated with spondylitis and sacroiliitis. Women tend to experience more atypical spondyloarthropathies than men.

> Wakefield D, Stahlberg TH, Toivanen A, et al. Serologic evidence of *Yersinia* infection in patients with anterior uveitis. *Arch Ophthalmol*. 1990;108:219–221.

Ankylosing spondylitis

This disorder varies from asymptomatic to severe and crippling. Symptoms of ankylosing spondylitis include lower back pain and stiffness after inactivity. Sacroiliac x-ray films may be difficult to interpret but should show sclerosis and eventual narrowing of the joint space. Ligamentous ossification is frequent. These films are best obtained by ordering a sacroiliac view that tunnels down the joint rather than a lumbosacral spine film, which is obtained by direct anteroposterior imaging and is less likely to clearly reveal sacroiliitis (Figs 7-4, 7-5). Similar disease is found in the pubic symphysis, where localized mineral loss and sclerosis erodes the subchondral bone.

HLA-B27 is found in up to 90% of patients with ankylosing spondylitis. The chance that an HLA-B27–positive patient will develop spondyloarthritis or eye disease is one in four, and family members may also have ankylosing spondylitis or iritis. Often, symptoms of back disease are lacking in persons with iritis who test positive. Certainly, not all HLA-B27–positive patients develop disease; most do not develop any form of autoimmune disease.

The ophthalmologist may be the first physician to suspect ankylosing spondylitis. Symptoms or family history of back problems together with HLA-B27 positivity suggest a diagnosis. Sacroiliac x-ray films should be obtained when indicated by a suggestive history in a patient with ocular disease consistent with HLA-B27 syndrome. Patients with ankylosing spondylitis should be informed of the risk of deformity and referred to an internist or a rheumatologist. Pulmonary apical fibrosis may develop; aortitis occurs in about 5% of cases and may be associated with aortic valvular insufficiency (Fig 7-6).

> Tay-Kearney M, Schwam BL, Lowder C, et al. Clinical features and associated systemic diseases of HLA-B27 uveitis. *Am J Ophthalmol*. 1996;121:47–56.

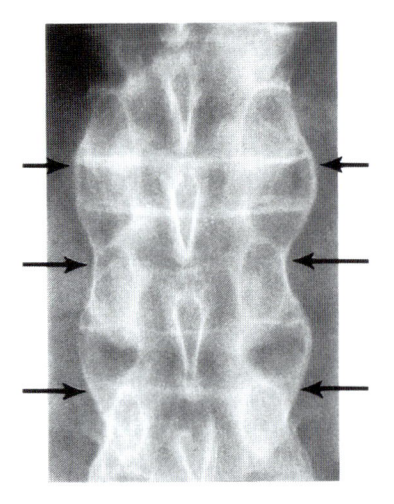

Figure 7-4 Ankylosing spondylitis x-ray film showing total fusion of vertebrae *(arrows)* and marked decalcification. *(Photograph courtesy of John D. Sheppard, Jr, MD.)*

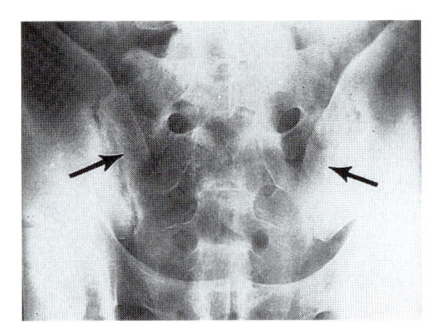

Figure 7-5 Ankylosing spondylitis with moderately severe sacroiliitis shown by tunnel view, with blurring of sacroiliac joint *(arrows).* *(Photograph courtesy of John D. Sheppard, Jr, MD.)*

Figure 7-6 Ankylosing spondylitis and aortitis with arterial wall destruction by fibrosis, thickening, and elastic fragmentation. *(Photograph courtesy of John D. Sheppard, Jr, MD.)*

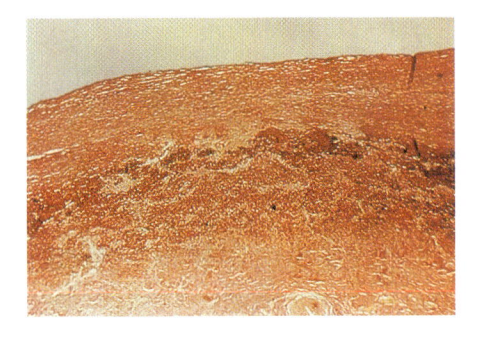

Wakefield D, Montanaro A, McCluskey P. Acute anterior uveitis and HLA-B27. *Surv Ophthalmol.* 1991;36:223–232.

Reiter syndrome

A classic triad of symptoms is diagnostic of Reiter syndrome:

- Nonspecific urethritis
- Polyarthritis
- Conjunctival inflammation, often accompanied by iritis

HLA-B27 is found in 85%–95% of patients, and prostatic fluid culture is negative. The condition occurs most frequently in young adult males, although 10% of patients are female.

Reiter syndrome may be triggered by episodes of diarrhea or dysentery without urethritis. *Chlamydia, Ureaplasma urealyticum, Shigella, Salmonella,* and *Yersinia* have all been implicated as triggering infections. Arthritis begins within 30 days of infection in

CHAPTER 7: Anterior Uveitis • 131

80% of patients. The knees, ankles, feet, and wrists are affected asymmetrically and in an oligoarticular distribution. Sacroiliitis is present in as many as 70% of patients.

Two conditions in addition to the classic triad are considered to be major diagnostic criteria:

- *Keratoderma blennorrhagicum:* a scaly, erythematous, irritating disorder of the palms and soles of the feet (Figs 7-7, 7-8)
- *Circinate balanitis:* a persistent, scaly, erythematous, circumferential rash of the distal penis

The keratoderma blennorrhagicum may resemble pustular psoriasis; this resemblance demonstrates the difficulty of distinguishing among the various seronegative spondyloarthropathies.

Numerous minor criteria are also useful in establishing a diagnosis of Reiter syndrome, according to the American Rheumatologic Association guidelines. These include plantar fasciitis (Fig 7-9), Achilles tendinitis (Fig 7-10), sacroiliitis, nailbed pitting, palate ulcers, and tongue ulcers.

Conjunctivitis is the most common eye lesion associated with Reiter syndrome. Conjunctivitis is usually mucopurulent and papillary. Punctate and subepithelial keratitis may also occur, occasionally leaving permanent corneal scars. Acute nongranulomatous iritis occurs in 5%–10% of patients. In some cases, the iritis becomes bilateral and chronic because of a permanent breakdown of the blood–aqueous barrier.

Inflammatory bowel disease

Ulcerative colitis and *Crohn disease (granulomatous ileocolitis)* are both associated with acute iritis. Between 5% and 12% of patients with ulcerative colitis and 2.4% of patients with Crohn disease develop acute anterior uveitis. Occasionally, bowel disease is asymptomatic and follows the onset of iritis. Of patients with inflammatory bowel disease, 20% may have sacroiliitis; of these patients, 60% are HLA-B27–positive. Patients with both

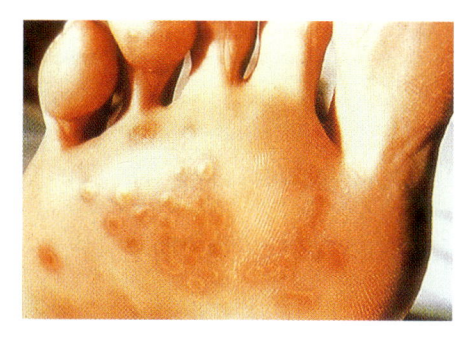

Figure 7-7 Reiter syndrome with keratoderma blennorrhagicum on the sole. *(Photograph courtesy of John D. Sheppard, Jr, MD.)*

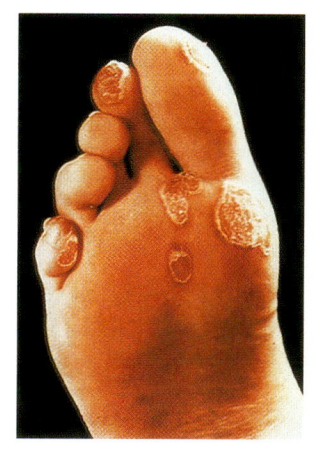

Figure 7-8 Reiter syndrome with pedal discoid keratoderma blennorrhagicum. *(Photograph courtesy of John D. Sheppard, Jr, MD.)*

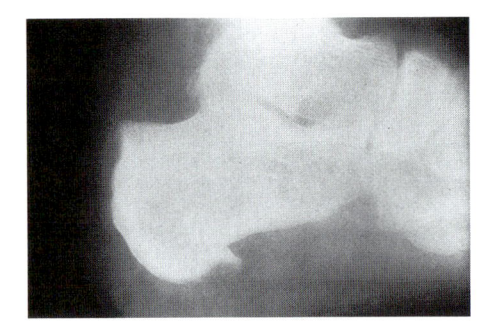

Figure 7-9 Reiter syndrome, x-ray view of calcific plantar fasciitis. *(Photograph courtesy of John D. Sheppard, Jr, MD.)*

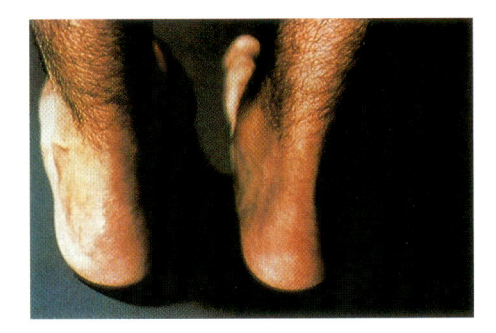

Figure 7-10 Reiter syndrome with chronic Achilles tendinitis. *(Photograph courtesy of John D. Sheppard, Jr, MD.)*

acute iritis and inflammatory bowel disease tend to have HLA-B27 as well as sacroiliitis. In contrast, patients with inflammatory bowel disease who develop sclerouveitis tend to be HLA-B27–negative, have symptoms resembling rheumatoid arthritis, and usually do not develop sacroiliitis.

> Salmon JF, Wright JP, Murray AD. Ocular inflammation in Crohn's disease. *Ophthalmology.* 1991;98:480–484.

Psoriatic arthritis

Acute iritis may occur in conjunction with psoriatic arthritis. Iritis is not associated with psoriasis without arthritis. Twenty percent of patients with psoriatic arthritis may have sacroiliitis, and inflammatory bowel disease occurs more frequently than would be expected by chance with psoriatic arthritis. Diagnosis is based on the findings of the typical cutaneous changes (Fig 7-11), terminal phalangeal joint inflammation (Fig 7-12), and ungual involvement (Figs 7-13, 7-14).

Treatment consists of mydriatic/cycloplegic agents as well as corticosteroids, which are usually given topically. In severe cases, periocular or systemic corticosteroids may be required, and chronic cases may require the use of immunosuppressive agents.

> Derhaag PJ, Linssen A, Broekema N, et al. A familial study of the inheritance of HLA-B27–positive acute anterior uveitis. *Am J Ophthalmol.* 1988;105:603–606.
>
> Rothova A, van Veenedaal WG, Linssen A, et al. Clinical features of acute anterior uveitis. *Am J Ophthalmol.* 1987;103:137–145.

Behçet Syndrome

Behçet syndrome is a generalized occlusive vasculitis of unknown cause (Fig 7-15). Its classic presentation is a triad consisting of

- Acute iritis with hypopyon (Fig 7-16)
- Aphthous stomatitis (cankerlike mouth ulcers) (Fig 7-17)
- Genital ulceration

Although Behçet syndrome may actually cause panuveitis, the syndrome is discussed with acute anterior uveitis because of the classic acute hypopyon iritis seen in Figure 7-16.

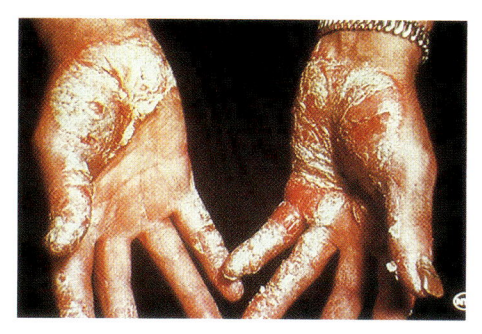

Figure 7-11 Psoriatic arthritis with classic erythematous, hyperkeratotic rash. *(Photograph courtesy of John D. Sheppard, Jr, MD.)*

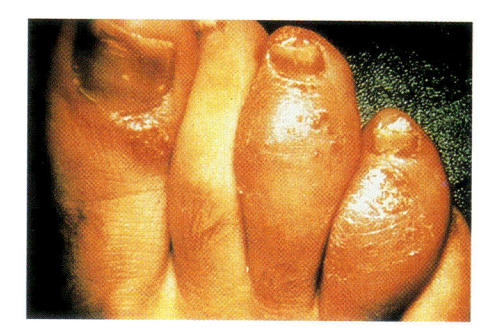

Figure 7-12 Psoriatic arthritis with sausage digits resulting from tissue swelling and distal interphalangeal joint inflammation. *(Photograph courtesy of John D. Sheppard, Jr, MD.)*

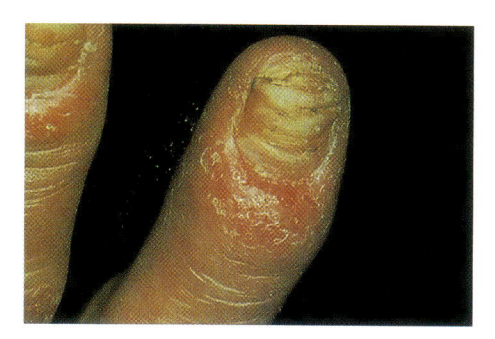

Figure 7-13 Psoriatic arthritis with typical destructive nail changes of subungual hyperkeratosis and onycholysis. *(Photograph courtesy of John D. Sheppard, Jr, MD.)*

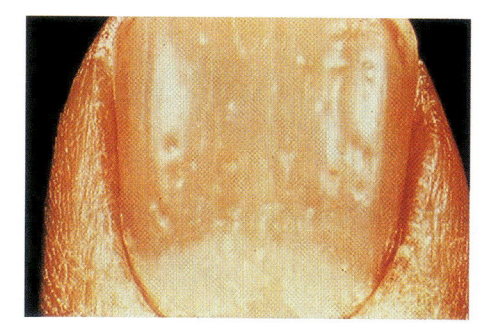

Figure 7-14 Psoriatic arthritis with typical nail-bed pitting changes. *(Photograph courtesy of John D. Sheppard, Jr, MD.)*

Behçet syndrome is rare in the United States; 1.8% of patients had the syndrome at one referral uveitis clinic. It is more common in countries stretching eastward from the eastern Mediterranean to Japan. At one Japanese uveitis clinic, 20% of patients had Behçet syndrome. The disease occurs most frequently in young adults.

A characteristic ocular feature of Behçet syndrome is recurrent acute iritis or chronic iridocyclitis that is often bilateral and associated with a transient hypopyon. More common than anterior involvement in men is a posterior involvement that includes retinal vasculitis (Fig 7-18) (occlusive arteritis and periphlebitis), retinal hemorrhages, macular edema, focal areas of retinal necrosis, ischemic optic neuropathy, and vitritis.

The characteristic mucous membrane lesions are orogenital ulcerations. Lesions elsewhere on the skin are the fourth typical feature of Behçet syndrome. The most common skin lesion is erythema nodosum on the legs, ankles, and elsewhere. Nondestructive recurrent arthritis-arthralgia may affect the wrists and ankles in 60% of patients. Ulcerative hemorrhages that can mimic inflammatory bowel disease may occur in the gastrointestinal tract. Central nervous system symptoms such as strokes, palsies, and a confusional state may develop in 25% of patients. Superficial thrombophlebitis is common.

The diagnosis is based on finding some or all of the four main signs: oral aphthous lesions, skin lesions, ocular lesions, and genital lesions. The *complete type* of Behçet syndrome shows all four main signs; the *incomplete type* shows either three main signs or typical ocular findings along with one main sign. The *suspect group* of patients display two main (nonocular) signs; the *possible group* shows only one main sign. The prevalence of HLA-B5 or subset B51 is increased among patients with Behçet syndrome.

While treatment of Behçet syndrome includes the initial use of oral corticosteroids, most authorities advocate the early institution of immunosuppressive medication, which has been shown to improve the long-term prognosis. Azathioprine, chlorambucil, and cyclosporine have all been found useful in this regard. One study has demonstrated a rapid resolution of intraocular inflammation following a single intravenous infusion of infliximab. Behçet syndrome is a chronic disorder that tends to recur over a period of 2–4 years and may lead to blindness if ischemic optic neuropathy and retinopathy are not adequately treated.

Hashimoto T, Takeuchi A. Treatment of Behçet's disease. *Curr Opin Rheumatol.* 1992;4:31–34.

Michelson JB, Friedlaender MH. Behçet's disease. *Int Ophthalmol Clin.* 1990;30:271–278.

Nussenblatt JB, Palestine AG, Chan CC, et al. Effectiveness of cyclosporine therapy for Behçet's disease. *Arthritis Rheum.* 1985;28:671–679.

Sfikakis PP, Theodossiadis PG, Katsiari CG, et al. Effect of infliximab on sight-threatening panuveitis in Behçet disease. *Lancet.* 2001;358:295.

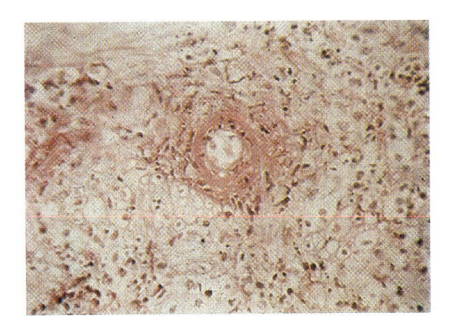

Figure 7-15 Behçet syndrome, histopathologic view of perivascular inflammation.

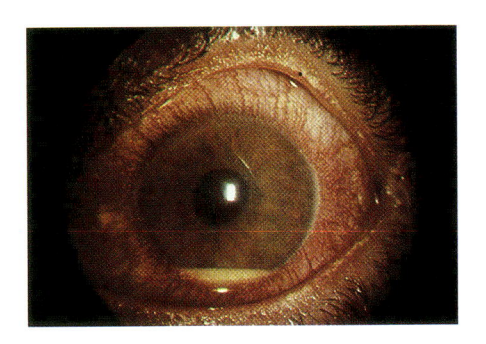

Figure 7-16 Behçet syndrome, hypopyon.

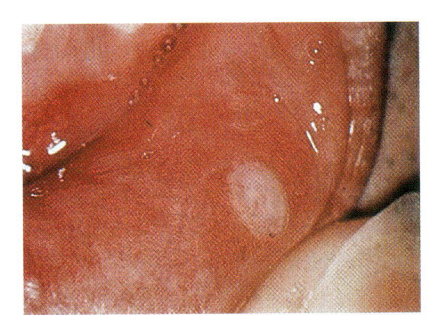

Figure 7-17 Behçet syndrome, mucous membrane ulcers.

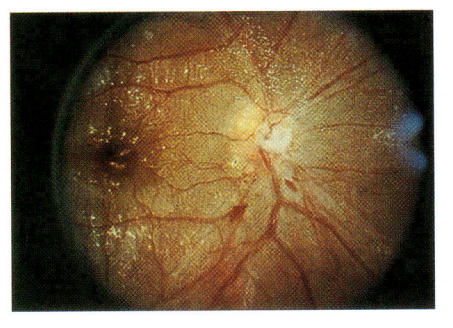

Figure 7-18 Behçet syndrome, retinal vasculitis.

Yazici H, Pazarli H, Barnes CG, et al. A controlled trial of azathioprine in Behçet's syndrome. *N Engl J Med.* 1990;322:281–285.

Glaucomatocyclitic Crisis (Posner-Schlossman Syndrome)

Glaucomatocyclitic crisis (Posner-Schlossman syndrome) usually manifests as a unilateral mild acute iritis. Symptoms are vague, such as discomfort, blurred vision, or haloes. Signs include markedly elevated IOP, corneal edema, fine KPs, low-grade cell and flare, and a slightly dilated pupil. Episodes last from several hours to several days, and recurrences are common over many years. Treatment is with topical corticosteroids and antiglaucoma medication, including, if necessary, carbonic anhydrase inhibitors. Pilocarpine probably should be avoided because it may exacerbate ciliary spasm.

Glaucomatocyclitic crisis, like Vogt-Koyanagi-Harada disease, which is discussed in Chapter 10, may be associated with the HLA-B54 gene locus. Because Posner-Schlossman syndrome is rare, it should be a diagnosis of exclusion, established only after other, more common syndromes such as herpetic uveitis have been ruled out.

Lens-Associated Uveitis

Uveitis may result from an immune reaction to lens material. This can occur following disruption of the lens capsule (traumatic or surgical) or from leakage of lens protein through the lens capsule in mature or hypermature cataracts (Figs 7-19 to 7-22).

This type of uveitis was once divided into several categories, including phacoanaphylactic endophthalmitis, phacotoxic uveitis, and phacolytic glaucoma. Some of these terms are misleading and do not accurately describe the disease process. For example, the term *phacoanaphylactic* is not appropriate since anaphylaxis involves immunoglobulin E (IgE), mast cells, and basophils, none of which is present in phacogenic uveitis. Also, the term *phacotoxic* is misleading, since there is no evidence that lens proteins are directly toxic to ocular tissues.

The exact mechanism of lens-induced uveitis, although unknown, is thought to represent an autoimmune reaction to lens protein. Experimental animal studies suggest that altered tolerance to lens protein leads to the inflammation, which usually has an abrupt onset but may occasionally occur insidiously. Patients previously sensitized to lens protein

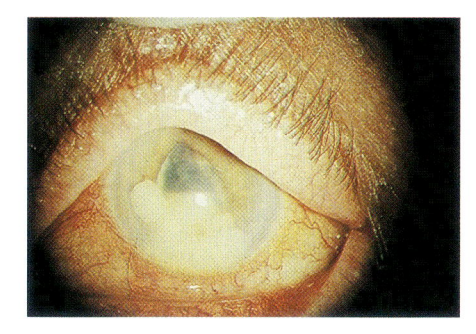

Figure 7-19 Phacoantigenic reaction following phacoemulsification.

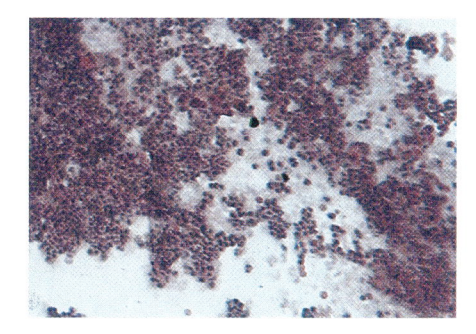

Figure 7-20 Phacoantigenic reaction, histopathology (aqueous tap). Note neutrophils *(blue)* around lens *(gray)*.

136 • Intraocular Inflammation and Uveitis

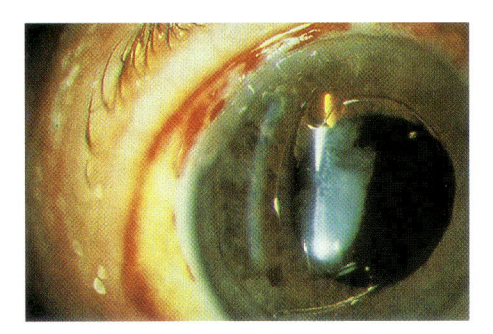

Figure 7-21 Low-grade postoperative uveitis in this patient could be secondary to retained lens cortex or the anterior chamber IOL. *(Photograph courtesy of John D. Sheppard, Jr, MD.)*

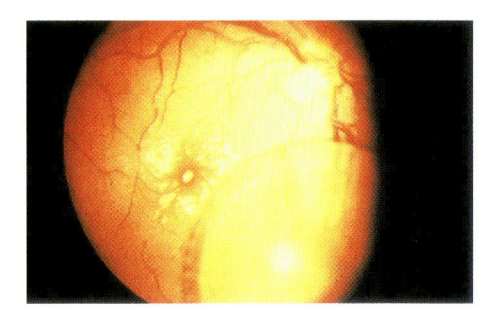

Figure 7-22 Traumatically dislocated nucleus atop the optic nerve produced progressively severe phacoantigenic uveitis and glaucoma, necessitating pars plana lensectomy and vitrectomy. *(Photograph courtesy of John D. Sheppard, Jr, MD.)*

(eg, after cataract extraction in the fellow eye) can experience inflammation within 24 hours after capsular rupture.

Clinically, patients show an anterior uveitis that may be granulomatous or nongranulomatous. Keratic precipitates are usually present and may be small or large. Anterior chamber reaction varies from mild (eg, postoperative inflammation where there is a small amount of retained cortex) to severe (eg, traumatic lens capsule disruption); hypopyon may be present. Posterior synechiae are common, and intraocular pressure is often elevated. Inflammation in the anterior vitreous cavity is common, but fundus lesions do not occur.

Histopathologically, a zonal granulomatous inflammation is centered at the site of lens injury. Neutrophils are present about the lens material with surrounding lymphocytes, plasma cells, epithelioid cells, and occasional giant cells.

Treatment consists of topical and, in severe cases, systemic corticosteroids, as well as mydriatic/cycloplegic agents. Surgical removal of all lens material is usually curative. When small amounts of lens material remain, corticosteroid therapy alone may be sufficient to allow resorption of the inciting material.

Phacolytic glaucoma

Phacolytic glaucoma involves an acute increase in IOP caused by clogging of the trabecular meshwork by lens protein and engorged macrophages. This form occurs with hypermature cataracts. The diagnosis is suggested by elevated IOP, lack of keratic precipitates, refractile bodies in the aqueous (representing lipid-laden macrophages), and lack of synechiae. Therapy includes pressure reduction, often with osmotic agents as well as topical medications, and prompt cataract extraction. Aqueous tap may reveal swollen macrophages.

Infectious endophthalmitis must be included in the differential diagnosis of postoperative inflammation and hypopyon. *Propionibacterium acnes* is a cause of delayed or late-onset endophthalmitis following cataract surgery, as are *Staphylococcus epidermidis* and *Candida* species. Infectious endophthalmitis is discussed in more detail in Chapter 11.

Apple DJ, Mamalis N, Steinmetz RL, et al. Phacoanaphylactic endophthalmitis associated with extracapsular cataract extraction and posterior chamber intraocular lens. *Arch Ophthalmol.* 1984;102:1528–1532.

Meisler DM. Intraocular inflammation and extracapsular cataract surgery. In: *Focal Points: Clinical Modules for Ophthalmologists.* San Francisco: American Academy of Ophthalmology; 1990;8:7.

Wohl LG, Kline OR Jr, Lucier AC, et al. Pseudophakic phacoanaphylactic endophthalmitis. *Ophthalmic Surg.* 1986;17:234–237.

IOL-Associated Postoperative Inflammation

IOL-associated uveitis may range from mild inflammation to the uveitis-glaucoma-hyphema (UGH) syndrome. Surgical manipulation results in breakdown of the blood–aqueous barrier, leading to vulnerability in the early postoperative period. IOL implantation can activate complement cascades and promote PMN chemotaxis, leading to cellular deposits on the IOL, synechiae formation, capsular opacification, and anterior capsule phimosis. Retained lens material from extracapsular cataract extraction may exacerbate the usual transient postoperative inflammation. Iris chafing caused by the edges or loops of IOLs on either the anterior or the posterior surface of the iris can result in mechanical irritation and inflammation. In particular, metal-loop lenses and poorly polished lenses can cause this reaction. The incidence of this type of complication with modern lenses is 1% or less of cases. The motion of an iris-supported or an anterior chamber IOL may cause intermittent corneal touch and lead to corneal endothelial damage or decompensation, low-grade iritis, peripheral anterior synechiae, recalcitrant glaucoma, and cystoid macular edema (Figs 7-23, 7-24). These lenses should be removed and exchanged when penetrating keratoplasty is performed.

The *uveitis-glaucoma-hyphema syndrome* still occurs today, although it has become much less common. The syndrome was caused in the past through irritation of the iris root by the warped footplates of poorly made rigid anterior chamber IOLs. Flexible

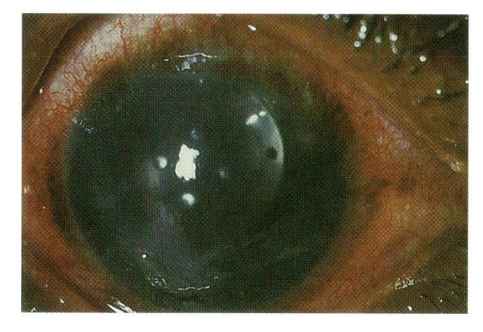

Figure 7-23 Pseudophakic bullous keratopathy and chronic iridocyclitis caused by iris-fixated anterior chamber IOL, with corneal touch, iris stromal erosion, and chronic recalcitrant cystoid macular edema. *(Photograph courtesy of John D. Sheppard, Jr, MD.)*

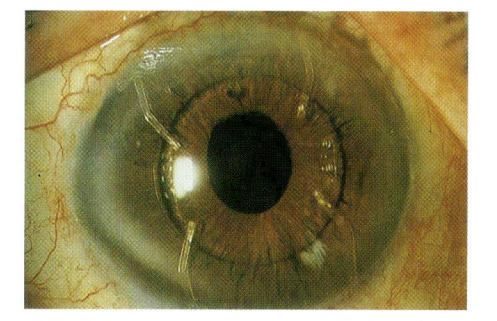

Figure 7-24 Fixed-haptic anterior chamber IOL (Azar 91Z) associated with peripheral and superior corneal edema, chronic low-grade iridocyclitis, peripheral anterior synechiae, global tenderness, and intermittent microhyphema. *(Photograph courtesy of John D. Sheppard, Jr, MD.)*

anterior chamber IOLs are less likely to cause uveitis-glaucoma-hyphema syndrome. Various polymers used in the manufacture of IOLs may activate complement and cause polymorphonuclear neutrophil chemotaxis and resultant inflammation. Retained lens material from extracapsular cataract extraction may exacerbate the usual transient postoperative inflammation.

> Auffarth GU, Wesendahl TA, Brown SJ, et al. Are there acceptable anterior chamber intraocular lenses for clinical use in the 1990s? An analysis of 4104 explanted anterior chamber intraocular lenses. *Ophthalmology*. 1994;101:1913–1922.

As a general rule, the more biocompatible the IOL material, the less likely it is to incite an inflammatory response. Irregular or damaged IOL surfaces as well as polypropylene haptics have been associated with enhanced bacterial and leukocyte binding and probably should be avoided in patients with uveitis. Several attempts have been made to modify the IOL surface to increase its biocompatibility. These modifications include molecular bonding of heparin to the surface of the PMMA lenses *(heparin surface modification)* and molecular surface passivation to minimize bacterial and leukocyte adherence.

Foldable implant materials also have been found to be well-tolerated in many patients with uveitis. Some studies have shown increased cellular deposition on silicone optics compared with acrylic or hydrogel optics, but others have shown no difference between the lens materials. In general, acrylic IOLs appear to have excellent biocompatibility, with low rates of cellular deposits and capsular opacification.

Randomized, controlled studies still need to be performed to determine the optimal IOL material in these patients. In any event, one of the most important factors in the success of cataract surgery in patients with uveitis is aggressive control of the intraocular inflammation in both the pre- and the postoperative periods. For further discussion and illustrations, see BCSC Section 11, *Lens and Cataract*.

> Rauz S, Stavrou P, Murray PI. Evaluation of foldable intraocular lenses in patients with uveitis. *Ophthalmology*. 2000;107:909–919.
> Ravalico G, Baccara F, Lovisato A, et al. Postoperative cellular reaction on various intraocular lens materials. *Ophthalmology*. 1997;104:1084–1091.

Herpetic Disease

Acute anterior uveitis is often associated with herpetic viral disease. BCSC Section 8, *External Disease and Cornea*, extensively discusses herpes simplex virus and herpes zoster virus (Figs 7-25, 7-26, 7-27). Usually, the uveal inflammation associated with these herpesviruses is a keratoiritis secondary to corneal disease. On occasion, the iritis may occur without noticeable keratitis. In many cases, the inflammation becomes chronic. Herpes zoster virus may be considered in the differential diagnosis of chronic unilateral iridocyclitis, even if the cutaneous component of the condition occurred in the past or was minimal even when present.

Varicella (chickenpox), which is caused by the same virus responsible for secondary varicella-zoster virus reactivation, is frequently associated with an acute, mild, nongranulomatous, self-limited, bilateral iritis or iridocyclitis. Cutaneous vesicles at the side of the tip of the nose *(Hutchinson's sign)* indicate nasociliary nerve involvement and a

CHAPTER 7: Anterior Uveitis • 139

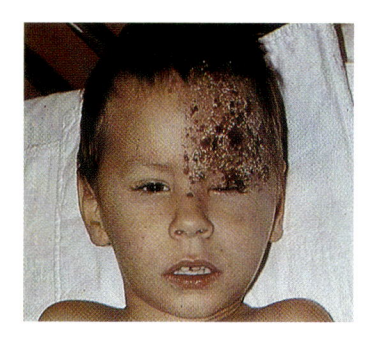

Figure 7-25 Herpes zoster virus, skin lesions.

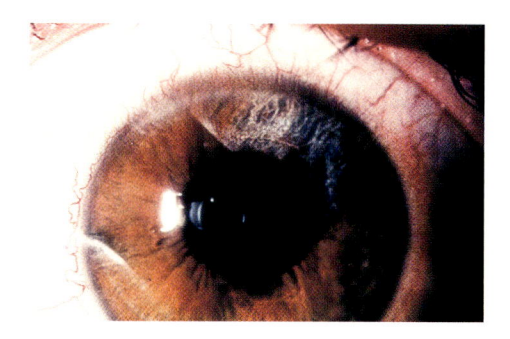

Figure 7-26 Iris stromal atrophy in a patient with herpes zoster iridocyclitis. *(Photograph courtesy of David Forster, MD.)*

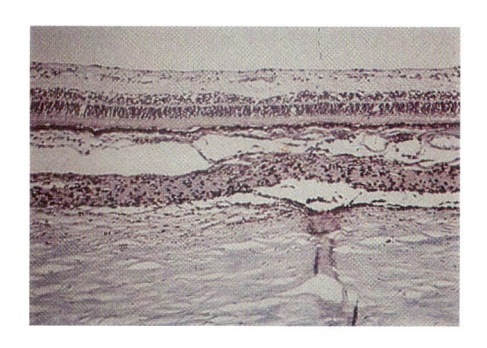

Figure 7-27 Herpes zoster virus, necrosis of long ciliary nerve.

greater likelihood that the eye will be affected. Most patients are asymptomatic, but as many as 40% of patients with primary herpes zoster virus infection may develop iritis when examined prospectively.

Patients with intraocular viral infections, particularly the herpes group infections, which also include cytomegalovirus, may occasionally develop stellate KPs. This morphology is also seen in Fuchs heterochromic iridocyclitis and toxoplasmosis. These stellate KPs usually assume a diffuse distribution, as opposed to the usual distribution in the inferior third of the cornea known as Arlt's triangle. In addition, the KPs are fine and fibrillar, often with a distinctly stellate pattern on high-magnification biomicroscopy. The identification of diffuse or stellate KPs is useful in the differential diagnosis of anterior segment inflammation, although not diagnostic of any particular condition. In patients with herpetic disease and concomitant keratopathy, however mild, anterior segment inflammation may also be associated with diffuse or localized decreased corneal sensation and neurotrophic keratitis.

Glaucoma is a frequent complication of herpetic uveitis and is thus a helpful diagnostic hallmark. Most inflammatory syndromes are usually associated with decreased IOP as a result of ciliary body hyposecretion. However, just as the herpesvirus can localize to corneal, cutaneous, or conjunctival tissues, herpetic reactivation may directly cause trabeculitis and thus increase IOP, often to as high as 50–60 mm Hg. In addition, inflammatory cells may contribute to trabecular obstruction and congestion. Hyphema may occur in herpetic uveitis.

Iris atrophy is also characteristic of herpetic inflammation and can be seen with either herpes simplex or herpes zoster. The atrophy may be patchy or sectoral (see Fig 7-26). Such atrophy is best demonstrated with retroillumination at the slit lamp.

Viral retinitis may occur with these entities, particularly in immunocompromised hosts. Vasculitis commonly occurs with herpes zoster ophthalmicus, and it may lead to anterior segment ischemia, retinal artery occlusion, and scleritis. Vasculitis in the orbit may lead to cranial nerve palsies.

Treatment for viral iritis usually includes topical corticosteroids and cycloplegic agents. Topical antiviral agents usually are ineffective in the treatment of herpetic uveitis but may be indicated in patients with herpes simplex keratouveitis to prevent dendritic keratitis during topical corticosteroid therapy. Systemic antivirals such as acyclovir, famciclovir, or valacyclovir are often beneficial in cases of severe uveitis. Initiation of oral antiviral therapy within the first few days after herpes zoster onset is now recommended. Patients with herpetic uveitis may require prolonged corticosteroid therapy with very gradual tapering. In fact, some patients with herpes zoster require chronic, albeit extremely low, doses of topical corticosteroids (as infrequent as one drop per week) to remain quiescent. Systemic corticosteroids are at times necessary. Long-term, low-dose antiviral therapy may be beneficial in patients with herpetic uveitis, but controlled studies are lacking. Consultation with an infectious disease specialist may be appropriate.

Barron BA, Gee L, Hauck WW, et al. Herpetic Eye Disease Study: a controlled trial of oral acyclovir for herpes simplex stromal keratitis. *Ophthalmology*. 1994;101:1871–1882.

Cunningham ET Jr. Diagnosis and management of herpetic anterior uveitis. *Ophthalmology*. 2001;107:2129–2130.

Parrish CM. Herpes simplex virus eye disease. In: *Focal Points: Clinical Modules for Ophthalmologists*. San Francisco: American Academy of Ophthalmology; 1997;15:2.

Sandor EV, Millman A, Croxson TS, et al. Herpes zoster ophthalmicus in patients at risk for the acquired immune deficiency syndrome (AIDS). *Am J Ophthalmol*. 1986;101:153–155.

Van der Lelij A, Ooijman FM, Lijlstra A, et al. Anterior uveitis with sectoral iris atrophy in the absence of keratitis: a distinct clinical entity among herpetic eye disease. *Ophthalmology*. 2000;107:1164–1170.

Wilhelmus KR, Gee L, Hauck WW, et al. Herpetic Eye Disease Study: a controlled trial of topical corticosteroids for herpes simplex stromal keratitis. *Ophthalmology*. 1994;101:1883–1895.

Other Viral Diseases

Acute iritis may occur in other infectious entities. The iritis in influenza, adenovirus, and infectious mononucleosis is mild and transient. Synechiae and ocular damage seldom occur. Iritis with adenovirus is usually secondary to corneal disease (see BCSC Section 8, *External Disease and Cornea*). Rarely, retinal periphlebitis may be seen in mononucleosis. Treatment beyond cycloplegia may not be necessary, although topical corticosteroids can be used. Iritis is unusual in mumps, although it may occur 4–14 days after onset. Papillitis or neuroretinitis appears 2–4 weeks after onset and lasts 2–3 weeks.

Drug-Induced Uveitis

Treatment with certain medications has been associated with the development of intraocular inflammation. Examples include rifabutin and cidofovir, both of which can cause acute anterior uveitis. Treatment is generally with topical corticosteroids and cycloplegic agents, if necessary. Recalcitrant cases may require cessation or tapering of the offending systemic medication.

> Moorthy RS, Valluri S, Jampol LM. Drug-induced uveitis [review]. *Surv Ophthalmol.* 1998;42:557–570.

Chronic Iridocyclitis

Inflammation of the anterior segment that lasts longer than 3 months is termed *chronic iridocyclitis,* and it may persist for years. This type of inflammation usually starts insidiously, with variable amounts of redness, discomfort, and photophobia. Some patients have no symptoms. The disease can be unilateral or bilateral, and the amount of inflammatory activity is variable. Cystoid macular edema is common.

Juvenile Rheumatoid Arthritis

Juvenile rheumatoid arthritis (JRA), also called *juvenile chronic arthritis* or *juvenile idiopathic arthritis,* is the most common systemic disorder associated with iridocyclitis in the pediatric age group. JRA is subdivided into three types:

- *Systemic onset (Still disease).* This type, usually seen in children under age 5, is characterized by fever, rash, lymphadenopathy, and hepatosplenomegaly. Joint involvement may be minimal or absent initially. This type accounts for approximately 20% of all cases of JRA, but ocular involvement is rare: fewer than 6% of patients with JRA have uveitis.
- *Polyarticular onset.* This group shows involvement of five or more joints in the first 6 weeks of the disease. It constitutes 40% of JRA cases overall but only 7%–14% of cases of JRA-associated iridocyclitis.
- *Pauciarticular onset.* This group includes the vast majority (80%–90%) of patients with JRA who have uveitis. Patients have involvement of four or fewer joints during the first 6 weeks of disease and may have no joint symptoms. This type is subdivided into two subsets. *Type 1* disease is seen primarily in girls under age 5 who typically test positive for antinuclear antibody (ANA); chronic iridocyclitis occurs in up to 25% of these patients. *Type 2* disease is seen in older boys, many of whom go on to develop evidence of seronegative spondyloarthropathy (75% are HLA-B27–positive). The uveitis in these patients tends to be acute and recurrent rather than chronic as in type 1.

Ocular involvement in JRA

The average age of onset of uveitis in patients with JRA is 6 years. Uveitis generally develops within 5–7 years of the onset of joint disease but may occur as long as 28 years

142 • Intraocular Inflammation and Uveitis

after the development of arthritis. There is usually little or no correlation between ocular and joint inflammation. Risk factors for the development of chronic iridocyclitis in patients with JRA include female gender, pauciarticular onset, and the presence of circulating ANA. Most patients test negative for rheumatoid factor.

The eye is often white and uninflamed. Symptoms include moderate pain, photophobia, and blurring, although some patients do not have pain. Often, the eye disease is found incidentally during a routine school physical examination. The signs of inflammation include fine KPs, band keratopathy, flare and cells, posterior synechiae, and cataract (Figs 7-28, 7-29). Patients in whom JRA is suspected should undergo ANA testing and should be evaluated by a pediatric rheumatologist, since the joint disease may be minimal or absent at the time the uveitis is diagnosed. The differential diagnosis in these patients includes sarcoidosis, the seronegative spondyloarthropathies, herpetic uveitis, and Lyme disease.

Prognosis

Because of the frequently asymptomatic nature of the uveitis in these patients, profound silent ocular damage can occur, and the long-term prognosis often depends on the extent

Figure 7-28 Juvenile rheumatoid arthritis, chronic iridocyclitis, cataract.

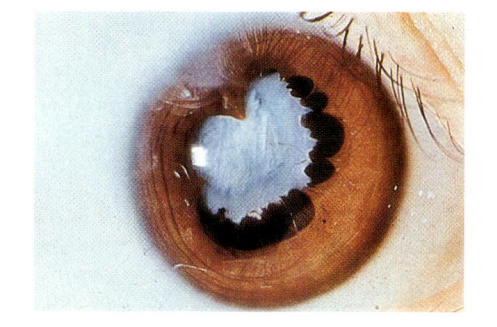

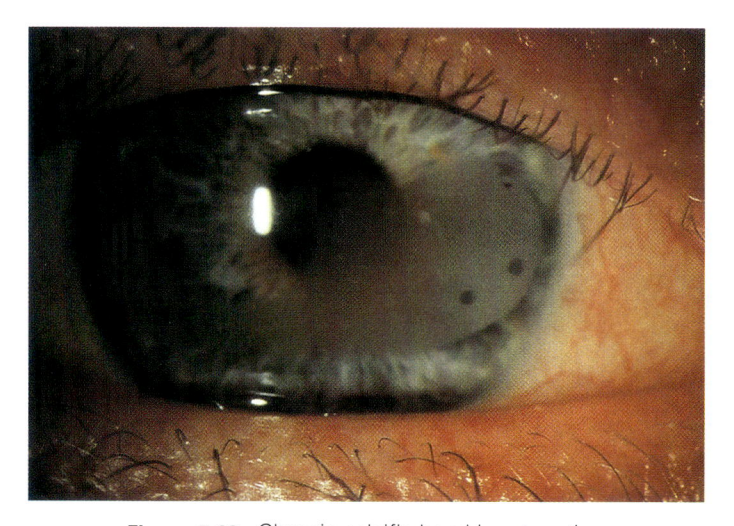

Figure 7-29 Chronic calcific band keratopathy.

of damage at the time of first diagnosis. Complications are frequent and often severe and include band keratopathy, cataract, glaucoma, vitreous debris, macular edema, chronic hypotony, and phthisis. Children with JRA, especially those who are ANA-positive or have pauciarticular disease, should undergo regular slit-lamp examinations. Table 7-1 outlines the recommended schedule for screening patients with JRA for uveitis, as developed by the American Academy of Pediatrics.

Management

The initial treatment consists of topical corticosteroids. More severe cases may require systemic or periocular corticosteroids. Steroid therapy is not indicated in patients with chronic aqueous flare in the absence of active cellular reaction. Short-acting mydriatic agents are useful in patients with chronic flare to keep the pupil mobile and to prevent posterior synechiae formation. Use of systemic NSAIDs may permit a lower dose of corticosteroids.

Because of the chronic nature of the inflammation, steroid-induced complications are common. The chronic use of systemic corticosteroids in children presents numerous problems, including growth retardation from premature closure of the epiphyses. In addition, there is evidence that even low-grade inflammation, if present for a prolonged period, can result in unacceptable ocular morbidity and visual loss. For these reasons, many of these children are now treated with weekly low-dose methotrexate. Numerous studies have shown that this treatment regimen can effectively control the uveitis, is generally well-tolerated, and can spare patients the complications of chronic corticosteroid use.

Patients with JRA-associated iridocyclitis present some of the most difficult management problems of all uveitis cases with respect to cataract removal. Conventional cataract extraction is associated with a high rate of complications in these patients. Great care must be taken, including the following steps:

- Control the inflammation adequately for at least 3 months prior to surgery
- Evaluate the angle and synechiae preoperatively
- Treat with adequate anti-inflammatory medications, including immunosuppressive therapy if indicated, in the perioperative period

At this time, most authorities agree that IOL implantation is generally contraindicated in younger children with JRA-associated iridocyclitis because of the severity of the inflammation in these patients, the higher incidence of fibrous reaction around the IOL, and the presence of cystoid macular edema. However, IOL implantation may be successful in selected adults or older children with JRA in whom the inflammation has been adequately controlled. Combined lensectomy-vitrectomy may improve the prognosis. The decision not to implant an IOL must be weighed against the difficulty in preventing amblyopia in a young child who is aphakic. Patients with band keratopathy should be treated (eg, scraping or chelation with sodium EDTA) and allowed to heal well before cataract surgery is attempted. See also Chapter 13 and BCSC Section 6, *Pediatric Ophthalmology and Strabismus,* Chapter 23.

Glaucoma should be treated with medical therapy initially, although surgical intervention is often necessary in severe cases. Standard filtering procedures are usually

Table 7-1 Recommended Screening Schedule for JRA Patients Without Known Iridocyclitis

JRA Subtype at Onset	Age of Onset <7 Years[1]	Age of Onset ≥7 Years[2]
Pauciarticular		
+ANA	Every 3–4 months[3]	Every 6 months
−ANA	Every 6 months	Every 6 months
Polyarticular		
+ANA	Every 3–4 months[3]	Every 6 months
−ANA	Every 6 months	Every 6 months
Systemic	Every 12 months	Every 12 months

[1] All patients are considered at low risk 7 years after the onset of their arthritis and should have yearly ophthalmologic examination indefinitely.
[2] All patients are considered at low risk 4 years after the onset of their arthritis and should have yearly ophthalmologic examinations indefinitely.
[3] If no uveitis 4 years after onset of arthritis, should have ophthalmologic examination every 6 months.

(Adapted from: American Academy of Pediatrics Section on Rheumatology and Section on Ophthalmology. Guidelines for ophthalmologic examinations in children with juvenile rheumatoid arthritis. *Pediatrics*. 1993; 92:295–296.)

unsuccessful, and the use of antifibrotic agents or aqueous drainage devices is usually required for successful control of the glaucoma.

> Cunningham ET Jr. Uveitis in children. *Ocul Immunol Inflamm*. 2000;8:251–261.
>
> Dana MR, Merayo-Lloves J, Schaumberg DA, et al. Visual outcomes prognosticators in juvenile rheumatoid arthritis–associated uveitis. *Ophthalmology*. 1997;104:236–244.
>
> Dinning WJ. Uveitis and juvenile chronic arthritis. In: *Focal Points: Clinical Modules for Ophthalmologists*. San Francisco: American Academy of Ophthalmology, 1990;8:5.
>
> Giannini EH, Brewer EJ, Kuzmina N, et al. Methotrexate in resistant juvenile rheumatoid arthritis. Results of the U.S.A.–U.S.S.R. double-blind placebo-controlled trial. The Pediatric Rheumatology Collaborative Study Group and The Co-operative Children's Study Group. *N Engl J Med*. 1992;326:1043–1049.
>
> Kanski JJ. Juvenile arthritis and uveitis. *Surv Ophthalmol*. 1990;34:253–267.
>
> Probst LE, Holland EJ. Intraocular lens implantation in patients with juvenile rheumatoid arthritis. *Am J Ophthalmol*. 1996;122:161–170.
>
> Weiss AH, Wallace CA, Sherry DD. Methotrexate for resistant chronic uveitis in children with juvenile rheumatoid arthritis. *J Pediatr*. 1998;133:266–268.

Fuchs Heterochromic Iridocyclitis (Fuchs Uveitis Syndrome)

Fuchs heterochromic iridocyclitis, or *Fuchs uveitis syndrome*, is an entity that is frequently overlooked. Between 2% and 3% of patients referred to various uveitis clinics have Fuchs heterochromic iridocyclitis. This condition is usually unilateral, and its symptoms vary from none to mild blurring and discomfort. Signs include

- Diffuse iris stromal atrophy with variable pigment epithelial layer atrophy (Fig 7-30)

- Small white stellate KPs scattered *diffusely* over the entire endothelium (Fig 7-31); diffusely distributed KPs also occur with herpetic keratouveitis
- Cells present in the anterior chamber as well as the anterior vitreous

Synechiae almost never form, but glaucoma and cataracts occur frequently (see Fig 7-30). Generally, fundus lesions are absent, but fundus scars and retinal periphlebitis have been reported on rare occasions. Macular edema seldom occurs.

The diagnosis is based on the distribution of KPs, lack of synechiae, lack of symptoms, and heterochromia. Often, the inflammation is discovered on a routine examination, such as when a unilateral cataract develops. Usually, but not invariably, the lighter-colored iris indicates the involved eye (Fig 7-32). In blue-eyed persons, however, the affected eye may become darker as the stromal atrophy progresses and the darker iris pigment epithelium shows through.

Patients generally do well with cataract surgery, and IOLs can usually be implanted successfully. However, some patients may suffer significant visual disability as a result of extensive vitreous opacification, even after uncomplicated cataract surgery with IOL implantation in the capsular bag. Pars plana vitrectomy should be carefully considered

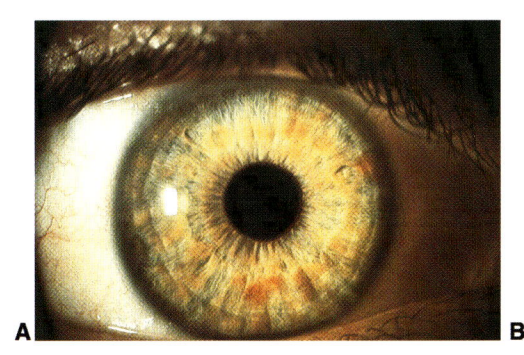

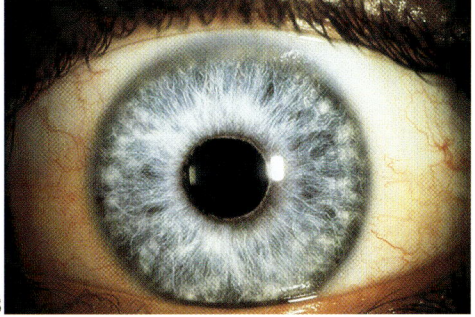

Figure 7-30 Heterochromia in Fuchs heterochromic iridocyclitis. **A,** Right eye. **B,** Left eye. Note the lighter iris color and stromal atrophy (moth-eaten appearance) in the left eye, which was the affected eye. *(Photographs courtesy of David Forster, MD.)*

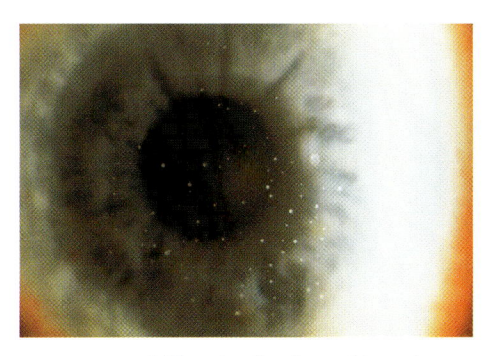

Figure 7-31 Diffusely distributed keratic precipitates in Fuchs heterochromic iridocyclitis. *(Photograph courtesy of David Forster, MD.)*

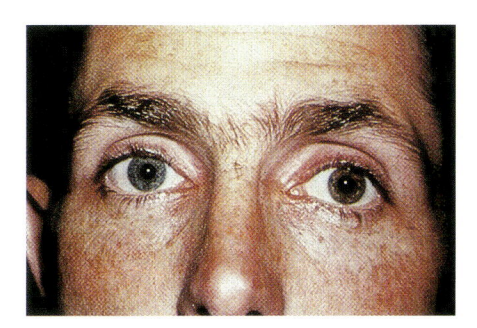

Figure 7-32 Heterochromia in Fuchs heterochromic iridocyclitis in a brown-eyed patient.

in such patients. Glaucoma control can be difficult. Abnormal vessels may bridge the angle on gonioscopy. These vessels may bleed during surgery, resulting in postoperative hyphema.

Few cases of Fuchs heterochromic iridocyclitis require therapy. The prognosis is good in most cases even though the inflammation persists for decades. Since topical corticosteroids can lessen the inflammation but typically do not resolve it, aggressive treatment to eradicate the cellular reaction is not indicated. Cycloplegia is seldom necessary. Histopathology shows plasma cells in the ciliary body, indicating that true inflammation occurs.

> Jones NP. Fuchs' heterochromic uveitis: a reappraisal of the clinical spectrum. *Eye.* 1991; 5:649–661.
>
> Liesegang TJ. Clinical features and prognosis in Fuchs' heterochromic uveitis syndrome. *Arch Ophthalmol.* 1982;100:1622–1626.

Idiopathic Iridocyclitis

In many patients with chronic iridocyclitis, the cause is unknown. Therapy, including cycloplegia, may be necessary before a specific diagnosis is possible. In some cases initially labeled as idiopathic, repeat diagnostic testing at a later date may reveal an underlying systemic condition.

CHAPTER 8

Intermediate Uveitis and Pars Planitis

Intermediate uveitis accounts for up to 15% of all cases of uveitis. It is characterized by ocular inflammation concentrated in the anterior vitreous and the vitreous base overlying the ciliary body and peripheral retina–pars plana complex. Anterior vitreous cellular reaction is apparent. Inflammatory cells may aggregate in the vitreous *(snowballs)*, where some coalesce *(snowmen)*. In some patients, inflammatory exudative accumulation on the inferior pars plana *(snowbanking)* seems to correlate with a more severe disease process. There may be associated retinal phlebitis. Anterior chamber reaction may occur, but in adults it is usually mild and attributed to spillover from the vitreous.

Intermediate uveitis is associated with various conditions, including sarcoidosis, multiple sclerosis (MS), Lyme disease, peripheral toxocariasis, syphilis, tuberculosis, primary Sjögren syndrome, and infection with human T-cell lymphoma virus 1. Intermediate uveitis of unknown cause, *pars planitis,* is the most common form, constituting approximately 85%–90% of cases.

Pars Planitis

Pars planitis, also known as *chronic cyclitis* and *peripheral uveitis,* most commonly affects persons 5 to 40 years of age. It has a bimodal distribution, affecting a younger group (5–15 years) and an older group (20–40 years). No overall gender predilection is apparent. The pathogenesis of pars planitis is not well understood and is thought to involve autoimmune reactions against the vitreous, peripheral retina, and ciliary body. An association between the HLA-DR15 allele, coding for one of the two HLA-DR2 subtypes, and pars planitis has been found. HLA-DR2 is also associated with MS, suggesting a common immunogenetic predisposition to both diseases.

Clinical Characteristics

Approximately 80% of cases are bilateral but can often be asymmetric in severity. In children, the initial presentation may consist of significant anterior chamber inflammation accompanied by redness, photophobia, and discomfort. The onset in teenagers and young adults may be more insidious, with the presenting complaint generally being floaters. Ocular manifestations include variable numbers of spillover anterior chamber cells, vitreous cells, snowballs (Fig 8-1), and pars plana snowbanks. Inferior peripheral retinal phlebitis with retinal venous sheathing is common. With chronic inflammation, cystoid macular edema often develops. Chronic, refractory cystoid macular edema develops in approximately 10% of patients. This is the major cause of visual loss in pars planitis. Ischemia from retinal phlebitis, combined with angiogenic stimuli from intraocular inflammation, can lead to neovascularization along the inferior snowbank in 5%–10% of cases. These neovascular complexes can bleed and result in vitreous hemorrhages, contract, and lead to peripheral tractional and rhegmatogenous retinal detachments; rarely, the complexes evolve into peripheral retinal angiomas. Retinal detachments occur in 10% of patients with pars planitis. With chronicity, posterior synechiae and band keratopathy may also develop. Other possible causes of visual loss associated with chronic inflammation include posterior subcapsular cataracts in 15% of cases, epiretinal membrane in 5%–10% of cases, and vitreous cellular opacification.

Differential Diagnosis

The differential diagnosis of pars planitis includes syphilis, Lyme uveitis, sarcoidosis, intermediate uveitis associated with MS, and toxocariasis. Lyme and syphilitic uveitis may simulate any anatomical subtype of uveitis. Lyme antibody titers may be particularly useful in endemic areas, especially in the presence of cutaneous and articular disease. Iridocyclitis and intermediate uveitis may occur in 5%–20% of patients with MS. Sarcoid uveitis presents as an intermediate uveitis in 7% of cases. Periphlebitis and retinal neovascularization frequently occur in sarcoidosis; however, anterior uveitis is much more common. Elevated levels of serum angiotensin-converting enzyme and chest radiographic findings can aid in differentiating sarcoidosis from pars planitis. Peripheral toxocara granuloma can mimic the unilateral pars plana snowbank in a child and should be ruled out. Serologic testing can be helpful in these cases.

Vitritis without other ocular findings is rarely suggestive of primary central nervous system lymphoma. These patients are much older at presentation than patients with pars planitis, usually in their seventh and eighth decades of life. Fuchs heterochromic irido-

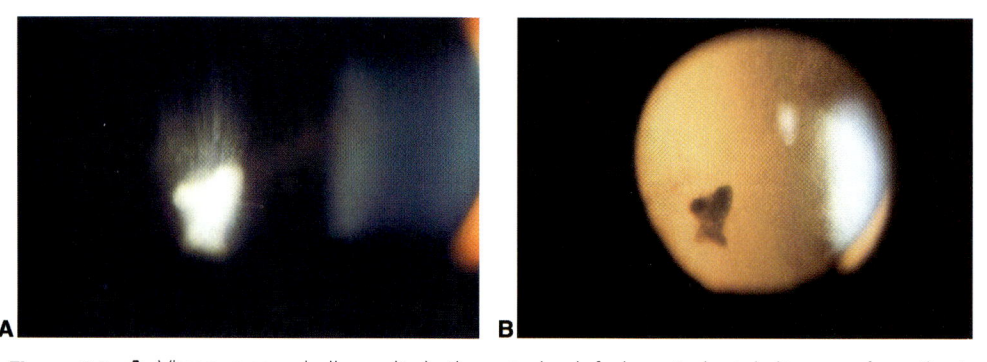

Figure 8-1 A, Vitreous snowball opacity in the anterior, inferior retrolental vitreous of a patient with pars planitis. **B,** Same vitreous snowball opacity in retroillumination, showing its location with respect to the lens. Note also the vitreous cellularity as evidenced by retroillumination. *(Photographs courtesy of Ramana S. Moorthy, MD.)*

cyclitis can produce mild to dense vitritis but has characteristic keratic precipitates and iris heterochromia.

Ancillary Tests and Histopathology

Diagnosis of pars planitis is based on classic clinical findings. Laboratory workup to rule out other causes of intermediate uveitis, including sarcoidosis, Lyme disease, and syphilis, is essential. Serum angiotensin-converting enzyme, chest radiography, Lyme antibody titers, and syphilis serologic investigations should be considered. Fluorescein angiography may show diffuse peripheral venular leakage, disc leakage, and cystoid macular edema. Ultrasound biomicroscopy may be used in cases of a small pupil or dense cataract to demonstrate peripheral exudates or membranes over the pars plana.

Histopathologic examination of eyes with pars planitis shows vitreous condensation and cellular infiltration in the vitreous base. The inflammatory cells consist mostly of macrophages, lymphocytes, and a few plasma cells. Pars planitis is also characterized by peripheral lymphocytic cuffing of venules and a loose fibrovascular membrane over the pars plana.

Prognosis

The clinical course of pars planitis may be divided into three categories. Approximately 10% of cases have a self-limited, benign course; 30% have a smoldering course with remissions and exacerbations; and 60% have a prolonged course without exacerbations. Pars planitis may remain active for many years and has occasionally been documented at more than 30 years. In most cases, the disease "burns out" after 5–15 years. If cystoid macular edema is treated until resolution and kept from returning by adequate control of inflammation, the long-term visual prognosis can be good, with nearly 75% of patients maintaining visual acuity of 20/50 or better.

Treatment

Therapy should be directed toward treating the underlying cause of the inflammation, if possible. For example, infectious causes such as Lyme disease, tuberculosis, and syphilis should be treated with appropriate antimicrobial agents. If an underlying condition is not identified, as in pars planitis, or if therapy of an associated condition consists of nonspecific control of inflammation, as with sarcoidosis, anti-inflammatory therapy should be implemented. Treatment is usually implemented if visual acuity is 20/40 or worse or if cystoid macular edema is present. Mild cases without cystoid macular edema may require no treatment. The classic four-step approach is used to treat patients with pars planitis.

Step 1

Periocular corticosteroids usually constitute the first line of therapy. These may be administered by local injection of depot corticosteroids, using the posterior sub-Tenon's route (see Chapter 6, Fig 6-6). Triamcinolone or methylprednisolone may be used. Injections are usually repeated every 2 or 3 weeks until four injections have been administered. Generally, the inflammation responds and the cystoid macular edema improves.

These injections may be repeated as necessary. Steroid-induced intraocular pressure elevation is less common when a posterior sub-Tenon's route is used but may still occur in 5% of patients, especially those with a history of glaucoma. Other complications of periocular corticosteroids include aponeurotic ptosis, enophthalmos, and, rarely, globe perforation. Cataract formation can occur with any form of corticosteroid therapy.

Systemic corticosteroid therapy may be implemented if local therapy is not effective. Systemic corticosteroids are generally reserved for the more severe or bilateral cases. Patients may be treated with an initial dosage of 1–1.5 mg/kg per day, with a gradual tapering every 2 to 4 weeks to doses of less than 15 mg/day. Ideally, the disease should be controlled with 5 mg or less of daily prednisone.

Intravitreal triamcinolone injections may also be performed in severe refractory cases. These injections carry a risk of retinal detachment, vitreous hemorrhage, endophthalmitis, and sustained intraocular pressure elevation and glaucoma. The injections should be given inferotemporally with caution in cases of pars planitis because of the presence of peripheral snowbank or retinal traction.

Step 2

If corticosteroid therapy fails, peripheral ablation of the pars plana snowbank with cryotherapy or indirect laser photocoagulation should be performed. Retreatment is sometimes necessary. Cryoablation or laser photocoagulation of the pars plana snowbank may be indicated, particularly if neovascularization is present. Peripheral scatter laser photocoagulation seems to be as effective as cryotherapy in treating inflammation and peripheral neovascularization and does not seem to increase the risk of rhegmatogenous retinal detachment. Cryotherapy probably should not be performed in the presence of a traction retinal detachment with peripheral neovascularization because of the increased risk of progressive traction and development of rhegmatogenous retinal detachment.

Step 3

If cryotherapy fails and systemic immunosuppressive therapy is contraindicated or not desired because of the risk of systemic side effects, pars plana vitrectomy with induction of posterior hyaloidal separation and peripheral laser photocoagulation to pars plana snowbank may be performed. Vitrectomy may be necessary to treat severe visual loss caused by dense vitreous cellular accumulation and veils, vitreal hemorrhage or traction, retinal detachment, and cystoid macular edema. Vitrectomy may reduce the need for high doses of maintenance oral corticosteroids in some patients. Separation of posterior hyaloid during vitrectomy may have a beneficial effect in reducing cystoid macular edema. Complications include retinal detachment, endophthalmitis, and cataract formation.

Step 4

If all other therapeutic modalities have failed, systemic immunomodulating agents such as methotrexate, cyclosporine, azathioprine, or cyclophosphamide may also be tried. Because of their severe side effect and complication profiles, these agents are generally considered last among the therapeutic options. Because patients with pars planitis are younger, methotrexate and cyclosporine are the preferred agents.

Complications

Complications of pars planitis include cataract, glaucoma, cystoid macular edema, retinal neovascularization, vitreous hemorrhage, and traction and rhegmatogenous retinal detachment. Cataracts occur in 15%–60% of cases. Cataract surgery with intraocular lens implantation may be complicated by low-grade smoldering inflammation, repeated opacification of posterior capsule despite capsulotomy, and chronic cystoid macular edema, even in burned-out cases of pars planitis. Combining pars plana vitrectomy with cataract extraction and intraocular lens implantation may reduce the risk of these complications. Glaucoma occurs in approximately 10% of patients with pars planitis. Both angle-closure and open-angle glaucoma can occur. Cystoid macular edema may occur in 50% of patients with intermediate uveitis and is a hallmark of pars planitis. Retinal neovascularization occurs in 5%–15% of patients with pars planitis. Neovascularization of the disc as well as a peripheral snowbank have been reported. Occasionally, vitreous hemorrhage is the presenting sign of pars planitis, especially in children. Less than 5% of patients with pars planitis develop vitreous hemorrhage, which can be effectively treated with pars plana vitrectomy. Traction and rhegmatogenous retinal detachments occur in 5%–15% of patients and require scleral buckling, sometimes combined with vitrectomy. Risk factors for rhegmatogenous retinal detachment include severe inflammation, performing cryotherapy at the time of vitrectomy, and presence of neovascularization of the pars plana snowbank.

> Böke WRF, Manthey KF, Nussenblatt RB. *Intermediate Uveitis. Developments in Ophthalmology 23.* Basel: Karger; 1992.
>
> Dugel PU, Rao NA, Ozler S, et al. Pars plana vitrectomy for intraocular inflammation–related cystoid macular edema unresponsive to corticosteroids: a preliminary study. *Ophthalmology.* 1992;99:1535–1541.
>
> Hikichi T, Trempe CL. Role of the vitreous in the prognosis of peripheral uveitis. *Am J Ophthalmol.* 1993;116:401–405.
>
> Hooper PL. Pars planitis. In: *Focal Points: Clinical Modules for Ophthalmologists.* San Francisco: American Academy of Ophthalmology; 1993;9:11.
>
> Kaplan HJ. Intermediate uveitis (pars planitis, chronic cyclitis)—a four step approach to treatment. In: Saari KM, ed. *Uveitis Update.* Amsterdam: Excerpta Medica; 1984:169–172.
>
> Malinowski SM, Pulido JS, Folk JC. Long-term visual outcome and complications associated with pars planitis. *Ophthalmology.* 1993;100:818–824.
>
> Michelson JB, Friedlaender MH, Nozik RA. Lens implant surgery in pars planitis. *Ophthalmology.* 1990;97:1023–1026.
>
> Mochizuki M, Tajima K, Watanabe T, et al. Human T-lymphotropic virus type 1 uveitis. *Br J Ophthalmol.* 1994;78:149–154.
>
> Park SE, Mieler WF, Pulido JS. Peripheral scatter photocoagulation for neovascularization associated with pars planitis. *Arch Ophthalmol.* 1995;113:1277–1280.
>
> Pederson JE, Kenyon KR, Green WR, et al. Pathology of pars planitis. *Am J Ophthalmol.* 1978;86:762–774.
>
> Potter MJ, Myckatyn SO, Maberley AL, et al. Vitrectomy for pars planitis complicated by vitreous hemorrhage: visual outcome and long-term follow-up. *Am J Ophthalmol.* 2001;131:514–515.
>
> Pulido JS, Mieler WF, Walton D, et al. Results of peripheral laser photocoagulation in pars planitis. *Trans Am Ophthalmol Soc.* 1998;96:127–141.

Raja SC, Jabs DA, Dunn JP, et al. Pars planitis: clinical features and class II HLA associations. *Ophthalmology.* 1999;106:594–599.

Rosenbaum JT, Bennett RM. Chronic anterior and posterior uveitis and primary Sjögren's syndrome. *Am J Ophthalmol.* 1987;104:346–352.

Multiple Sclerosis

Patients with MS may develop variants of intermediate uveitis. Retinal periphlebitis may occur in 5%–20% of patients with MS. Conversely, 15% of patients with intermediate uveitis may eventually develop MS. Periphlebitis in MS is not clearly associated with optic neuritis, systemic exacerbations, or disease severity. Intermediate uveitis may precede MS by 5–10 years.

The immunopathogenesis of MS is not well understood but appears to involve humoral, cellular, and immunogenetic components directed against myelin. Both patients with intermediate uveitis and those with MS appear to share the HLA-DR2 haplotype. Immunocytologic studies have shown some cross-reactivity between myelin-associated glycoprotein and Müller cells.

The severity of intermediate uveitis in MS appears to be milder than in idiopathic cases. Macular edema is less common. Most patients develop mild vitritis with periphlebitis. Treatment of the uveitis may not be necessary. It is unclear whether treatment of MS with interferon has any effect on intermediate uveitis.

Bregerbc LIH, Leopold IH. The incidence of uveitis in multiple sclerosis. *Am J Ophthalmol.* 1966;62:540–545.

Nissenblatt MJ, Masciulli L, Yaran DL, et al. Pars planitis—a demyelinating disease? *Arch Ophthalmol.* 1981;99:697.

Zierhut M, Foster CS. Multiple sclerosis, sarcoidosis and other diseases in patients with pars planitis. *Dev Ophthalmol.* 1992;23:41–47.

CHAPTER 9

Posterior Uveitis

Posterior uveitis is defined as ocular inflammation primarily involving the retina or choroid, or both (Fig 9-1). The overlying vitreous can be involved with the inflammatory process, and cells or collections of cells may be seen in the vitreous or on the posterior vitreous face. Patients with posterior uveitis complain of floaters, decreased acuity, metamorphopsia, scotomata, or a combination thereof. Ocular examination reveals focal, multifocal, or diffuse areas of retinitis or choroiditis, the clinical appearances of which may appear similar; thus, diagnosis through pattern recognition is often challenging. A differential diagnosis is required and includes both infectious and noninfectious conditions. Infectious causes include viruses, bacteria, fungi, protozoa, and helminths. The noninfectious group includes conditions of possible immunologic or allergic origin, unknown causes, and masquerade conditions such as endophthalmitis and neoplasms.

The approach to the diagnosis of posterior uveitis should include an accurate and complete medical history and a review of systems to detect any associated systemic disorders that may be responsible for the uveitis. A history of underlying systemic disease such as AIDS, corticosteroid or other immunosuppressive therapy, antibiotic therapy, intravenous drug use, or hyperalimentation is common in patients with endogenous bacterial, fungal, or viral ocular disease. In patients with systemic collagen vascular diseases, dermatologic, joint, pulmonary, gastrointestinal, or genitourinary complaints may be associated with the ocular inflammation. These systemic findings are often essential clues to diagnosis.

Figure 9-1 Posterior uveitis. *(Reproduced with permission from Cunningham ET Jr. Diagnosis and management of anterior uveitis. In: Focal Points: Clinical Modules for Ophthalmologists. San Francisco: American Academy of Ophthalmology; 2002;20:1. Illustration by Walter Denn.)*

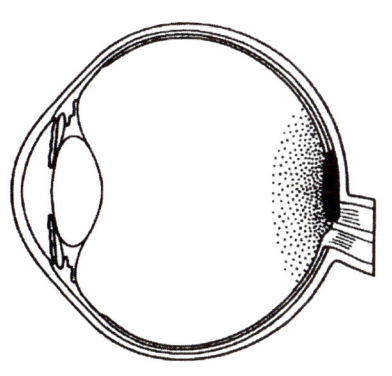

**Posterior uveitis
(retinitis, choroiditis, papillitis)**

The clinician should describe the biomicroscopic and fundus appearance of these disorders as accurately as possible. Certain syndromes or infectious agents cause only a retinitis, choroiditis, retinochoroiditis, or chorioretinitis. Cytomegalovirus causes a brushfire retinitis, toxoplasmosis produces a focal retinochoroiditis, and histoplasmosis presents as a multifocal chorioretinitis. The clinician should also be specific when describing retinal vasculitis. Patients with acute retinal necrosis develop a retinal arteriolitis, whereas the vasculitis in birdshot retinochoroidopathy primarily involves the venules. This differentiation may help diagnostically.

Ancillary laboratory testing and diagnostic procedures are often indicated in patients with posterior uveitis. These tests are discussed in Chapter 6. Perhaps the most useful test in evaluating posterior forms of uveitis is fluorescein angiography, which can provide critical information not available from biomicroscopic or fundus examination that can greatly assist in the diagnosis and management. Cystoid macular edema, retinal vasculitis, secondary choroidal or retinal neovascularization, and areas of retinal or choroidal inflammation can all be detected using angiography. Several of the white dot syndromes have a characteristic and pathognomonic appearance on fluorescein angiography. B-scan ultrasonography is also useful in posterior uveitis, particularly in patients with significant media opacification. Ultrasonographic studies can detect vitreous debris, retinal detachment, and choroidal thickening. Diagnostic vitrectomy may provide information to clarify the cause by antibody titer, culture, cytologic study, and the polymerase chain reaction. In patients with severe, sight-threatening forms of posterior uveitis, or in cases not responding to empiric therapies, retinal or chorioretinal biopsy may be indicated to help establish a tissue diagnosis.

Syndromes with primarily posterior segment involvement are included in this chapter; diagnoses routinely producing both anterior and posterior segment involvement are addressed in Chapter 10, which discusses panuveitis. However, the astute diagnostician must realize that these categories exist for convenience only and that many uveitis syndromes may present with a wide variety of clinical manifestations.

Infectious Diseases

Viral Disease

Acute retinal necrosis (ARN) syndrome and progressive outer retinal necrosis (PORN)

ARN is a fulminant, necrotizing viral infection of the retina. The disease is bilateral (BARN) in 33% of patients, and onset of contralateral involvement may be delayed up to 26 years after initial presentation. ARN/BARN is not an etiologic diagnosis. Varicella-zoster virus, herpes simplex virus type 2, and cytomegalovirus have all been associated with this syndrome. It affects adolescents to older adults. Patients are typically healthy and not debilitated, although ARN may occur in patients with AIDS.

ARN is diagnosed by clinical appearance. Patients present with an acute loss of vision. Anterior segment inflammation may range from minor to severe, and vitreous cellular exudation is heavy. Within 2 weeks, the patient experiences the classic triad of occlusive retinal arteriolitis, vitritis, and a multifocal yellow-white peripheral retinitis (Figs 9-2, 9-3). Scattered retinal hemorrhages may be present but are not characteristic or extensive. The peripheral retinal lesions progress rapidly and coalesce to form a confluent 360° creamy retinitis. The posterior pole tends to be spared.

Unlike other forms of viral retinitis, most patients with ARN are not immunosuppressed, and systemic antiviral agents may be useful. Intravenous acyclovir (1500 mg/m^2 per day in three divided doses over 10–14 days) is the treatment of choice to inhibit further viral replication. Oral acyclovir should be continued for 2–4 months following the intravenous induction. Antiviral therapy may reduce the incidence of contralateral disease (BARN). After 24–48 hours of antiviral therapy, corticosteroids can be introduced to treat the active vitritis. Aspirin or other anticoagulation agents may be used to treat an associated hypercoagulable state with uncertain results. Intravitreal ganciclovir (200 µg/0.1 mL) can assist in the induction phase of therapy in certain patients (see Chapter 14).

PORN is a unique form of necrotizing herpetic retinitis occurring in patients with advanced stages of AIDS. In contrast to ARN, the posterior pole may be involved early in the course of the disease, inflammatory cells are absent from the vitreous, and vasculitis is minimal (Fig 9-4). Visual prognosis is poor because of macular involvement and the ineffectiveness of antiviral agents.

Multiple posterior retinal breaks and combined traction-rhegmatogenous retinal detachments occur in up to 75% of patients with ARN (Fig 9-5). Prophylactic laser photocoagulation applied to areas of healthy retina at the border of the lesions may prevent retinal detachment. Laser surgery should be performed after the retinal infection has subsided. Early vitrectomy combined with endolaser photocoagulation has been proposed to eliminate the role of vitreous traction on the necrotic retina. Internal repair through vitrectomy techniques and use of silicone oil may be more successful at reattaching the retina than standard scleral buckle procedures because of the extensive vitreous scarring and multiple posterior retinal tears. Although the condition tends to resolve slowly over 1–2 months, the visual prognosis is poor; 65% of patients have worse than 20/200 acuity

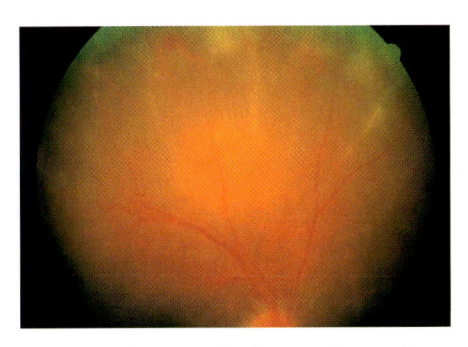

Figure 9-2 Acute retinal necrosis, vitritis, arteriolitis, and multiple peripheral "thumbprint" areas of retinitis. *(Photograph courtesy of E. Mitchel Opremcak, MD.)*

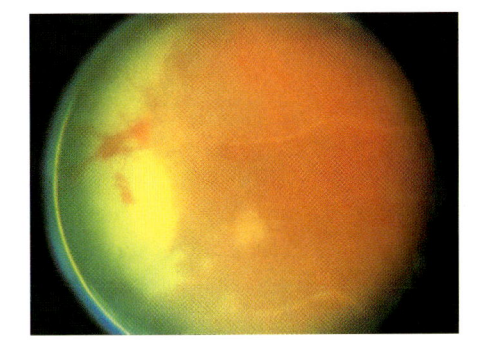

Figure 9-3 Acute retinal necrosis, confluent peripheral retinitis. *(Photograph courtesy of E. Mitchel Opremcak, MD.)*

156 • Intraocular Inflammation and Uveitis

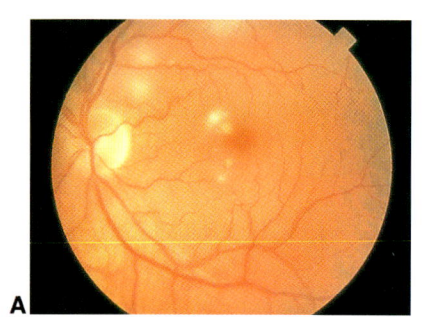

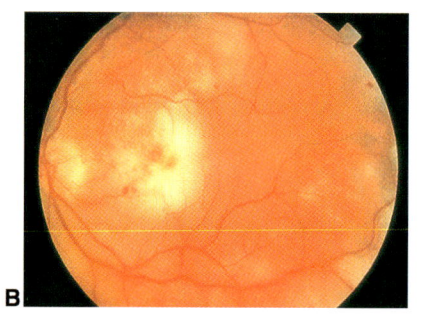

Figure 9-4 A, Multifocal areas of white retinitis in a patient with PORN. **B,** Fundus photograph taken 5 days later showing rapid disease progression and confluence of the areas of the viral retinitis. *(Photographs courtesy of E. Mitchel Opremcak, MD.)*

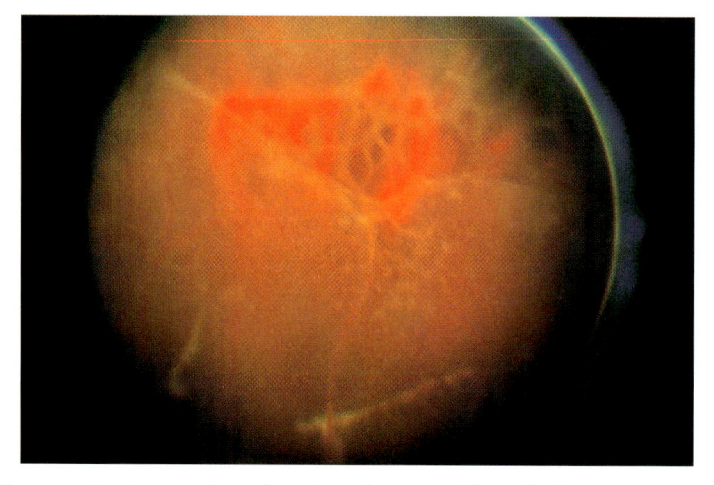

Figure 9-5 Acute retinal necrosis, retinal detachment with multiple, posterior retinal breaks. *(Photograph courtesy of E. Mitchel Opremcak, MD.)*

as a result of the extensive retinal necrosis and retinal detachment. See also BCSC Section 12, *Retina and Vitreous*.

> Blumenkranz M, Clarkson J, Culbertson WW, et al. Visual results and complications after retinal reattachment in the acute retinal necrosis syndrome. The influence of operative technique. *Retina*. 1989;9:170–174.
> Holland GN and the Executive Committee of the American Uveitis Society. Standard diagnostic criteria for the acute retinal necrosis syndrome. *Am J Ophthalmol*. 1994;117:663.

Cytomegalovirus

Cytomegalovirus (CMV) is a double-stranded DNA virus in the Herpesvirus family. Clinical disease occurs in neonates and immunocompromised patients with leukemia, lymphoma, conditions requiring immunosuppressive agents, and AIDS. Congenital CMV retinitis occurring in neonates is often associated with other systemic manifestations. Signs and symptoms include fever, thrombocytopenia, anemia, pneumonitis, and hepatosplenomegaly. Fundus examination reveals multifocal areas of brushfire retinitis. Cataract formation can occur in these children. With resolution of the retinitis, both pigmented and atrophic lesions are present, and optic nerve atrophy may also occur.

Signs and symptoms of acquired disease include yellow-white areas of retinal necrosis, hemorrhages, vascular sheathing, and attenuation. Microaneurysms and capillary nonperfusion have also been described. Late in the disease course, rhegmatogenous retinal detachments with multiple breaks may be present in the areas of retinal necrosis. Massive periretinal proliferation and late development of new holes can occur.

Diagnosis of congenital disease is suggested by the clinical appearance of the lesions coupled with the findings of viral inclusion bodies in urine, saliva, and subretinal fluid and the associated systemic disease findings. The complement fixation test for cytomegalic inclusion disease is of value 5–24 months after the loss of the maternal antibodies transferred during pregnancy. Diagnosis of acquired disease is based on the findings of focal retinitis in the setting of systemic immunosuppression.

The disease frequently causes significant retinal destruction and rhegmatogenous retinal detachment (Fig 9-6). The histopathologic features of both congenital and acquired disease are primary coagulative necrotizing retinitis and secondary diffuse choroiditis. Infected retinal cells show cytomegalic changes associated with large eosinophilic intranuclear inclusions and small multiple basophilic cytoplasmic inclusions (Fig 9-7). Viral inclusions may also be seen in the RPE and vascular endothelium. Electron microscopy of infected retinal tissue reveals viral particles with typical morphology of the herpes family of viruses. Chapter 14 discusses cytomegalovirus and its management more extensively.

Epstein-Barr virus

EBV is an encapsulated, double-stranded DNA virus in the herpes family that is ubiquitous: 90% of the population has acquired antibodies by the third decade of life. EBV has a tropism for B lymphocytes resulting in B-cell activation and mononuclear proliferation. Specific antibodies develop that are directed toward viral capsid antigens during the course of infection, and these antibodies are diagnostically helpful. EBV nuclear antigens and other viral proteins stimulate anti–EBV nuclear antigen antibodies as well as antibodies against early diffuse (EA-D) and restricted (EA-R) antigens.

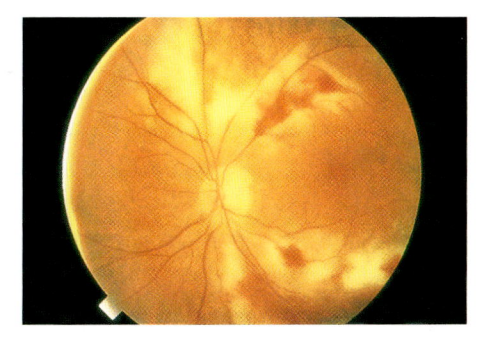

Figure 9-6 Cytomegalovirus retinitis. *(Photograph courtesy of E. Mitchel Opremcak, MD.)*

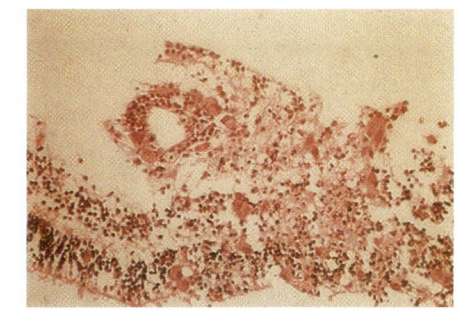

Figure 9-7 Histopathologic view of cytomegalovirus retinitis. Note giant *(megalo)* cells with inclusions in necrotic retina.

EBV infection has been associated with asymptomatic childhood illnesses, infectious mononucleosis, nasopharyngeal carcinoma, Burkitt lymphoma, Hodgkin disease, and Sjögren syndrome. Macular edema, retinal hemorrhages, chorioretinitis, punctate outer retinitis, and a multifocal choroiditis and panuveitis have been reported during the course of infectious mononucleosis and other EBV infections.

The diagnosis is suggested by fundus lesions developing during infectious mononucleosis or serologic testing supporting active or persistent EBV infection. The differential diagnosis for the various retinal findings is extensive, and other causes of posterior uveitis should be considered.

Therapy for EBV infection is supportive, and oral acyclovir may limit viral replication. As with all herpesviruses, a latent infection is established following initial exposure, introducing the possibility of recurrent or chronic illness.

Raymond LA, Wilson CA, Linnemann CC Jr. Punctate outer retinitis in acute Epstein-Barr virus infection. *Am J Ophthalmol.* 1987;104:424–426.

Rubella

Rubella virus, an enveloped, single-stranded RNA virus, is the etiologic agent for German measles. Rubella may involve the retina in both congenital and acquired forms of the disease. German measles presents with a viral prodrome of malaise and fever and evolves into a characteristic maculopapular skin rash that begins on the trunk and spreads to the extremities over 3–5 days. Acquired rubella has been reported to cause conjunctivitis, keratitis, iritis, and, rarely, a bilateral retinitis and exudative retinal detachment. Retinitis is more frequently seen in infants with maternal rubella syndrome contracted during the first trimester of pregnancy (approximately 25%–50%). Although cataract (15%), glaucoma (10%), and anterior segment inflammatory signs with atrophy of the iris and posterior synechiae may be present, the most prominent findings occur in the posterior pole.

Histopathologic studies of the lens reveal retention of cell nuclei in the embryonic nucleus, as well as anterior and posterior cortical degeneration. Poor development of the dilator muscle, necrosis of the iris pigment epithelium, and chronic nongranulomatous inflammation are present in the iris. The RPE displays alternating areas of atrophy and hypertrophy. The anterior chamber angle appears similar to the way it looks in congenital glaucoma.

Vitreous haze seen on ocular examination seldom prevents a view of the retina, where unilateral or bilateral pigmentary changes result in a *salt-and-pepper fundus*. Pigmentation is generally fine and powdery (Fig 9-8); however, rather large, more discrete areas of pigmentation may be seen as well. The blood vessels are normal, and the optic nerve may be slightly pale. Despite a loss of the foveal light reflex and the prominent RPE changes, neither vision nor electrophysiologic testing (ie, electroretinogram) are typically affected. In rare instances, subretinal neovascularization with significant visual loss may complicate the usually benign course.

The pathognomonic retinal appearance and the history of maternal exposure to rubella suggest the diagnosis. Other stigmata of congenital rubella syndrome may also be present, including deafness, cardiac defects, cataract, and strabismus (Fig 9-9). Viral

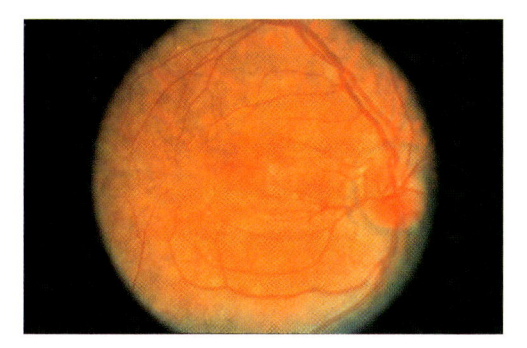

Figure 9-8 Congenital rubella syndrome with fine salt-and-pepper pigmentation. *(Photograph courtesy of E. Mitchel Opremcak, MD.)*

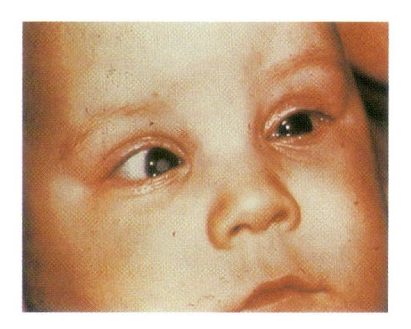

Figure 9-9 Congenital rubella syndrome patient with cataract, esotropia, mental retardation, congenital heart disease, and deafness. *(Photograph courtesy of John D. Sheppard, Jr, MD.)*

antibody studies may be confirmatory. Although usually present at birth, the process may develop postnatally.

Measles (rubeola)

Measles virus is an enveloped, extremely contagious RNA virus that causes worldwide pandemics every 2–3 years. Immunization has reduced the frequency of the disease in the United States, and measles is now quite rare. Measles virus can cause both congenital and acquired disease. Fundus changes similar to congenital rubella retinopathy have been reported in children whose mothers developed measles (rubeola) during pregnancy. The virus is transmitted from the pregnant woman to her fetus through the placenta. Measles retinitis has also been reported to occur following an acquired infection. Macular edema, neuroretinitis, attenuated retinal vessels, and macular star formation occur. No effective treatment is known, and the visual prognosis varies.

Subacute sclerosing panencephalitis virus (SSPE)

This slow viral infection of the central nervous system can cause a distinct maculopathy. SSPE is caused by a variant of the measles virus with a mutation of the viral envelope M protein. It affects school-age children 6–7 years after the measles-like infection. The slow virus infection of the cerebrum, the cerebellum, and the eye causes an encephalitis with behavioral changes, mental deterioration, progressive neurologic deficits, and cortical blindness. Disc edema, papillitis, and optic atrophy can be found in 30%–75% of cases. The most consistent finding is a maculopathy that begins as a focal area of macular edema and evolves into a localized white retinal infiltrate that may be associated with macular hemorrhage. Late in the course of the disease, the retinitis resolves, leaving focal gliosis of the macula.

SSPE should be considered in any school-age child with slowly progressive deterioration of mental function, behavioral changes, and visual dysfunction. The optic nerve and macular findings do not coincide with the other CNS symptoms and may precede other neurologic signs. Extremely high titers of measles antibodies and brain biopsy confirm the diagnosis. SSPE is a progressively fatal disease. Treatment is supportive, and visual prognosis is grave.

Robb RM, Watters GV. Ophthalmic manifestations of subacute sclerosing panencephalitis. *Arch Ophthalmol.* 1970;83:426–435.

Fungal Diseases

Ocular histoplasmosis syndrome (OHS)

This multifocal chorioretinitis is epidemiologically linked to *Histoplasma capsulatum,* a dimorphic fungus with both yeast and filamentous forms. The yeast form is the cause of systemic and ocular disease. OHS is frequently diagnosed in endemic areas of the United States such as the Ohio–Mississippi River valleys. However, sporadic cases are seen in other areas as well. Primary infection occurs after inhalation of the fungal spores into the lungs. Dissemination to the spleen, liver, and choroid follows the initial pulmonary infection. Acquired histoplasmosis is usually asymptomatic or may result in a benign illness, typically during childhood.

So-called *histo spots* first appear in the eye during adolescence, but maculopathy does not usually develop until 20–50 years of age, with an average of 41 years. Pathologically, the first lesion seems to be a granuloma in the choroid. This choroiditis may subside and leave a scar with depigmentation of the pigment epithelium, or it may result in breaks in Bruch's membrane and the pigment epithelium with an associated lymphocytic infiltration. Focal areas of choroiditis result in RPE proliferation and secondary subretinal neovascularization originating from the choroid. Lacking tight junctions, these neovascular complexes may leak fluid, lipid, and blood, resulting in loss of macular function. HLA-B27 has been associated with macular lesions but is not associated with the other ocular manifestations of OHS.

The diagnosis of OHS is based on the clinical triad of disseminated atrophic histo spots, peripapillary pigment changes, and maculopathy characterized by a pigment ring with detachment of the overlying sensory retina, usually with hemorrhage (Fig 9-10). The maculopathy typically begins at the site of a histo scar in the disc–macula area. Linear equatorial streaks can be seen in 5% of patients (Fig 9-11). Vitreous cells are *not*

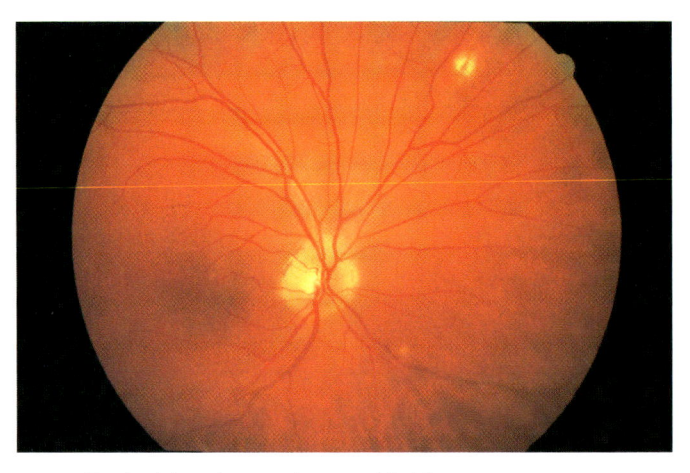

Figure 9-10 Ocular histoplasmosis: atrophic histo spots. *(Photograph courtesy of E. Mitchel Opremcak, MD.)*

seen in OHS, and symptoms seldom accompany the peripheral, atrophic histo spots. These spots represent focal, healed, punched-out lesions resulting from a variable amount of scarring in the choroid and adjacent outer layers of retina. The visual distortion and profound reduction in central vision following macular involvement bring the patient to the ophthalmologist.

Symptomatic areas of choroiditis may be treated with oral or regional corticosteroids (Fig 9-12). In the early stages of the fluorescein angiogram, active choroiditis blocks the dye and appears hypofluorescent. In later frames, the choroidal lesions stain and become hyperfluorescent. In contrast, areas of active choroidal neovascularization appear hyperfluorescent early in the angiogram and intensify throughout the study. The choroidal neovascularization is clinically important only if it lies in the disc–macula area; if it is outside the superotemporal and inferotemporal vascular arcades, the membrane does not reduce vision and therefore requires no treatment. However, if this membrane is located 1–200 µm from the center of the foveal avascular zone (juxtafoveal location) or 20–2500 µm from the center (extrafoveal location), laser photocoagulation is indicated to prevent further loss of vision (Fig 9-13).

In a collaborative multicenter study, the Macular Photocoagulation Study Group showed a beneficial effect with argon blue-green photocoagulation. A six-line loss of vision was more common in untreated patients (50%) than in laser-treated patients (22%) over a 24-month period. Krypton red or argon green wavelengths may give better visual results with less retinal injury than argon blue-green photocoagulation. Patients with active subretinal neovascular membrane located under the foveal avascular zone may benefit from submacular surgery and removal of the membrane (Fig 9-14). Photocoagulation and the potential role of photodynamic therapy are discussed in greater detail in BCSC Section 12, *Retina and Vitreous*.

Without treatment, 59% of patients with maculopathy end up with a visual acuity of 20/200 or worse. Massive subretinal exudation and hemorrhagic retinal detachments may occur and result in permanent loss of macular function. If histo spots appear in the macular area, the patient has a 25% chance of developing maculopathy within 3 years. If no histo spots are present, the chances fall to 2%. Macular disease is highly variable; some cases resolve spontaneously with a return to normal vision.

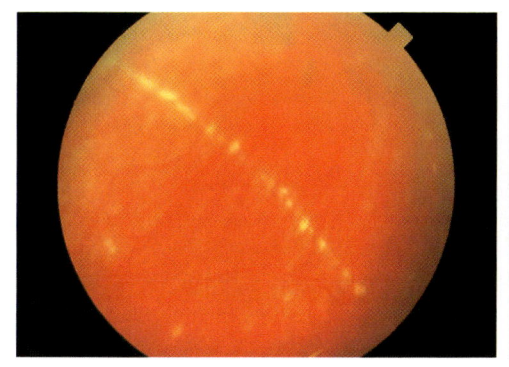

Figure 9-11 Ocular histoplasmosis: linear equatorial streaks. *(Photograph courtesy of E. Mitchel Opremcak, MD.)*

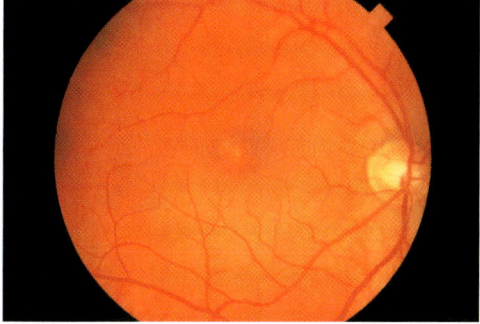

Figure 9-12 Ocular histoplasmosis: macular choroiditis with multiple yellow elevated lesions. *(Photograph courtesy of E. Mitchel Opremcak, MD.)*

162 • Intraocular Inflammation and Uveitis

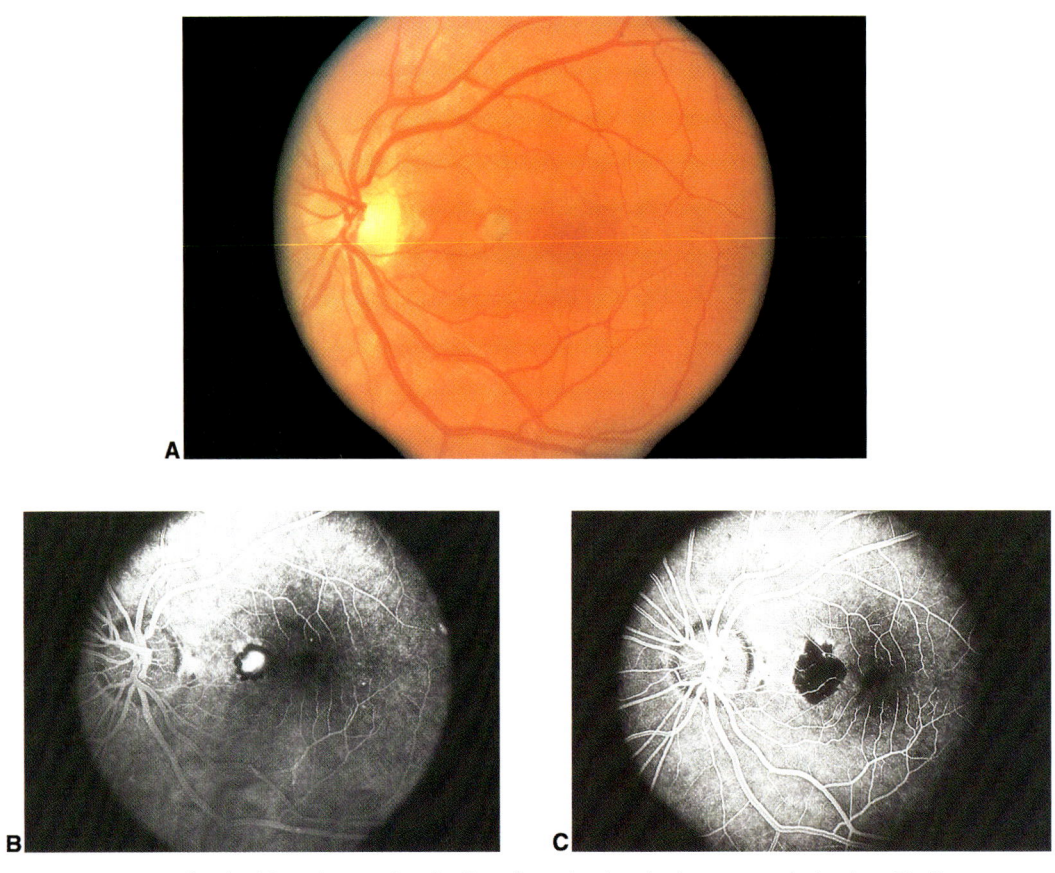

Figure 9-13 Ocular histoplasmosis. **A,** Extrafoveal subretinal neovascularization. **B,** Fluorescein angiogram of an extrafoveal subretinal neovascular membrane. **C,** Fluorescein angiogram of subretinal neovascular membrane following laser photocoagulation. *(Photographs courtesy of E. Mitchel Opremcak, MD.)*

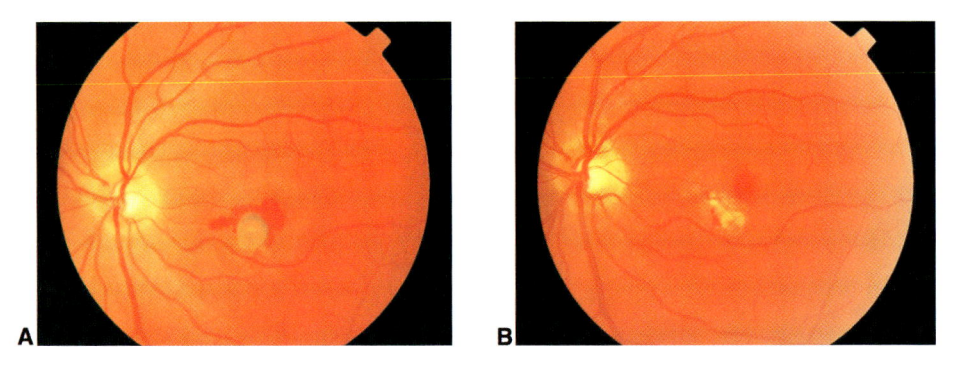

Figure 9-14 Ocular histoplasmosis. **A,** Subfoveal neovascularization. **B,** Subfoveal neovascular membrane following submacular surgical removal. *(Photographs courtesy of E. Mitchel Opremcak, MD.)*

The differential diagnosis of OHS includes angioid streaks, choroidal rupture, and idiopathic choroidal neovascularization. The atrophic spots and maculopathy of myopic degeneration and the maculopathy of age-related macular disease may also be confused with OHS.

> Campochiaro PA, Morgan KM, Conway BP, et al. Spontaneous involution of subfoveal neovascularization. *Am J Ophthalmol.* 1990;109:668–675.
> Macular Photocoagulation Study Group. Argon laser photocoagulation for ocular histoplasmosis: results of a randomized clinical trial. *Arch Ophthalmol.* 1983;101:1347–1357.
> Sabates FN, Lee KY, Ziemianski MC. A comparative study of argon and krypton laser: photocoagulation in the treatment of presumed ocular histoplasmosis syndrome. *Ophthalmology.* 1982;89:729–734.
> Thomas MA, Kaplan HJ. Surgical removal of subfoveal neovascularization in the presumed ocular histoplasmosis syndrome. *Am J Ophthalmol.* 1991;111:1–7.

Coccidioidomycosis (Coccidioides immitis)

Coccidioidomycosis is a disease caused by the dimorphic soil fungus *C immitis*. It is endemic in the San Joaquin Valley and southwestern United States. Inhalation of spores results in pulmonary infection and secondary dissemination to the central nervous system and eye. Intraocular manifestations are uncommon but include a granulomatous iridocyclitis and multifocal chorioretinitis. Serologic testing for anticoccidioidal antibodies and skin testing for exposure to coccidioidin can support a clinical diagnosis. Amphotericin B is the most effective therapy for active infection. Visual prognosis is determined by the location of the chorioretinal lesions.

Cryptococcosis (Cryptococcus neoformans)

This fungal disease primarily affects immunocompromised patients. *C neoformans* has a worldwide distribution and is found in contaminated soil. Inhalation of the aerosolized fungus results in pulmonary infection and secondary dissemination to the central nervous system. Ocular infection may occur via direct spread through the optic nerve or via hematogenous spread. Ocular manifestations include papilledema, choroiditis, retinitis, uveitis, and endophthalmitis. A clinical diagnosis includes a high degree of suspicion and can be supported by the demonstration of the organism via India ink stains or culture of the organism from CSF. Intravenous amphotericin B and oral flucytosine are required to halt disease progression. Prognosis is poor for visual recovery once the optic nerve or posterior pole is involved.

Candidiasis (Candida albicans)

Although candidiasis is still uncommon, the incidence of ocular inflammatory disease caused by *C albicans* has increased notably as a result of the widespread use of immunosuppressive therapy, hyperalimentation, and intravenous drugs. Rarely, *Candida* retinitis is seen in AIDS patients following intravenous drug use (Figs 9-15, 9-16). *Candida* endophthalmitis occurs in 10%–37% of patients with candidemia if they are not receiving antifungal therapy. Ocular involvement drops to 3% in patients who are receiving treatment for their disease.

The organism spreads through metastasis to the choroid. Fungal replication results in secondary retinal and vitreous involvement. Symptoms of ocular candidiasis include

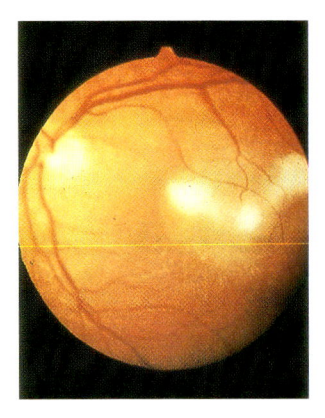

Figure 9-15 *Candida* retinitis.

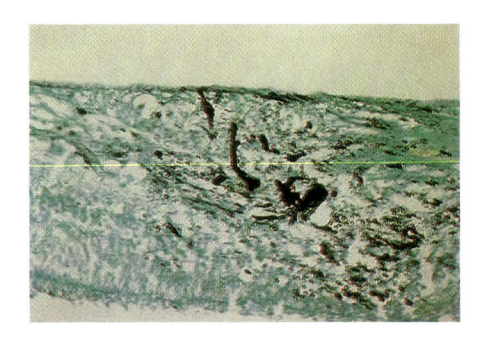

Figure 9-16 Pathology of *Candida* retinitis. Note fungi *(black)* in Gomori's methenamine silver stain of retina.

decreased vision or perception of floaters, depending on the location of the lesions. Mimicking toxoplasmic choroiditis, posterior pole lesions appear yellow white with fluffy borders, ranging in size from small cotton-wool spots to several disc diameters wide. The lesions originate in the retina and result in exudation into the vitreous. Peripheral lesions may resemble pars planitis.

Diagnosis of ocular candidiasis can be confirmed by positive blood cultures obtained during candidemia. The physician should be alert to the possible diagnosis of candidiasis in hospitalized patients with indwelling intravenous catheters or those receiving hyperalimentation or systemic therapy with antibiotics, steroids, and antimetabolites. Symptomatic or newly diagnosed, untreated cases of candidemia should prompt examination for ocular involvement. These patients should undergo two dilated fundus examinations 1–2 weeks apart to detect metastatic ocular disease.

Treatment of ocular candidiasis includes intravenous, periocular, and intraocular administration of antifungal agents such as amphotericin B and ketoconazole. Oral flucytosine, fluconazole, or rifampin may be administered in addition to intravenous amphotericin B. If the infectious process breaks through the retina into the vitreous cavity, intravitreal antifungal agents and vitrectomy should be considered. Prompt treatment of peripherally located lesions promotes a favorable prognosis. However, early treatment of central lesions seldom salvages useful vision because of damage to central photoreceptors. Consultation with an infectious disease specialist may be extremely helpful.

Protozoal Diseases

Toxoplasmosis

Toxoplasma gondii is an obligate intracellular parasitic protozoon that causes a necrotizing retinochoroiditis (Fig 9-17). It exists in three forms:

- Oocyst, or soil form (10–12 μm)
- Tachyzoite, or active infectious form (4–8 μm) (Fig 9-18)
- Tissue cyst, or latent form (10–200 μm), containing as many as 3000 bradyzoites

CHAPTER 9: Posterior Uveitis • 165

T gondii is an intestinal parasite found in cats. The oocysts of the organism are shed in cat feces that may then be ingested by rodents or birds that can in turn serve as reservoirs or intermediate hosts for the parasite. Insect vectors may also transmit *T gondii* from cat feces to human food sources, including plants and herbivorous animals.

Humans probably acquire the infection most frequently by eating raw or undercooked meat that contains tissue cysts; avoidance of steak tartar and similar foods could probably prevent many infections. While the risk of acquiring toxoplasmosis during pregnancy is low (0.2%–1%), women who do acquire the disease have a 40% transplacental transmission rate to the fetus with potential ocular, CNS, and systemic complications. Women who test positive for exposure to toxoplasmosis prior to pregnancy and women in whom a latent retinal toxoplasmosis lesion reactivates do not transmit the disease to the fetus because of maternal antibodies. BCSC Section 6, *Pediatric Ophthalmology and Strabismus,* discusses maternal transmission of toxoplasmosis in greater detail. Nonimmune pregnant women without serologic evidence of prior exposure to toxoplasmosis should take sanitary precautions when cleaning up after cats and avoid undercooked meats. Patients with AIDS are also particularly vulnerable (Fig 9-19); see the discussion in Chapter 14.

Toxoplasmosis may account for 7%–15% of all cases of uveitis. Because the disease can destroy visually important structures of the eye, it is important for the ophthalmol-

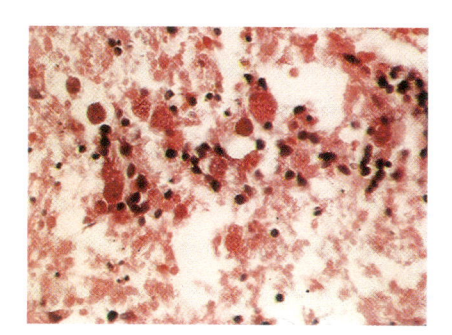

Figure 9-17 *Toxoplasma*, histopathologic view. Note cysts in necrotic retina.

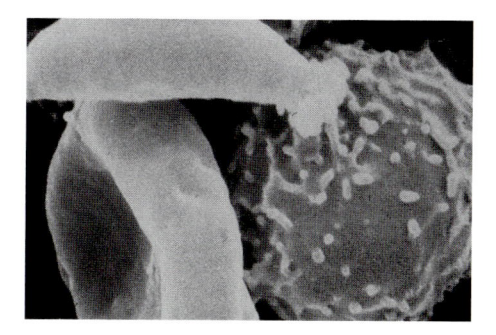

Figure 9-18 Scanning electron microscope view of toxoplasmal tachyzoite parasitizing a macrophage while a red blood cell looks on. *(Photograph courtesy of John D. Sheppard, Jr, MD.)*

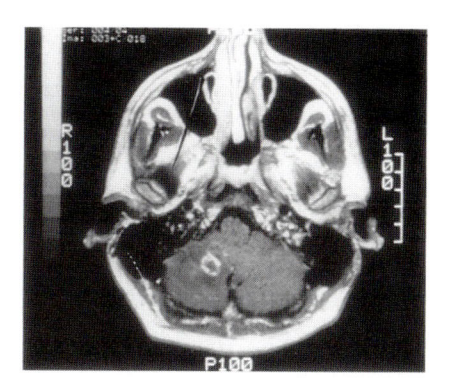

Figure 9-19 CNS toxoplasmosis presenting with ataxia in a patient with AIDS: cerebellar lesion in enhanced CT scan. *(Photograph courtesy of John D. Sheppard, Jr, MD.)*

ogist to recognize its lesions and to appreciate its potential for morbidity. Timely diagnosis is important, as toxoplasmosis responds to antimicrobial therapy and is thus a potentially treatable form of posterior uveitis.

Depending largely on the location of the lesion, the patient's complaints are unilateral floating spots or blurred vision. Generally, the anterior segment is not inflamed at the onset of the disease, and the patient shows a white, comfortable-looking eye. Occasionally, however, a granulomatous anterior uveitis, often with elevated IOP, occurs, especially in recurrent disease.

Vitreous opacities are generally obvious on ocular examination by both direct and indirect ophthalmoscopic examination. A whitish yellow, slightly raised, fuzzy lesion can usually be seen in the fundus, often next to a chorioretinal scar (Figs 9-20, 9-21). These lesions occur more commonly in the posterior pole than elsewhere in the fundus and are occasionally seen immediately adjacent to the optic nerve head. They may sometimes be mistaken for optic papillitis. Retinal vessels in the vicinity of an active lesion may show perivasculitis with diffuse venous sheathing and segmental arterial sheathing. This is the classic clinical complex of ocular toxoplasmosis.

The characteristic lesion is an exudative focal retinitis. The anterior layers of the retina are often singled out as the preferred site for proliferation of *T gondii*; however, a deep retinal form of ocular toxoplasmosis also exists. Punctate outer retinal toxoplasmosis (PORT) is a variant of toxoplasmosis that presents in the posterior pole with multiple small lesions, often adjacent to a pigmented old scar. Vitritis is minimal in PORT. Patients complain of decreased central activity early in the course of PORT and often fail to notice floating spots until the anterior layers of the retina and the posterior hyaloid membrane become involved (Fig 9-22).

Diagnosis The following conditions permit diagnosis of ocular toxoplasmosis:

- Observation of characteristic fundus lesion (focal necrotizing retinochoroiditis)
- Detection of the presence of anti-*Toxoplasma* antibodies in the patient's serum
- Reasonable exclusion of other infectious diseases that might cause necrotizing lesions of the fundus, principally syphilis, cytomegalovirus, and fungus

The *Toxoplasma* dye test of Sabin and Feldman, the hemagglutination test, or the indirect immunofluorescent antibody test all provide approximately the same information. How-

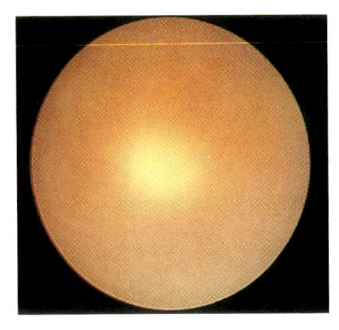

Figure 9-20 *Toxoplasma* retinochoroiditis, "headlight in the fog."

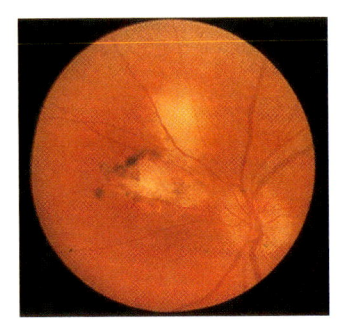

Figure 9-21 *Toxoplasma*, satellite retinitis around old scar.

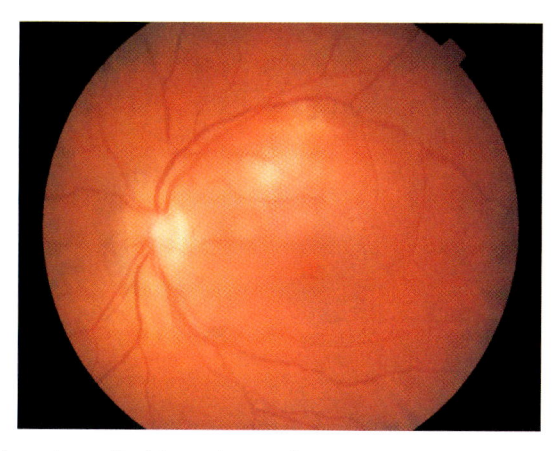

Figure 9-22 Punctate outer retinal toxoplasmosis. *(Photograph courtesy of E. Mitchel Opremcak, MD.)*

ever, the enzyme-linked immunosorbent assay (ELISA) may offer more sensitivity and specificity and has largely replaced the other assays.

It should be remembered that the serum titers of any of these tests may be extremely low in patients with ocular toxoplasmosis and no other systemic signs of toxoplasmal disease. Any titer of serum antibodies is significant if the patient has a fundus lesion that is compatible with ocular toxoplasmosis. Tests on the aqueous humor have been used to confirm the presence of toxoplasmal disease in doubtful cases. Such tests are most significant when the titer of antibodies is higher in the aqueous humor than in the serum.

Although the diagnosis of ocular toxoplasmosis is primarily based on the physical examination, negative antitoxoplasma antibodies must alert the ophthalmologist to another diagnosis. The clinician interpreting the standard IgG antibody test must remember that laboratories generally perform the test at a dilution of 1:8 or greater, even though a positive antibody reaction may be found at dilutions of 1:4 or less. These extremely low antibody titers may still indicate a previous exposure to toxoplasmosis but are also more likely to be falsely positive as a result of nonspecific reactions.

Most patients with toxoplasmal infections in the United States are presumed to have contracted the disease in utero and to have a congenital infection (Figs 9-23, 9-24). In countries where patients are more likely to have consumed toxoplasmal cysts as adults, acquired toxoplasmosis may be found as well. An acquired infection may often be more fulminating than a congenital infection, in which established maternal antibody titers may play a greater role. An acquired toxoplasmal infection is diagnosed by a positive IgM antibody titer. The IgM antibody titer will no longer be detectable 2–6 months following initial infection, even during a relapse of acquired toxoplasmosis.

Treatment Small lesions in the retinal periphery not associated with a significant decrease in vision or vitritis may not require treatment. These lesions can be observed for 3 weeks to 6 months for spontaneous resolution in patients with mild symptoms. The anterior uveitis associated with toxoplasmosis may be treated with topical corticosteroids and cycloplegic agents. Patients with prominent vitritis or vision-threatening lesions in the posterior pole or adjacent to the optic nerve should be treated with antiprotozoal agents.

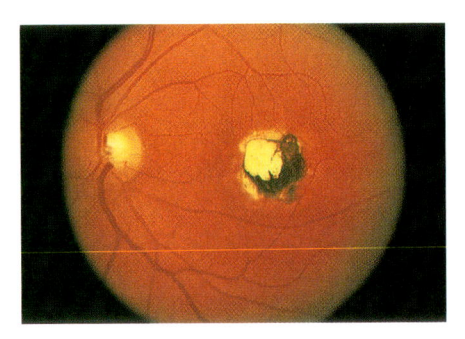

Figure 9-23 Congenital quiescent, mature, hyperpigmented toxoplasmal macular scar. Patient has 20/400 acuity. *(Photograph courtesy of John D. Sheppard, Jr, MD.)*

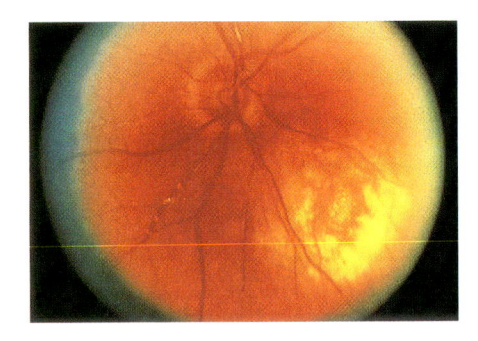

Figure 9-24 Recently acquired large, nonpigmented, inactive toxoplasmal retinal scar. *(Photograph courtesy of John D. Sheppard, Jr, MD.)*

The standard treatment for ocular toxoplasmosis consists of pyrimethamine (Daraprim) and sulfonamide therapy. A loading dose of 150 mg of pyrimethamine is followed by 25 mg daily for 6 weeks, with a loading dose of 4 g of triple sulfa or sulfadiazine, followed by 1 g of the same medication four times a day for 6 weeks. Therapy with pyrimethamine and sulfonamides produces disappointing or unreliable results in older massive lesions of the fundus that have been present for several months. Potential side effects of sulfa compounds include skin rash, kidney stones, and Stevens-Johnson syndrome.

Many ophthalmologists currently use trimethoprim/sulfamethoxazole (Bactrim, Septra) as an alternative to sulfadiazine because sulfadiazine is more expensive and very difficult to obtain. Folinic acid generally prevents the leukopenia and thrombocytopenia that may result from pyrimethamine therapy. Leukocyte and platelet counts should be monitored weekly. Folinic acid is now available in an oral preparation and administered as a 5-mg tablet (leucovorin calcium) once daily. Clindamycin, 300 mg four times a day, has been effective in the management of acute lesions when used alone or in combination with other agents. However, pseudomembranous colitis has been reported with clindamycin therapy. Pregnant women with acquired toxoplasmosis require special consideration, as the most effective antimicrobial agents are potentially toxic to the fetus. The ophthalmologist should consult with the obstetrician when considering the use of such agents. Spiramycin is considered the safest agent and may be combined with sulfadiazine during the first two trimesters and with pyrimethamine in the last months of pregnancy.

Newer agents are becoming available for the treatment of toxoplasmosis. Atovaquone is a cysticidal agent with the potential to eradicate even the encysted form of the parasite. This medication is highly fat-soluble and is extremely well tolerated, even in systemically ill, immunocompromised patients. Recurrences have been observed in patients treated with this agent, however, and it has not been proven in the clinical setting to prevent subsequent attacks of toxoplasmosis. Further investigation is required before atovaquone is established as a front-line treatment for ocular toxoplasmosis.

Many ophthalmologists think that maintenance suppression of toxoplasmal disease lowers the incidence of recurrent retinitis, particularly in immunocompromised patients.

Agents that are candidates for chronic suppressive therapy include trimethoprim/sulfamethoxazole and doxycycline. No adequate clinical trials have proven the effectiveness of prophylactic suppressive regimens, however.

Corticosteroids must be used with great caution and only with concomitant administration of antimicrobial agents. Oral corticosteroids to quell acute inflammatory lesions that threaten the destruction of the macula or the optic nerve may be given in the form of prednisone, 60–100 mg per day, 24–48 hours after initiating antibiotic therapy. Periocular injections of depot corticosteroids should be avoided: corticosteroids administered by this route may be immunosuppressive, resulting in an uncontrolled proliferation of the organism, acute retinal necrosis, and disastrous clinical results (Fig 9-25).

Photocoagulation therapy and cryotherapy have enjoyed limited success, although overly vigorous treatment with these modalities has resulted in ophthalmic disasters and neither has completely prevented recurrences. Retinal neovascularization may be seen with toxoplasmosis, and photocoagulation of neovascular lesions may prevent loss of vision secondary to vitreous hemorrhages. Pars plana vitrectomy may be helpful when inflammatory vitreous membranes, epiretinal membranes, or traction retinal detachments produce significant visual symptoms and perpetuate the inflammatory process.

> Dodds EM. Ocular toxoplasmosis: clinical presentations, diagnosis, and therapy. In: *Focal Points: Clinical Modules for Ophthalmologists.* San Francisco: American Academy of Ophthalmology; 1999;19:10.
>
> Engstrom RE Jr, Holland GN, Nussenblatt RB, et al. Current practices in the management of ocular toxoplasmosis. *Am J Ophthalmol.* 1991;111:601–610.
>
> Gormley PD, Pavesio CE, Minnasian D, et al. Effects of drug therapy on *Toxoplasma* cysts in an animal model of acute and chronic disease. *Invest Ophthalmol Vis Sci.* 1998;39:1171–1175.
>
> Lam S, Tessler HH. Quadruple therapy for ocular toxoplasmosis. *Can J Ophthalmol.* 1993; 28:58–61.
>
> Lopez JS, de Smet MD, Masur H, et al. Orally administered 566C80 for treatment of ocular toxoplasmosis in a patient with the acquired immunodeficiency syndrome. *Am J Ophthalmol.* 1992;113:331–333.
>
> Opremcak EM, Scales DK, Sharpe MR. Trimethoprim-sulfamethoxazole therapy for ocular toxoplasmosis. *Ophthalmology.* 1992;99:920–925.
>
> Rothova A. Ocular involvement in toxoplasmosis. *Br J Ophthalmol.* 1993;77:371–377.
>
> Rutzen AR, Smith RE, Rao NA. Recent advances in the understanding of ocular toxoplasmosis. *Curr Opin Ophthalmol.* 1994;5:3–9.

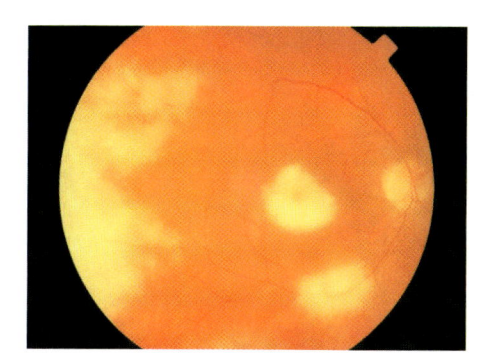

Figure 9-25 Toxoplasmosis, acute retinal necrosis following periocular corticosteroid injection. *(Photograph courtesy of E. Mitchel Opremcak, MD.)*

Helminthic Diseases

Toxocariasis

Ocular toxocariasis is a rare but well-known cause of unilateral ocular disease in children and young adults caused by *Toxocara canis*. One series found antibody testing in a kindergarten population as high as 30%. Clinically, however, toxocariasis is seen only occasionally. A study of enucleated globes showed that 2% of 1100 globes of children under 15 years of age harbored the causative organism.

T canis, a common canine intestinal parasite found in up to 50% of healthy dogs, may invade humans through the ingestion of ova-contaminated soil or vegetables. The ova reach the human intestine and produce larvae, which then invade the intestinal wall, penetrate the blood vessels and lymphatic system, and reach the liver and lungs. Once in the liver and lungs, the larvae can be disseminated to many organs, including the eye.

The disease is usually unilateral. Toxocariasis produces three recognizable ocular syndromes:

- Leukocoria from chronic endophthalmitis (Fig 9-26)
- Localized granuloma (Fig 9-27)
- Peripheral granuloma (Fig 9-28)

Table 9-1 lists the characteristics of each syndrome. In all forms, the eye may be asymptomatic or may present with minimal redness and photophobia. Strabismus from reduced vision in the affected eye may be the presenting complaint.

Aqueous cytologic investigation may show eosinophils (Fig 9-29). Because of the specificity of the serum ELISA, this test is helpful in identifying patients with ocular toxocariasis. The presence of any antibody titer (even in undiluted serum) may be significant. The antibody titer in intraocular fluids of patients with this disorder is higher than that found in the serum. Ova and parasites are not found in stool specimens in ocular toxocariasis.

Chronic endophthalmitis may result in loss of vision and subsequent enucleation. The location of the granuloma determines the visual deficit. Peripheral granulomas usually cause heterotropia of the macula and some loss of central vision, but the globe remains intact. Corticosteroids, both systemic and periocular, can be used in the active inflammatory phase of the syndrome. Thiabendazole, while useful for systemic toxo-

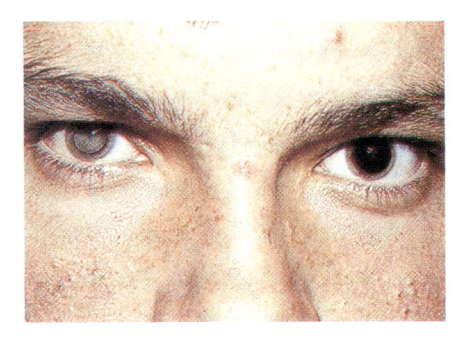

Figure 9-26 *Toxocara*, leukocoria.

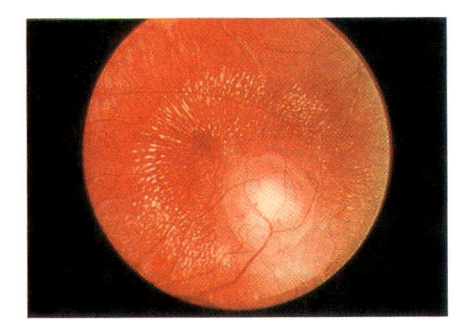

Figure 9-27 *Toxocara*, macular granuloma.

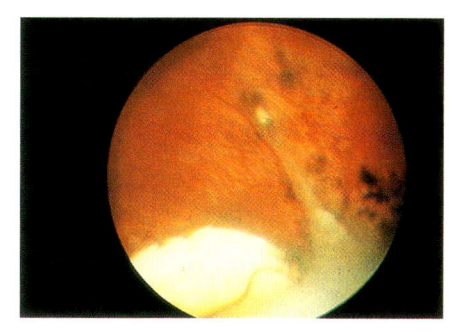

Figure 9-28 *Toxocara*, peripheral granuloma.

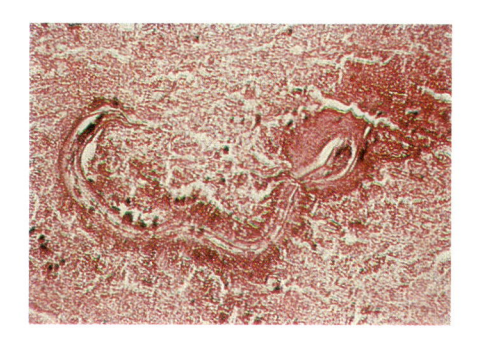

Figure 9-29 *Toxocara*, eosinophilic vitreous abscess, organism in center of abscess.

Table 9-1 Ocular Toxocariasis

Syndrome	Age of Onset	Characteristic Lesion
Chronic endophthalmitis	2–9	Chronic unilateral uveitis, cloudy vitreous cyclitic membrane
Localized granuloma	6–14	Present in the macula and peripapillary region Solitary, white, elevated in the retina: minimal reaction; 1–2 disc diameters in size
Peripheral granuloma	6–40	Peripheral hemispheric masses with dense connective tissue strands in the vitreous cavity that may connect to the disc Rarely bilateral

cariasis, has not been effective in treating the ocular disease and may make the ocular disease worse. Vitrectomy may reduce vitreous traction and clear the media.

Biglan AW, Glickman LT, Lobes LA Jr. Serum and vitreous *Toxocara* antibody in nematode endophthalmitis. *Am J Ophthalmol.* 1979;88:898–901.

Cysticercosis

This condition is a common cause of ocular inflammation in Mexico, Central and South America, and Africa. *Cysticercus cellulosae*, the larva of *Taenia solium*, is the most common tapeworm to invade the eye. The eggs of the *T solium* mature, and the larvae penetrate the intestinal mucosa and are spread hematogenously to the eye. Larvae may be seen in the vitreous or subretinal space in 13%–46% of infected patients. A viable larva with the protoscolex can often be seen undulating in these spaces. Death of the larvae produces a severe inflammatory reaction. Pathological studies show a zonal granulomatous inflammation surrounding the necrotic larva.

Observation of a *Cysticercus* organism within the eye is diagnostic (Figs 9-30, 9-31); an ELISA for antibodies to types of *Taenia* may be helpful. Larvae can be surgically removed from the vitreous and subretinal space via vitrectomy and subretinal surgical techniques. Praziquantel (50 mg/kg/day) and laser photocoagulation can kill the larvae, but these treatments may be associated with worsening ocular disease and panuveitis.

Kraus-Mackiw E, O'Connor GR, eds. *Uveitis, Pathophysiology and Therapy.* 2nd ed. New York: Thieme; 1986.

Smith RE, Nozik RA. *Uveitis: A Clinical Approach to Diagnosis and Management.* 2nd ed. Baltimore: Williams & Wilkins; 1989:125–128.

Diffuse unilateral subacute neuroretinitis (DUSN)

This condition, also called *unilateral wipe-out syndrome,* is caused by a motile nematode, probably the raccoon ascarid *Baylisascaris procyonis.* An immunologic or toxic reaction to the worm or worm by-products appears to cause the DUSN. The average age of patients is 14 years, with a range of 11 to 65 years.

DUSN is a biphasic condition. Patients first note a unilateral decrease in acuity. Early in the course of the disease the fundus develops multiple, postequatorial, evanescent crops of grayish white dots (400–1500 μm) with a mild vitritis and retinal vasculitis (Fig 9-32). Careful ophthalmoscopy reveals a motile nematode (400–2000 μm). In the second phase of the disease, the RPE, retina, and optic nerve develop a unilateral wipe-out with optic atrophy, extensive pigmentary disruption, and arteriolar attenuation (Fig 9-33). Rarely, a small retinal granuloma may be associated with the worm's demise.

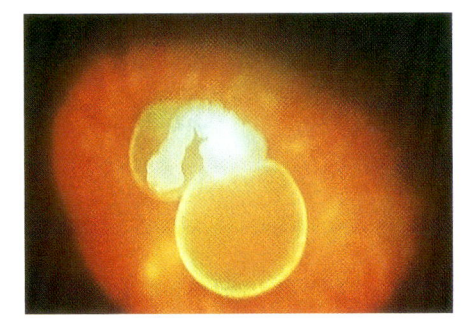

Figure 9-30 Intraocular cysticercus.

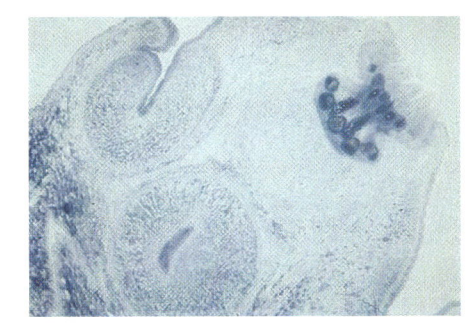

Figure 9-31 Pathology of cysticercus, showing protoscolex, or head of larva.

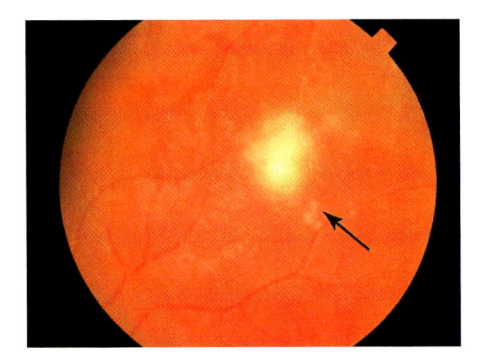

Figure 9-32 Diffuse unilateral subacute neuroretinitis. Note the multiple white retinal lesions and the S-shaped subretinal nematode *(arrow). (Photograph courtesy of E. Mitchel Opremcak, MD.)*

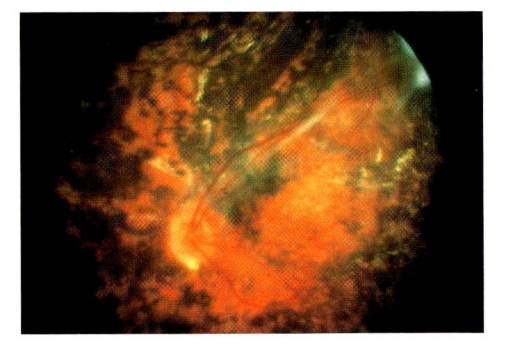

Figure 9-33 DUSN, or unilateral wipe-out. *(Photograph courtesy of E. Mitchel Opremcak, MD.)*

The diagnosis is based on clinical findings. Laser photocoagulation in the early phases of the disease can prevent disease progression and is not associated with worsening ocular disease following the death of the worm (Fig 9-34).

> Goldberg MA, Kazacos KR, Boyce WM. Diffuse unilateral subacute neuroretinitis. Morphometric, serologic, and epidemiologic support for *Baylisascaris* as a causative agent. *Ophthalmology.* 1993;100:1695–1701.

Immunologic Diseases

Collagen Vascular Diseases

Systemic lupus erythematosus

Systemic lupus erythematosus (SLE) is a collagen vascular disease with multisystemic and protean manifestations. Most patients (90%) are women of child-bearing age. The pathogenesis of SLE is not completely understood, but it is thought to be an autoimmune disorder resulting in the formation of autoantibodies including the antinuclear antibodies and immune complexes. Systemic symptoms include malaise, fever, arthritis, rash, pleurisy, and oral ulcers. Renal disease and neurologic complications are common.

The eye is involved in 50% of SLE cases through keratitis, scleritis, and, rarely, uveitis. The most common ocular manifestations are in the retina:

- Cotton-wool spots form as a result of the microvascular disease (Fig 9-35).
- Retinal arteriolitis and vascular occlusion may occur, resulting in ischemic retina and secondary retinal neovascularization and vitreous hemorrhage (Fig 9-36).
- The choroid can develop choroidal infarction, choroiditis, subretinal exudation, and choroidal neovascularization (Fig 9-37).

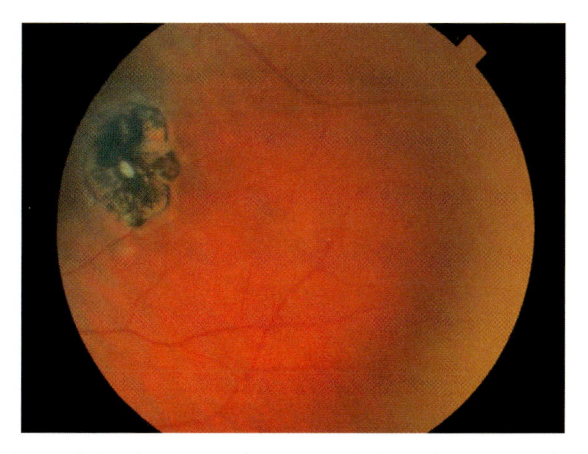

Figure 9-34 Retinal scar following laser photocoagulation of a nematode in DUSN. *(Photograph courtesy of E. Mitchel Opremcak, MD.)*

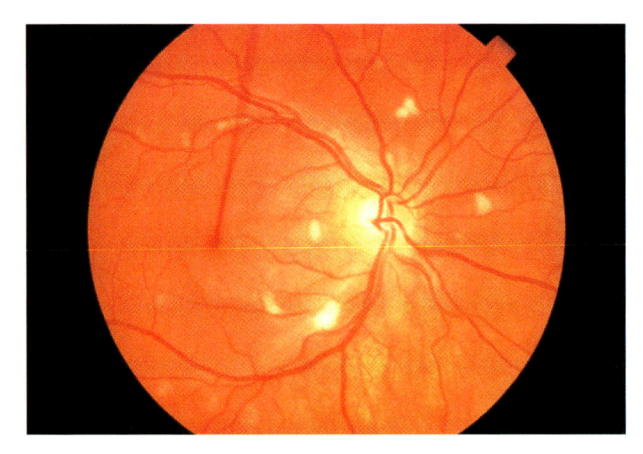

Figure 9-35 Systemic lupus erythematosus, multiple cotton-wool spots. *(Photograph courtesy of E. Mitchel Opremcak, MD.)*

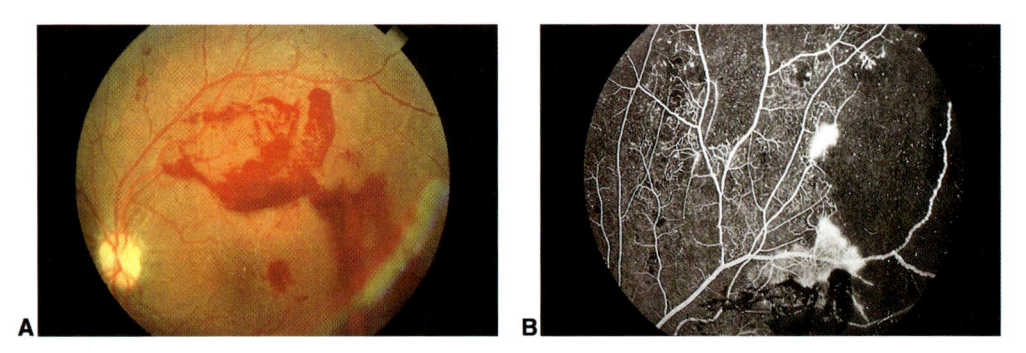

Figure 9-36 A, Ischemic retinal vasculitis and neovascularization in systemic lupus erythematosus. **B,** Fluorescein angiogram of the same patient as in **A** showing capillary nonperfusion. *(Photographs courtesy of E. Mitchel Opremcak, MD.)*

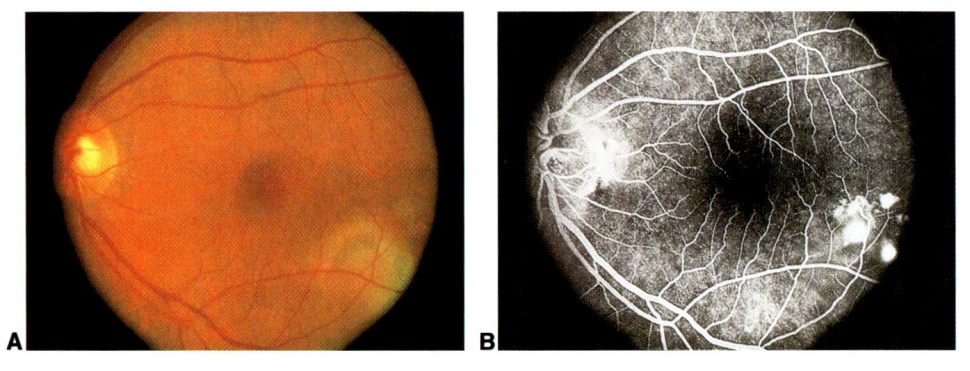

Figure 9-37 A, Multifocal choroiditis in systemic lupus erythematosus. **B,** Fluorescein angiogram showing multifocal areas of hyperfluorescence. *(Photographs courtesy of E. Mitchel Opremcak, MD.)*

It is important to separate these findings from the effects on the retina of SLE-induced hypertension and nephritis, which may result in arteriolar narrowing, retinal hemorrhage, and disc edema.

The presence of 4 of 14 major symptoms, signs, and laboratory results permits clinical diagnosis. A positive antinuclear antibody test, anemia, proteinuria, and urinary casts support the diagnosis. Treatment involves control of the underlying SLE through use of NSAIDs, corticosteroids, and immunosuppressive agents. The ischemic retina and proliferative changes that occur in SLE can be treated with panretinal photocoagulation. The presence of retinal vasculitis and neovascularization may indicate CNS involvement and occult cerebral vasculitis.

Jabs DA, Hanneken AM, Schachat AP, et al. Choroidopathy in systemic lupus erythematosus. *Arch Ophthalmol*. 1988;106:230–234.

Vine AK, Barr CC. Proliferative lupus retinopathy. *Arch Ophthalmol*. 1984;102:852–854.

Polyarteritis nodosa (PAN)

This multisystemic disease is associated with a necrotizing vasculitis. The disease affects adults in the age range of 40–60. Immune complexes are found deposited within the walls of medium- to small-sized arterioles; an autoimmune response is the postulated disease mechanism. Patients with PAN note fatigue, fever, weight loss, and arthralgia. The heart, kidneys, liver, GI tract, and CNS are affected by the multifocal necrotizing vasculitis. The disease has serious and potentially fatal complications related to renal and CNS injury.

The eye is involved in 20% of cases. Scleritis, iritis, and vitritis can be present, and the most common findings are retinal vasculitis, cotton-wool spots, and retinal hemorrhages (Fig 9-38). Central retinal artery occlusion and optic atrophy may also be noted.

PAN should be considered in the differential diagnosis of any case involving multiple systemic complaints and retinal vasculitis, specifically a necrotizing arteriolitis. Tissue biopsy confirms the diagnosis. Without treatment, the 5-year mortality rate is 90%. Corticosteroids reduce this rate to 50%. Appropriate systemic immunosuppression with cyclophosphamide results in a 5-year survival rate of 80% and resolution of the retinal vasculitis.

Akova YA, Jabbur NS, Foster CS. Ocular presentation of polyarteritis nodosa: clinical course and management with steroid and cytotoxic therapy. *Ophthalmology*. 1993;100:1775–1781.

Wegener granulomatosis

This multisystemic autoimmune disorder results in a granulomatous necrotizing vasculitis. The disease is uncommon and may occur between the ages of 8 and 80 years. It characteristically affects the upper and lower respiratory tract: sinusitis, epistaxis, cough, saddle-nose deformity, and renal disease are systemic manifestations.

The eye is involved in 50% of cases in the form of proptosis, orbital pseudotumor, and scleritis. Posterior scleritis may cause visual loss and ocular pain with exudative retinal detachment. Retinal vasculitis and true retinitis have been reported in 10%–20% of patients with Wegener granulomatosis (Fig 9-39).

Tissue biopsy establishes the histologic diagnosis. Antineutrophilic cytoplasmic antibodies are detected in this disease, and this test is useful in patients presenting with retinal vasculitis and respiratory complaints. Treatment includes oral corticosteroid and

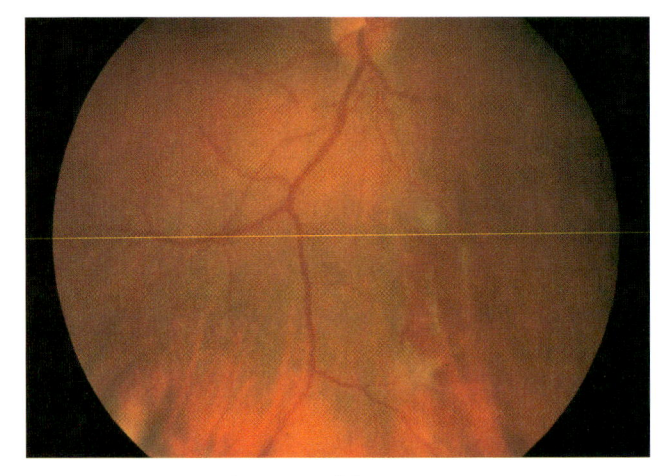

Figure 9-38 Polyarteritis nodosa, retinal vasculitis. *(Photograph courtesy of E. Mitchel Opremcak, MD.)*

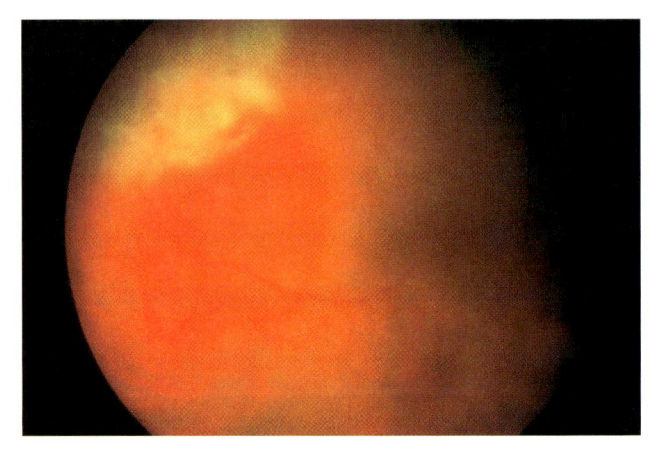

Figure 9-39 Wegener granulomatosis, retinitis. *(Photograph courtesy of E. Mitchel Opremcak, MD.)*

immunosuppressive regimens. Without therapy, the 1-year mortality rate is 80%. With cyclophosphamide and corticosteroid treatment, 90% of patients attain complete remission and resolution of the ocular manifestations.

> Bullen CL, Liesegang TJ, McDonald TJ, et al. Ocular complications of Wegener's granulomatosis. *Ophthalmology.* 1983;90:279–290.

Retinochoroidopathies

Retinochoroidopathies are a collection of disorders of unknown cause with characteristic clinical presentations involving inflammation of the choroid, choriocapillaris, RPE, and sensory retina. Common symptoms include blurred vision and scotomata. Anterior segment inflammation is usually absent, and vitreous cellular reaction is usually minimal. During the early stages, single or multiple white, yellow, or gray areas appear deep to the

Table 9-2 **White Dot Syndromes**

	Age	Sex	Pathology	Laterality	Size	Morphology	Location	Color	A/C	VIT	FA	EOG	ERG	Prognosis	Etiology	Treatment
ARPE	29 (16–40)	=	RPE	75% Uni	Small	Bull's-eye lesion	Macula	Black Halo	–	–	No leak Bull's-eye lesion	↓	↑	Good	Virus?	None
MEWDS	26 (14–47)	F > M (4:1)	RPE Retina	80% Uni	100–200 μm	Granular Macula	Perifoveal	White	–	+	Early "Wreath"	↓	↓	Recover	Virus 50%	None
OHS	41 (20–50)	=	C-R	62% Bi	200–700 μm	Punched out	Triad	White Green	–	–	Stain SRNVM	OK	OK	Variable	Histoplasmosis	Laser Steroids
PIC	27	F	Choroid	Bi	100–300 μm	Discrete	Posterior pole	Yellow pigment scar	–	–/+	Block Stain	OK	OK	Poor if SRNVM	? Myopia	Steroids
MCP	33	F > M (3:1)	Choroid RPE	80% Bi	50–350 μm	Punched out	Multifocal	Yellow pigment ring	52%	98%	Early Stain		↑↓	Poor	EBV?	Steroids Acyclovir?
SFU	(14–34)	F 100%	Subret	Bi	Large Small	Stellate Fibrous	Multifocal	White Yellow	–/+	+	Black Stain	↓	↓	Poor	B cell	Immunosuppressives/ steroids Acyclovir
Birdshot	50 (35–70)	F > M (2:1)	Choroid RPE	Bi	100–300 μm	Ovoid	Posterior equator	Creamy, no pigment	30%	100%	Vessel Leak Mac/ON		↓	Chronic	S-Ag CMI	CSA
APMPPE	29	=	RPE Choroid	Bi	Large	Placoid	Posterior pole	White Scar	+	50%	Block Stain	↓	↓	80% Good	50% Viral	None Steroids
Serpiginous	45	=	Choroid RPE	Bi	Large	Serpiginous	Disc Macula	Yellow Gray	–	30%	Loss of choriocapillaris	↓		Poor	?	None Immunosuppressives

retina. Later, pigment may be deposited at the periphery of the lesions (Table 9-2). The diagnosis is one of exclusion, ruling out infectious causes of multifocal choroiditis or retinitis. Fluorescein angiography often demonstrates classic photographic and angiographic patterns that may aid diagnosis.

Acute posterior multifocal placoid pigment epitheliopathy (APMPPE)

This uncommon condition is thought to follow a prodromal influenza-like illness in adolescents and young adults. Wheather APMPPE results from primary disease of the pigment epithelium or is caused by obstruction of choroidal circulation with a secondary pigment epithelial reaction remains controversial. Patients complain of decreased vision. Characteristically, there is minimal anterior segment inflammation. Vitreous cells and disc edema may occur along with multiple cream-colored, plaquelike, homogeneous lesions beneath the retina, probably at the level of the pigment epithelium or choriocapillaris. These lesions are usually one disc diameter or less in size but may be confluent, and the margins are slightly blurred (Fig 9-40). Over 2–6 weeks, the lesions fade, leaving a permanent geographic-shaped alteration in the pigment epithelium, which consists of alternate depigmentation and pigment clumping. Rarely, cerebral vasculitis may cause associated life-threatening complications.

Diagnosis of APMPPE is based on the characteristic clinical presentation, especially if preceded by a viruslike systemic illness. In the acute stages of the disease, fluorescein angiography shows early hypofluorescence in the lesion areas and late hyperfluorescent staining (Figs 9-41, 9-42). The differential diagnosis includes serpiginous (geographic) choroidopathy. APMPPE is an acute, usually nonrecurrent disease; serpiginous choroidopathy is insidious and relentlessly progressive. A variant of APMPPE may have features of both diseases, being chronic or recurrent with progressive destruction of the retina and loss of central acuity.

There is no evidence that corticosteroids or any other medications are beneficial. Most patients recover normal visual acuity of 20/40 or better over a period of weeks to months. However, if the fovea is involved, visual acuity may remain at the 20/200 level.

Williams DF, Mieler WF. Long-term follow-up of acute multifocal posterior placoid pigment epitheliopathy. *Br J Ophthalmol.* 1989;73:985–990.

Acute retinal pigment epitheliitis (ARPE)

ARPE, or Krill disease, is an acute self-limiting inflammation of the RPE. The cause is unknown. ARPE generally occurs between the ages of 16 and 40 years. Patients are otherwise healthy and complain of a sudden unilateral loss of central acuity. Fundus examination shows subtle small hyperpigmented lesions at the level of the RPE (Fig 9-43). Two to four clusters of two to six dots appear in the posterior pole. Fluorescein angiography demonstrates a target or honeycomb pattern with hyperpigmented centers and a halo of hyperfluorescence around each lesion. No treatment is required, as the visual symptoms and retinal lesions subside over 6–12 weeks.

Deutman AF. Acute retinal pigment epitheliitis. *Am J Ophthalmol.* 1974;78:571–578.

CHAPTER 9: Posterior Uveitis • 179

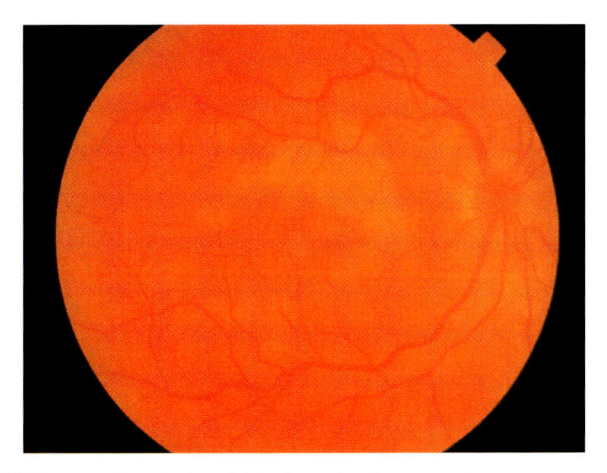

Figure 9-40 APMPPE, multifocal placoid lesions in the macula. *(Photograph courtesy of E. Mitchel Opremcak, MD.)*

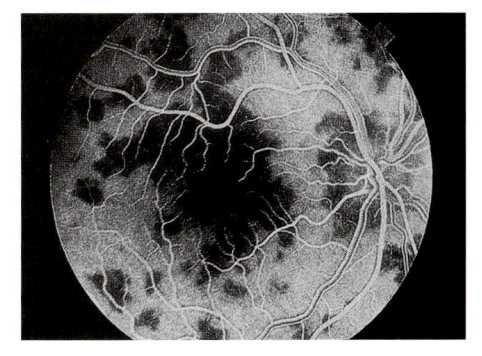

Figure 9-41 APMPPE, fluorescein angiogram showing early blocking of the choroidal circulation. *(Photograph courtesy of E. Mitchel Opremcak, MD.)*

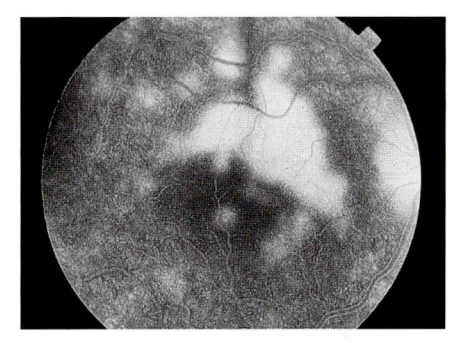

Figure 9-42 APMPPE, late-phase angiogram showing staining. *(Photograph courtesy of E. Mitchel Opremcak, MD.)*

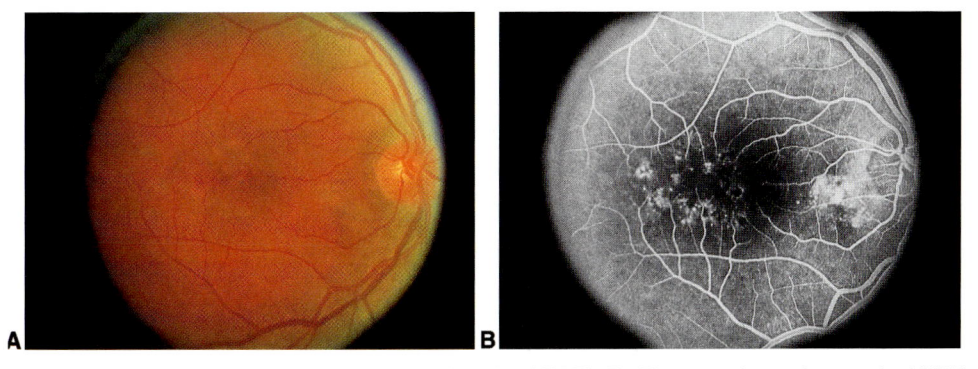

Figure 9-43 A, Acute retinal pigment epitheliitis (ARPE). **B,** Fluorescein angiogram in ARPE showing honeycomb lesions at the level of the RPE. *(Photographs courtesy of E. Mitchel Opremcak, MD.)*

Acute zonal occult outer retinopathy (AZOOR)

AZOOR is a newly described syndrome defined by a rapid loss of retinal function in one or several areas of the retina. Clinical examination reveals large peripheral scotomata, photopsias, mild vitritis (50%), and minimal retinal findings. Late in the course of the disease, retinal degeneration consisting of mild RPE pigmentary changes may be found. ERG abnormalities help establish the diagnosis in suspected cases. Cancer-associated retinopathy and retinitis pigmentosa should be considered in the differential diagnosis. The prognosis for central acuity is good, with stabilization of the field loss within 6 months. Corticosteroids have been used in patients with significant vitritis.

> Gass JDM. Acute zonal occult outer retinopathy. Donders Lecture: The Netherlands Ophthalmological Society, Maastricht, Holland, June 19, 1992. *J Clin Neuroophthalmol.* 1993; 13:79–97.

Birdshot retinochoroidopathy (vitiliginous chorioretinitis)

This uncommon condition occurs in adults past the fourth decade of life, usually females. Decreased vision, nyctalopia, and disturbance of color vision are the primary symptoms. Anterior segment inflammation may be minimal or lacking. Although the exact pathophysiologic mechanism is unknown, autoimmunity is postulated to play an important role in this disorder. Patients with birdshot retinochoroidopathy have been shown to have retinal autoantigen reactivity and a strong HLA association; the disease process responds to cyclosporine and other immunosuppressive agents. Vitritis is commonly noted on biomicroscopy. Fundus examination reveals characteristic, multifocal, postequatorial cream-colored or depigmented lesions scattered throughout the fundus, as if the fundus had been hit by birdshot from a shotgun (Fig 9-44). The spots appear to be at the level of the pigment epithelium. Retinal phlebitis and attenuated and sheathed retinal vessels are sometimes present. Disc edema, optic atrophy, narrowing of retinal vasculature, cystoid macular edema, and surface-wrinkling retinopathy may be present.

The diagnosis is suggested by retinal vascular leakage on fluorescein angiography with pronounced perifoveal capillary leakage and cystoid macular edema (Figs 9-45,

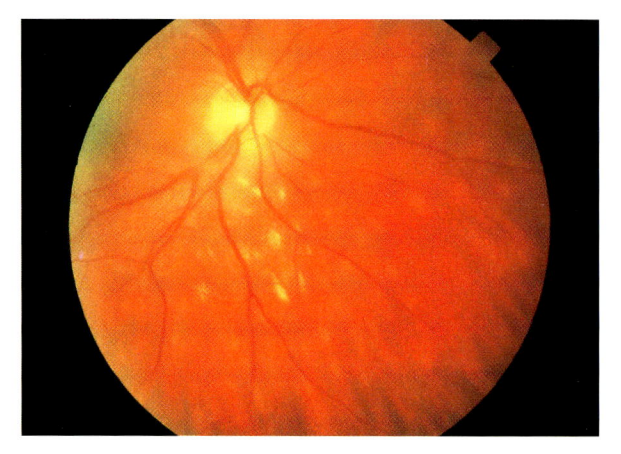

Figure 9-44 Birdshot chorioretinitis with multiple postequatorial, cream-colored ovoid lesions. *(Photograph courtesy of E. Mitchel Opremcak, MD.)*

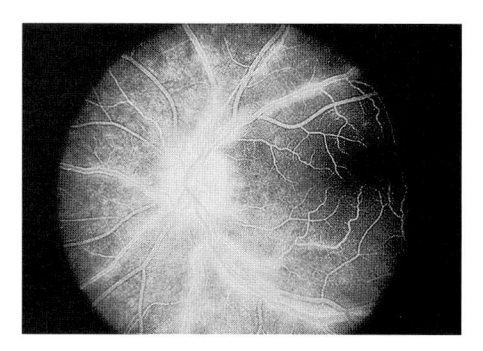

Figure 9-45 Fluorescein angiogram showing diffuse retinal phlebitis. *(Photograph courtesy of E. Mitchel Opremcak, MD.)*

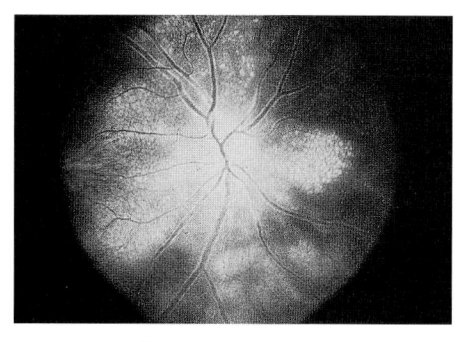

Figure 9-46 Fluorescein angiogram showing cystoid retinal edema in birdshot chorioretinitis. *(Photograph courtesy of E. Mitchel Opremcak, MD.)*

9-46). The electroretinogram is reduced or extinguished. Optic nerve edema is present in some cases, and subretinal choroidal neovascularization may occur. HLA-A29 has been detected in 80%–96% of patients, in contrast with the incidence of HLA-A29 in the unaffected population, which is approximately 7%.

Birdshot retinochoroidopathy characteristically responds poorly or incompletely to oral NSAIDs, corticosteroids, and second-generation immunosuppressive agents. Periocular steroids can assist in controlling cystoid macular edema, and the disease appears to respond favorably to cyclosporine preparations. Dosages ranging from 2 to 5 mg/kg/day are associated with resolution of the vitreous inflammatory cells and retinal edema and can stabilize the development of new retinal lesions. Birdshot retinochoroidopathy is a chronic disease with exacerbations and remissions. Some patients experience eventual optic atrophy or cystoid macular degeneration; others maintain or recover good vision. Epiretinal membranes are not uncommon.

> Bloch-Michel E, Frau E. Birdshot retinochoroidopathy and HLA-A29+ and HLA-A29– idiopathic retinal vasculitis: comparative study of 56 cases. *Can J Ophthalmol.* 1991;26:361–366.
>
> Brucker AJ, Deglin EA, Bene C, et al. Subretinal choroidal neovascularization in birdshot retinochoroidopathy. *Am J Ophthalmol.* 1985;99:40–44.
>
> Nussenblatt RB, Mittal KK, Ryan S, et al. Birdshot retinochoroidopathy associated with HLA-A29 antigen and immune responsiveness to retinal S-antigen. *Am J Ophthalmol.* 1982; 94:147–158.
>
> Ryan SJ, Maumenee AE. Birdshot retinochoroidopathy. *Am J Ophthalmol.* 1980;89:31.

Multiple evanescent white dot syndrome (MEWDS)

This idiopathic inflammatory condition of the retina occurs in women (90%) between the ages of 14 and 47 years. Patients typically complain of a unilateral (80%) decrease in visual acuity. Fundus examination shows multiple small (100–200 µm) outer retinal white dots in the posterior pole (Fig 9-47). The macula appears granular in the acute phase of the disease, a pathognomonic finding. Electrophysiologic studies show early abnormalities in receptor potential amplitudes. Rarely, MEWDS can be recurrent. The visual prognosis is excellent, as MEWDS resolves spontaneously within 1–2 months without therapy.

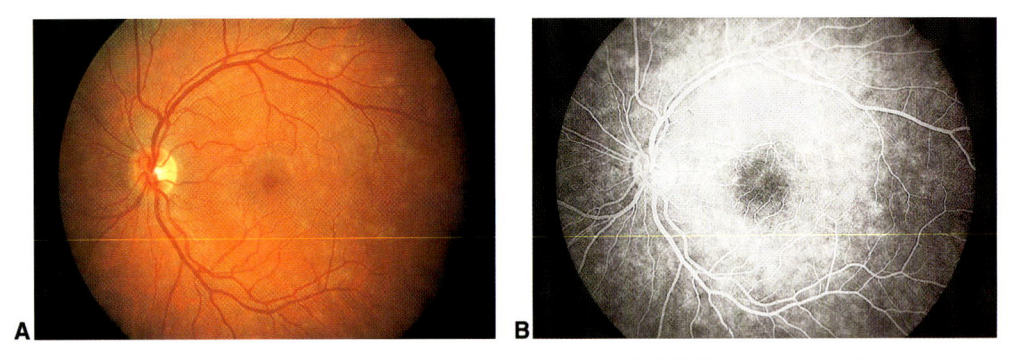

Figure 9-47 A, Multiple evanescent white dot syndrome (MEWDS). **B,** Fluorescein angiogram showing wreath sign. *(Photographs courtesy of E. Mitchel Opremcak, MD.)*

MEWDS has been associated with *acute macular neuroretinopathy (AMN)* and the *syndrome of prolonged enlargement of the blind spot.* AMN is a rare disorder causing paracentral scotomata and a characteristic reddish brown, wedge-shaped lesion in the macula. In the syndrome of prolonged enlargement of the blind spot, patients note a scotoma and on visual field testing show an enlargement of the physiologic blind spot. Treatment is not required, as patients recover over a 7-week period.

> Gass JD, Hamed LM. Acute macular neuroretinopathy and multiple evanescent white dot syndrome occurring in the same patients. *Arch Ophthalmol.* 1989;107:189–193.
>
> Jampol LM, Sieving PA, Pugh D, et al. Multiple evanescent white dot syndrome. I. Clinical findings. *Arch Ophthalmol.* 1984;102:671–674.

Punctate inner choroiditis (PIC)

PIC is an idiopathic inflammatory disorder of the choroid that typically occurs in myopic women between the ages of 18 and 37. Patients with PIC note a bilateral loss of central acuity. Cells are absent in the vitreous, but small (100–300 µm) punctate yellow inner choroidal lesions are found in the posterior pole (Fig 9-48). The lesions block early and stain late on the fluorescein angiogram (Figs 9-49, 9-50). Cases can be mild, as the disease clears in 4–6 weeks. Oral and regional corticosteroids have been used without adverse effect. Choroidal neovascular membranes can develop in 17%–40% of patients. Corticosteroids and laser photocoagulation should be considered in selected cases. PIC, multifocal choroiditis, and panuveitis syndrome and the subretinal fibrosis and uveitis syndrome have many similarities and may represent the clinical spectrum of one disease.

> Watzke RC, Packer AJ, Folk JC, et al. Punctate inner choroidopathy. *Am J Ophthalmol.* 1984;98:572–584.

Serpiginous choroidopathy

This geographic or helicoid choroidopathy is uncommon, affecting adults in the fourth to sixth decades of life. Blurred vision is the primary symptom. The vitreous varies from clear to mildly cellular. A serpiginous (pseudopodial) or geographic (maplike) pattern of scars may present in the posterior fundus. The edges of these lesions may be active, with a yellow-gray and edematous appearance (Fig 9-51). As active areas become atrophic over

CHAPTER 9: Posterior Uveitis • 183

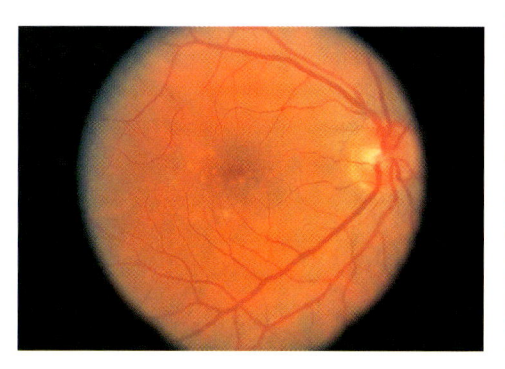

Figure 9-48 Punctate inner choroiditis (PIC). *(Photograph courtesy of E. Mitchel Opremcak, MD.)*

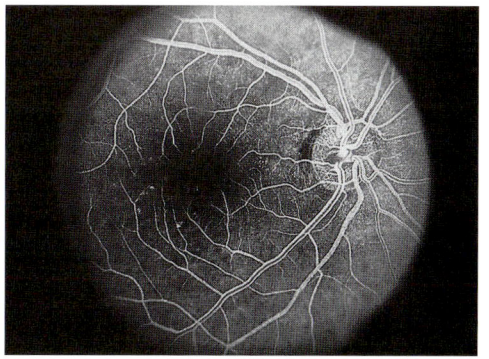

Figure 9-49 PIC, fluorescein angiogram showing blocked fluorescence early in the study. *(Photograph courtesy of E. Mitchel Opremcak, MD.)*

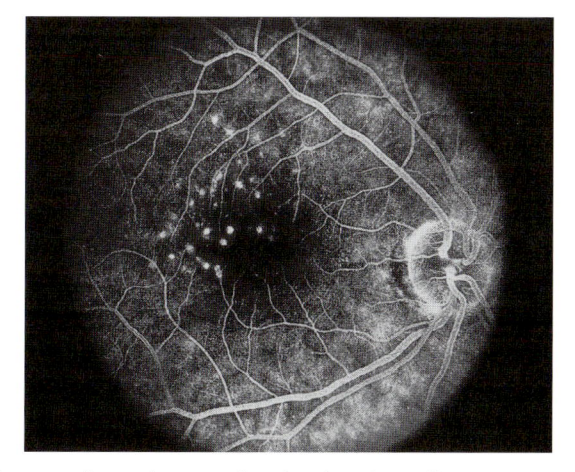

Figure 9-50 PIC, fluorescein angiogram showing late hyperfluorescence. *(Photograph courtesy of E. Mitchel Opremcak, MD.)*

weeks to months, new lesions can occur elsewhere or contiguously in a snakelike pattern. Occasionally, vascular sheathing is reported along with RPE detachment and neovascularization of the disc.

Diagnosis is suggested by the characteristic clinical picture and indolent course. Fluorescein angiography shows initial blockage of choroidal flush by the areas of active disease (Fig 9-52). When the disease is inactive, the affected pigmented areas transmit fluorescein but do not stain. Some cases appear inflammatory; others appear atrophic.

Corticosteroids and even immunosuppressives have been advocated, but there is no good evidence that they alter the course of the disease. Sub-Tenon's corticosteroids, oral cyclosporine, and oral acyclovir have been advocated for macula-threatening disease. The disease may progress relentlessly despite aggressive therapies. Photocoagulation at the border of the lesions has been unsuccessful in halting the progression. If the macula is involved, central visual acuity will be impaired. If the usual centrifugal movement of the

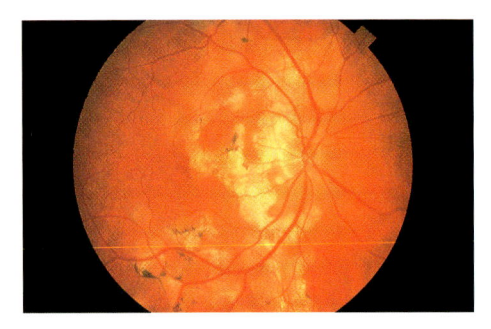

Figure 9-51 Serpiginous choroiditis. *(Photograph courtesy of E. Mitchel Opremcak, MD.)*

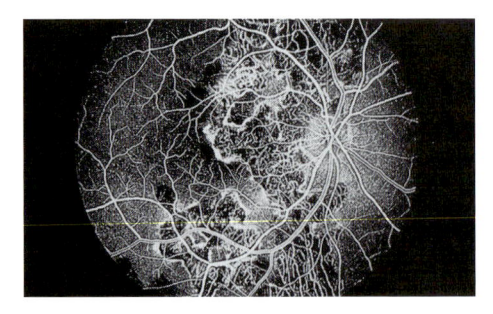

Figure 9-52 Fluorescein angiogram shows blocked fluorescence in the area of active disease. *(Photograph courtesy of E. Mitchel Opremcak, MD.)*

lesions from disc to periphery bypasses the macula, the prognosis tends to be good. Choroidal neovascularization may rarely occur.

> Wojno T, Meredith TA. Unusual findings in serpiginous choroiditis. *Am J Ophthalmol.* 1982;94:650–655.

Subretinal fibrosis and uveitis syndrome (SFU)

This panuveitis predominantly affects women between the ages of 14 and 34 years. The cause remains unknown. Histopathological investigation of chorioretinal biopsy specimens demonstrates primarily B cells and plasma cells. Patients are otherwise healthy and note a bilateral decrease of visual acuity. Early in the disease, patients present with bilateral vitritis and multifocal choroiditis. Later in the course, the choroidal lesions evolve into large stellate subretinal fibrotic lesions (Figs 9-53, 9-54). SFU responds poorly to most forms of treatment, and the visual prognosis is poor. Steroids and immunosuppressive agents have been used with little success (Figs 9-55, 9-56).

> Kim MK, Chan CC, Belfort R Jr, et al. Histopathologic and immunohistopathologic features of subretinal fibrosis and uveitis syndrome. *Am J Ophthalmol.* 1987;104:15–23.

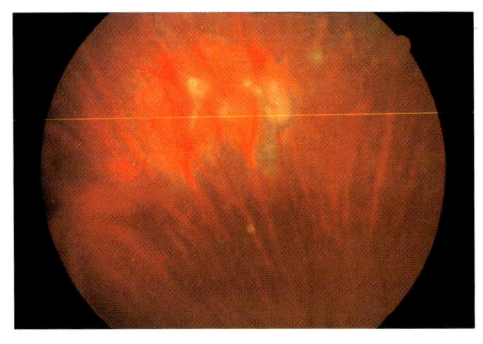

Figure 9-53 Subretinal fibrosis and uveitis syndrome (SFU), fundus photograph showing multifocal white subretinal lesions. *(Photograph courtesy of E. Mitchel Opremcak, MD.)*

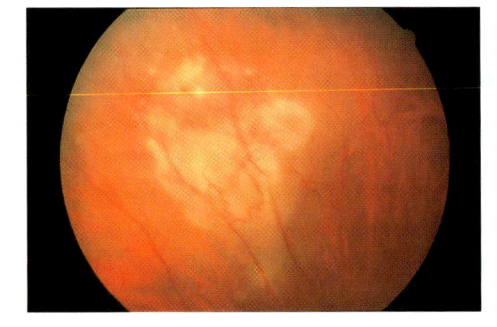

Figure 9-54 SFU, fundus photograph from the same patient, showing progressive subretinal fibrosis. *(Photograph courtesy of E. Mitchel Opremcak, MD.)*

CHAPTER 9: Posterior Uveitis • 185

Multifocal choroiditis and panuveitis syndrome (MCP)

MCP is an idiopathic inflammation of the choroid, retina, and vitreous more often noted in women. The cause is unknown. Patients present with bilateral vitritis (82%) and multifocal choroiditis. The lesions are small (50–350 µm) and yellowish when active (Fig 9-57). Peripapillary pigment scarring that resembles histoplasmosis scars appears. Macular lesions may be associated with subretinal neovascular membranes.

The diagnosis is one of exclusion, as many other conditions may cause multifocal choroiditis and panuveitis. Sarcoidosis, syphilis, tuberculosis, and other white dot syndromes of the retina need to be considered (see Table 9-2). Oral or regional corticosteroids help control the choroidal and vitreous inflammation. The disease is often chronic, and macular function may be impaired by cystoid macular edema or subretinal neovascularization.

Dreyer RF, Gass JD. Multifocal choroiditis and panuveitis: a syndrome that mimics ocular histoplasmosis. *Arch Ophthalmol.* 1984;102:1776–1784.

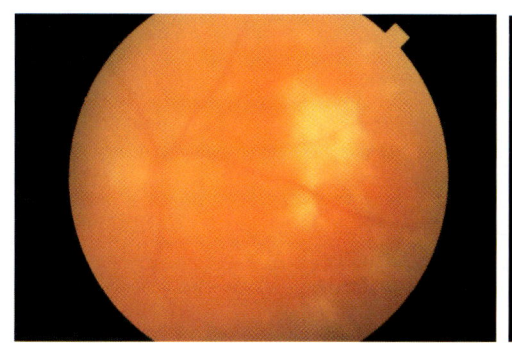

Figure 9-55 SFU, fundus photograph before treatment. *(Photograph courtesy of E. Mitchel Opremcak, MD.)*

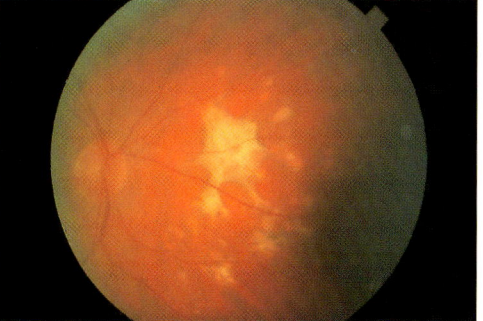

Figure 9-56 Same patient in remission following immunosuppressive therapy. *(Photograph courtesy of E. Mitchel Opremcak, MD.)*

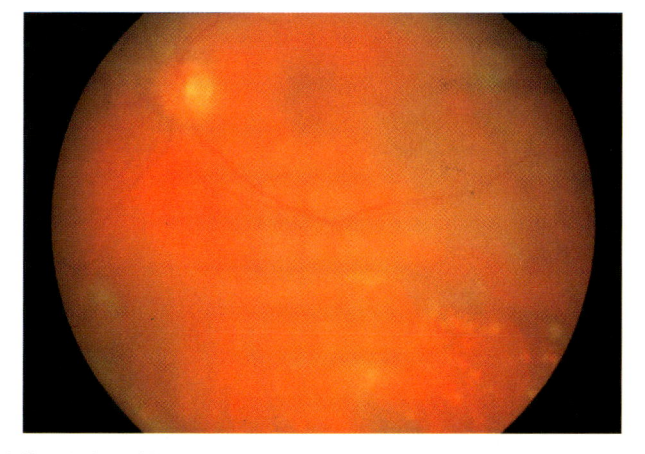

Figure 9-57 Multifocal choroiditis and panuveitis syndrome (MCP). *(Photograph courtesy of E. Mitchel Opremcak, MD.)*

CHAPTER 10

Panuveitis

Many systemic entities associated with uveitis are likely to cause diffuse inflammation leading to concomitant iridocyclitis and posterior uveitis. These include tuberculosis (the "great imitator") and spirochetal diseases such as Lyme disease and syphilis (the "great masquerader"), as well as sarcoidosis, sympathetic ophthalmia, and Vogt-Koyanagi-Harada disease. Many cases of Behçet syndrome, juvenile rheumatoid arthritis, lens-associated uveitis, and severe cases of toxoplasmosis or toxocariasis could also be considered panuveitis. These diseases are also discussed in earlier chapters in the context of anterior or posterior uveitis (see Chapters 7 and 9). BCSC Section 1, *Update on General Medicine,* also discusses syphilis, tuberculosis, and Lyme disease.

Although *panuveitis,* or *diffuse uveitis,* may originate as iritis or as choroiditis, usually these syndromes eventually involve all of the uvea, as well as other major ocular structures, including the cornea, trabecular meshwork, sclera, and optic nerve. Generally, panuveitis is bilateral, although one eye may be affected first and the severity is not necessarily symmetric.

Infectious Diseases

Bacterial Disease

Syphilis

This sexually transmitted or bloodborne bacterial infection is associated with multiple ocular manifestations. The disease is caused by *Treponema pallidum,* a highly coiled, helical bacterium with a long, 30-hour replication cycle. The incidence of syphilis is increasing. Syphilis accounts for 1%–3% of all uveitis cases; 5%–10% of all patients with secondary syphilis develop uveitis. The disease is one of the great masqueraders in medicine and must be considered a possible cause in all cases of uveitis.

Syphilitic uveitis is one of the few types of uveitis that can be cured, even in patients with AIDS. Delay in diagnosis of syphilitic chorioretinitis can lead to permanent visual loss that might have been avoided with early treatment. Syphilis can affect persons from any socioeconomic group, especially those with active sex lives with many different partners and patients with AIDS.

Congenital syphilis Keratouveitis from acute interstitial keratitis occurs in congenital syphilis between the ages of 5 and 25 years (Fig 10-1). Keratouveitis is thought to be an allergic response to *T pallidum* in the cornea. Symptoms are intense pain and photo-

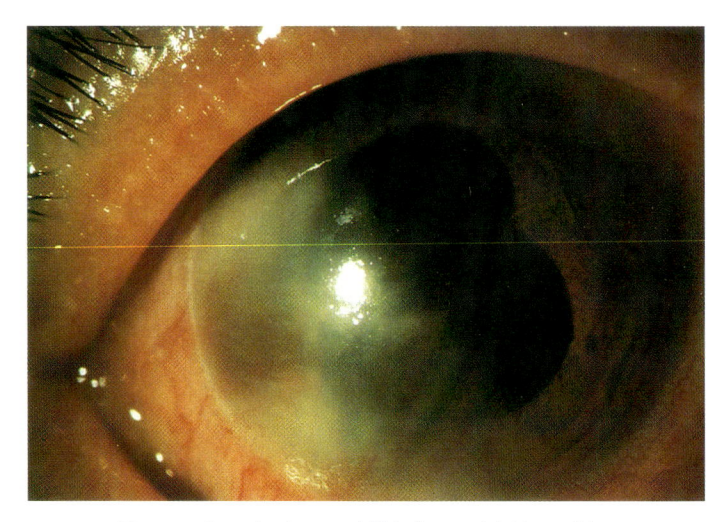

Figure 10-1 Active syphilitic interstitial keratitis.

phobia, and signs include a diffusely opaque cornea with reduced vision, even to light perception. Blood vessels invade the cornea, and when they meet in the center of the cornea after several months, the inflammation subsides and the cornea partially clears. Late stages show deep ghost (nonperfused) stromal vessels and opacities. The iritis accompanying interstitial keratitis is difficult to observe because of corneal haze; however, secondary guttata and hyaline strands projecting into the angle provide evidence of iritis. Glaucoma may also occur.

Congenital syphilis may also result in a bilateral salt-and-pepper fundus, which may affect the peripheral retina, the posterior pole, or a single quadrant. The changes are not progressive and may be associated with normal vision. Less commonly described variant signs associated with congenital disease include a bilateral secondary degeneration of pigment epithelium, with narrowing of vessels of the choroid and retina, and a pale optic disc with sharp margins and morphologically variable deposits of pigment. These findings may mimic retinitis pigmentosa.

Secondary syphilis Secondary syphilis, occurring 6 weeks to 6 months after primary disease, is characterized by a skin rash involving the palms and soles, fever, weight loss, and arthralgias. Ocular involvement may present with pain, redness, and photophobia or with blurred vision and floaters. A granulomatous or nongranulomatous anterior uveitis may be present. The iritis can be associated with iris roseola, vascularized papules (iris papulosa), larger yellow-red nodules (iris nodosa), and gummata. Focal or multifocal choroiditis can be seen during this stage, and exudates may appear around the disc and along the retinal arterioles. Arteritis and a perivasculitis may occur, along with ill-defined areas of retinitis and exudative retinal detachments (Figs 10-2, 10-3). In the later stages of secondary syphilis, extensive gliosis, atrophy, and pigment proliferation are present. The clinical picture may resemble retinitis pigmentosa. Neuroretinitis with papillitis and periarterial sheathing also occur.

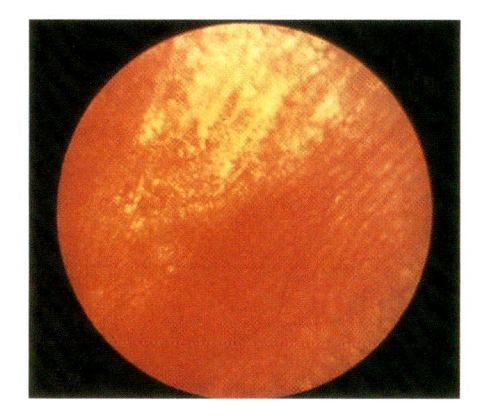

Figure 10-2 Syphilitic uveitis, acute retinitis.

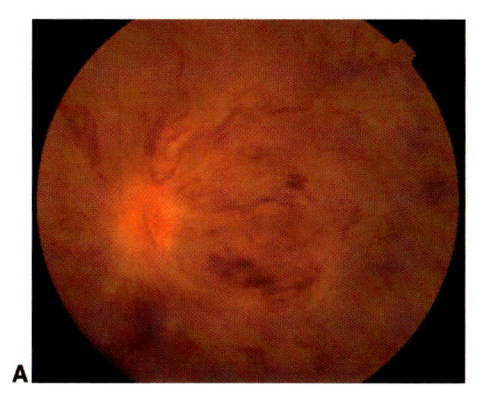

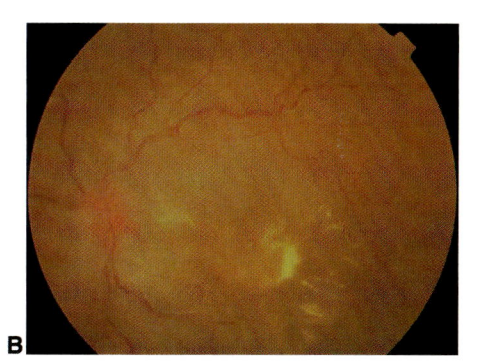

Figure 10-3 A, Acute syphilitic chorioretinitis. Note diffuse disc edema, retinal edema, and choroidal edema in the posterior pole. **B,** Healed chorioretinitis after 2 weeks of intravenous penicillin therapy. Note subretinal hard exudate that is organizing, reduction in disc edema, and reduction in choroidal inflammation. *(Photographs courtesy of Ramana S. Moorthy, MD.)*

Patients with syphilis who are immunocompromised or who have AIDS often have atypical or more fulminant ocular disease patterns. Optic neuritis and neuroretinitis are more common as an initial presentation in these patients, and disease recurrences are noted even after appropriate antibacterial therapy.

Diagnosis Syphilis is diagnosed on the basis of positive serologic results. The nontreponemal tests such as the Venereal Disease Research Laboratory (VDRL) or rapid plasma reagin (RPR) alone are insufficient, and a treponemal test such as the fluorescent treponemal antibody absorption (FTA-ABS) or the microhemagglutination assay–*T pallidum* (MHA-TP) must be used. A positive VDRL or RPR result indicates active disease and exposure to the bacteria. Both the VDRL and RPR results return to normal with effective therapy. In patients with uveitis and positive serologic results, asymptomatic neurosyphilis must be ruled out by a lumbar puncture. Any patient with syphilitic uveitis should undergo spinal fluid examination.

In latent syphilis, VDRL and FTA-ABS results are positive; cerebrospinal fluid (CSF) results are negative. In tertiary syphilis or in neurosyphilis, CSF serologic and serum

FTA-ABS results are positive, but the serum VDRL result may be low or negative. The presenting ocular complaint is usually blurred vision. Gumma of the iris and Argyll Robertson pupil are both characteristic in this stage of the disease (see BCSC Section 5, *Neuro-Ophthalmology*, for a description of this sign). Posterior pole lesions may develop in the late secondary stages of syphilis, but the presence of chorioretinitis usually indicates CSF involvement or neurosyphilis. Half of these lesions are bilateral, and the signs involve midzonal choroiditis. Vitreous haze, flame-shaped hemorrhages with fibrosis, and chorioretinal atrophy develop during the progress of inflammation (Fig 10-4). Diffuse neuroretinitis with papillitis and periarterial sheathing may also occur.

Treatment Once a diagnosis of syphilitic chorioretinitis has been established, systemic therapy is indicated. Different therapeutic regimens are used for ocular syphilis. Results of CSF serologic tests, protein, and cell count are important in determining the amount and duration of therapy. Ocular inflammation secondary to syphilis should be regarded and treated as neurosyphilis because of its anatomical and embryologic development with the CNS and the analogous blood–ocular barrier. The only proven effective therapy for this form of syphilis in both normal and immunocompromised patients is

- Penicillin G, 2–5 million units IV every 4 hours for 10–14 days, or
- Penicillin G procaine, 2–4 million units given IM every day with probenecid, 500 mg every 4 hours for 10–14 days

Patients with penicillin allergy may be treated with doxycycline 200 mg PO twice a day or erythromycin 500 mg PO four times a day for 15 days.

Once effective antibiotic therapy has started, ocular inflammation typically subsides. Topical, regional, or oral corticosteroids may be used to quiet anterior or posterior segment inflammation. Follow-up for patients with chorioretinitis and abnormal CSF requires spinal fluid examination every 6 months until cell count, protein, and VDRL results return to normal.

Aldave AJ, King JA, Cunningham ET Jr. Ocular syphilis [review]. *Curr Opin Ophthalmol.* 2001;12:433–441.

Gass JD, Braunstein RA, Chenoweth RG. Acute syphilitic posterior placoid chorioretinitis. *Ophthalmology.* 1990;97:1288–1297.

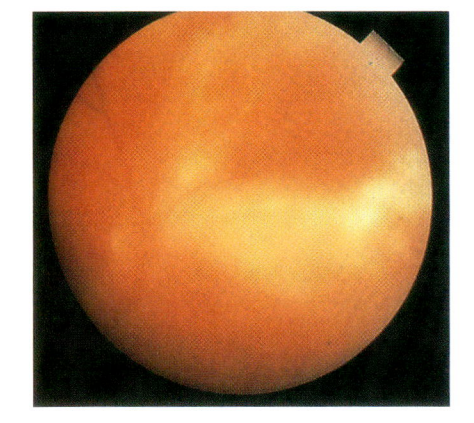

Figure 10-4 Acute syphilitic retinitis.

Hart G. Syphilis tests in diagnostic and therapeutic decision making. *Ann Intern Med.* 1986;104:368–376.

McLeish WM, Pulido JS, Holland S, et al. The ocular manifestations of syphilis in human immunodeficiency virus type 1–infected host. *Ophthalmology.* 1990;97:196–203.

Passo MS, Rosenbaum JT. Ocular syphilis in patients with human immunodeficiency virus infection. *Am J Ophthalmol.* 1988;106:1–6.

Tamesis RR, Foster CS. Ocular syphilis. *Ophthalmology.* 1990;97:1281–1287.

Lyme disease

Lyme disease is a tickborne spirochetal illness caused by *Borrelia burgdorferi.* Animal reservoirs for *B burgdorferi* include rodents, deer, birds, cats, and dogs. The spirochete is transmitted to humans through the bite of a tick, *Ixodes dammini* (eastern United States) or *Ixodes pacificus* (western United States). Spirochetemia follows the tick bite. Lyme disease is the most prevalent vectorborne illness in the United States, with seasonal outbreaks, especially in early summer and midautumn.

The clinical manifestations of Lyme disease have been divided into three stages:

- *Stage I,* occurring during the first month after infection, is characterized by skin, eye, and constitutional symptoms. Erythema chronicum migrans, an elevated annular erythematous skin lesion with central clearing, can occur at the site of the tick bite (Figs 10-5, 10-6). Follicular conjunctivitis may be present, and headache, stiff neck, malaise, myalgias, arthralgias, and fever may occur.
- *Stage II,* 1–4 months after infection, can be manifested by neurologic abnormalities and musculoskeletal disease, as well as by cardiac and ocular involvement. Neurologic disease, which occurs in 30%–40% of patients, can take the form of Bell palsy, encephalitis, or meningitis. Musculoskeletal disease, arthritis, tendinitis, and joint effusions can be present at this stage (Fig 10-7). Myocarditis or heart block appears in 8% of patients. Ocular manifestations in stage II Lyme disease include keratitis, iritis, intermediate uveitis, vitritis, panophthalmitis, and optic neuritis (Figs 10-8, 10-9).
- *Stage III,* with onset 5 months or more after infection, is characterized by chronic atrophic skin changes, keratitis, chronic meningitis, chronic arthritis, and adult respiratory distress syndrome.

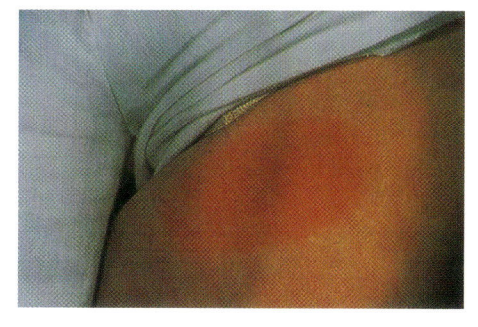

Figure 10-5 Erythema chronicum migrans: a single dense erythematous lesion. *(Photograph courtesy of Alan B. MacDonald, MD.)*

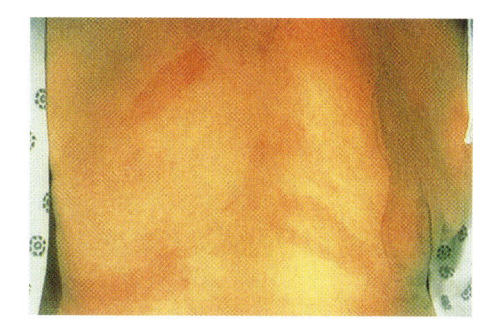

Figure 10-6 Erythema chronicum migrans: multiple bull's-eye lesions. *(Photograph courtesy of Alan B. MacDonald, MD.)*

192 • Intraocular Inflammation and Uveitis

Figure 10-7 Lyme disease arthritis. *(Photograph courtesy of Alan B. MacDonald, MD.)*

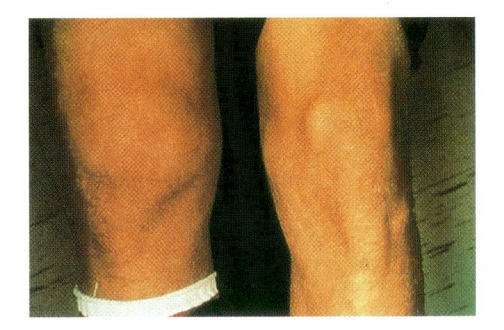

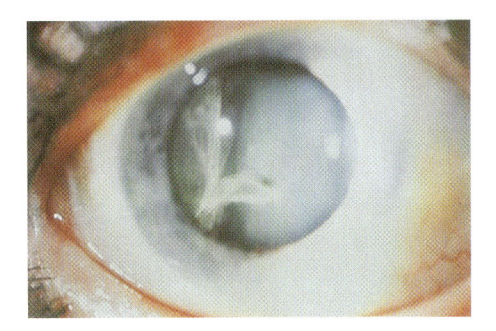

Figure 10-8 Dense anterior vitreous debris causing floaters and blurring in ocular Lyme disease. *(Photograph courtesy of William W. Culbertson, MD.)*

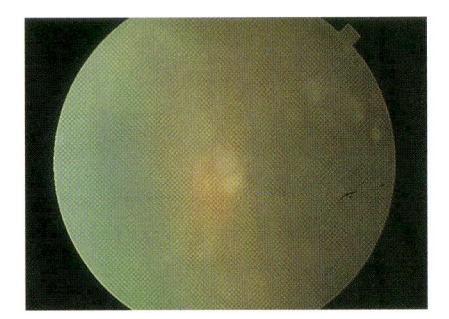

Figure 10-9 Grade III vitreous opacification in Lyme vitritis, as seen by indirect ophthalmoscopy, is reminiscent of severe pars planitis. *(Photograph courtesy of John D. Sheppard, Jr, MD.)*

Ocular involvement in Lyme disease occurs during all stages. An early sign is follicular conjunctivitis that is morphologically similar to that caused by other mechanisms (see BCSC Section 8, *External Disease and Cornea*, for further discussion and illustrations). The most characteristic intraocular manifestation of Lyme disease appears to be a chronic iridocyclitis and vitritis. Some cases of intermediate uveitis may be caused by *B burgdorferi*.

Laboratory diagnosis of Lyme disease is suboptimal, with a high frequency of both false-positive and false-negative results. Lyme immunofluorescent antibody titer, enzyme-linked immunosorbent assay for IgM and IgG, and Western blot testing should be ordered.

Because many cases of recalcitrant CNS Lyme disease have been well documented, antibiotic therapy of suspected Lyme disease should be aggressive. It is far easier to eradicate Lyme disease in its earlier stages with an oral course of antibiotic therapy alone than it is to eradicate established CNS disease, even with long-term IV antibiotics such as ceftriaxone. A patient with Lyme disease involving the eye must be considered to have CNS infection.

Recommended therapy for early Lyme disease consists of tetracycline, erythromycin, or penicillin. Duration of therapy is determined by clinical response. At present, IV ceftriaxone or penicillin is advised for neurologic or neuro-ophthalmologic Lyme disease.

Aaberg TM. The expanding ophthalmologic spectrum of Lyme disease. *Am J Ophthalmol.* 1989;107:77–80.

Winterkorn JM. Lyme disease: neurologic and ophthalmic manifestations. *Surv Ophthalmol.* 1990;35:191–204.

Winward KE, Smith JL, Culbertson WW, et al. Ocular Lyme borreliosis. *Am J Ophthalmol.* 1989;108:651–657.

Leptospirosis

The spirochete responsible for leptospirosis is commonly found around sewer water, rats, and urine. There are 170 serotypes of pathogenic bacteria in this genus. The disease is a zoonosis that humans acquire through exposure to secretions from infected animals. Plumbers and sewer workers are at increased risk.

Leptospira organisms gain access to humans through breaks in the skin or mucous membranes. The leptospiremia results in dissemination of the bacteria throughout the body, including the eye. Systemic manifestations include headache, chills, fever, and muscle ache. Kidney and liver disease are common, resulting in jaundice and azotemia. Ocular manifestations include anterior uveitis, sometimes with hypopyon, retinal periphlebitis, and panuveitis.

A high degree of clinical suspicion aids diagnosis. Medically unresponsive uveitis in a patient with systemic illness and a history of exposure to contaminated water or sick animals should prompt laboratory testing for leptospirosis antibodies. Leptospirosis may cause a positive RPR or FTA-ABS result. Intravenous penicillin, 2.4–3.6 million units per day; tetracycline, 2 g/day PO in four divided doses; or doxycycline, 100 mg twice daily for 10–14 days, have been used to treat this disease.

Rathinam SR, Rathnam S, Selvaraj S, et al. Uveitis associated with an epidemic outbreak of leptospirosis. *Am J Ophthalmol.* 1997;124:71–79.

Tuberculosis

Once considered the most common cause of uveitis, tuberculous ocular disease is now rarely found in clinics in the United States. Recently, however, the incidence of pulmonary and extrapulmonary tuberculosis (TB) has increased, in part because of the spread of AIDS. The incidence of tuberculous uveitis may vary from one location to another, and certain populations are at greater risk:

- Health care professionals
- Recent immigrants from endemic areas
- Immunosuppressed patients
- Indigent populations

These demographics must be considered in a differential diagnosis that includes ocular TB.

The TB bacillus is highly aerobic, with an affinity for highly oxygenated tissues. Thus, tuberculous lesions frequently appear in the apices of the lungs as well as in the choroid, which has the highest blood flow rate in the body.

Both direct infection and delayed hypersensitivity reactions have been implicated in the pathogenesis of tuberculous uveitis. Mycobacterial cell wall components are potent immunoadjuvants, used experimentally, for instance, in Freund's complete adjuvant.

194 • Intraocular Inflammation and Uveitis

Both granulomatous and nongranulomatous anterior uveitis with or without keratitis have been ascribed to TB. Yellow-white nodules in the choroid, ranging in size from ⅙ to 2 disc diameters with indistinct borders, may be present in association with miliary TB (Fig 10-10). Other manifestations include

- Larger, solitary masses, several disc diameters in size
- Retinal vasculitis, especially periphlebitis
- Vascular occlusion
- Dense vitritis
- Papillitis

Typically, patients with chronic ocular TB have chronic iridocyclitis, with or without posterior segment disease. These patients experience a waxing-and-waning course, with long-term degradation in the blood–aqueous barrier, accumulation of vitreous opacities, and cystoid macular edema (Figs 10-11, 10-12). Patients who follow an adequate regimen of antituberculous agents often experience gradual improvement until they cease to have chronic recurrent iritis or acute exacerbations of their disease.

A positive PPD or documented skin test conversion is useful in the diagnosis. Some patients have only second-strength (250 tuberculin units, or TU) PPD positivity and yet are found histopathologically to have TB bacilli in their eyes. These patients may also have a normal-appearing chest radiograph. Thus, if the first-strength (1 TU) and standard

Figure 10-10 Choroidal tubercle (miliary tuberculosis).

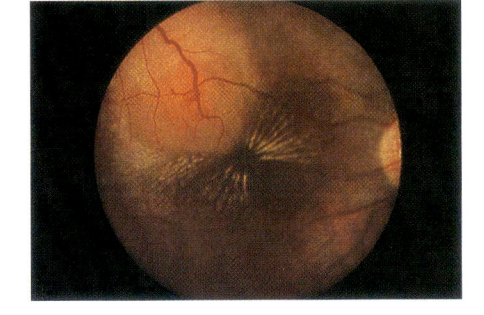

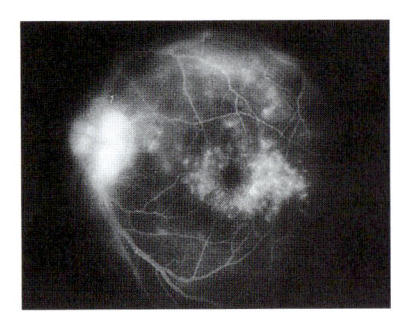

Figure 10-11 Chronic tuberculous uveitis with disc edema, vasculitis, periphlebitis, and cystoid macular edema. *(Photograph courtesy of John D. Sheppard, Jr, MD.)*

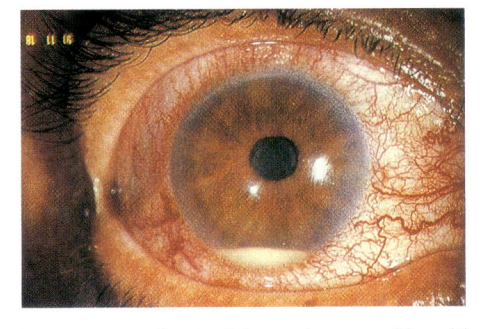

Figure 10-12 Acute tuberculous uveitis with hypopyon, posterior synechiae, vitritis, retinal vasculitis, and cystoid macular edema. *(Photograph courtesy of John D. Sheppard, Jr, MD.)*

intermediate-strength (5 TU) skin test results are negative, a second-strength PPD may be important.

While interpreting positive tuberculin skin tests in standard or second strength, the clinician must also consider the possibility of atypical mycobacterial infection, which is particularly common among rural populations and patients who have lived on a farm. This possibility, of course, complicates the diagnosis of ocular TB. Moreover, false-positive PPD results may be seen in patients born overseas who might have received a bacille Calmette-Guérin (BCG) childhood vaccination and in patients with bladder carcinoma who have been treated with intraluminal BCG injections.

Antibiotic therapy is clearly called for in patients with uveitis, a recently converted TB skin test result, a positive chest radiograph, and positive bacterial cultures. Multiple-agent therapy is suggested because of the increasing incidence of resistance to isoniazid, as well as compliance problems associated with long-term therapy. The extremely slow growth rate of TB contributes to the acquisition of drug resistance. Populations at particularly high risk for resistant organisms, now known as *multidrug-resistant tuberculosis (MDRTB)*, require three or more agents, such as isoniazid, rifampin, and pyrazinamide. MDRTB is found in previously noncompliant patients on single-agent therapy, migrant or indigent populations, immunocompromised patients, and recent immigrants from countries in which isoniazid and rifampin are available over the counter. The clinician may welcome the assistance of an infectious disease specialist or pulmonologist in treating these patients.

Less clear is the management approach to a patient with a diagnosis of possible or probable TB and uveitis. These patients are culture-negative and have a normal-appearing chest radiograph. A diagnosis of extrapulmonary TB may be entertained in the setting of medically unresponsive uveitis and a recent TB skin test conversion. Serum lysozyme and angiotensin-converting enzyme levels may be elevated, supporting the clinical impression.

Corticosteroids are often necessary in conjunction with antimicrobial therapy. Because steroids administered without concomitant antituberculous agents may lead to progressive worsening of tuberculous ocular disease, any patient who may have tuberculous disease should undergo testing before institution of intensive steroid therapy. Often, patients given topical steroids for what turns out to be tuberculous iritis may improve temporarily, only to worsen severely in the long run (Fig 10-13).

Barnes PF, Bloch AB, Davidson PT, et al. Tuberculosis in patients with human immunodeficiency virus infection. *N Engl J Med.* 1991;324:1644–1650.

Psilas K, Aspiotis M, Petroutsos G, et al. Antituberculosis therapy in the treatment of peripheral uveitis. *Ann Ophthalmol.* 1991;23:254–258.

Rosenbaum JT, Wernick R. The utility of routine screening of patients with uveitis for systemic lupus erythematosus or tuberculosis. A Bayesian analysis. *Arch Ophthalmol.* 1990;108:1291–1293.

Helminthic Diseases

Onchocerciasis

One of the leading causes of blindness in the world, onchocerciasis is endemic in many areas across Africa below the Sahara and in isolated foci in Central and South America. It is rarely seen or diagnosed in the United States. Worldwide, at least 18 million people

196 • Intraocular Inflammation and Uveitis

Figure 10-13 Long-standing, undiagnosed tuberculous uveitis with aphakia, dense pupillary membrane, posterior synechiae, cystoid macular edema, and chronic vitritis despite intensive steroid therapy. *(Photograph courtesy of John D. Sheppard, Jr, MD.)*

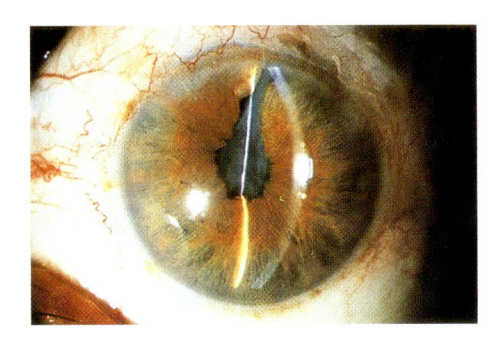

are infected, and of these, 1–2 million are blind. In hyperendemic areas, everyone over the age of 15 is infected, and half will become blind before they die.

Humans are the only host for *Onchocerca volvulus*, the filarial parasite that causes the disease. The infective larvae of *O volvulus* are transmitted through the bite of female blackflies of the *Simulium* genus. The flies breed in fast-flowing streams; hence, the disease is commonly called *river blindness*. The larvae develop into mature adult worms that form subcutaneous nodules. The adult female releases millions of microfilariae that migrate throughout the body, particularly to the skin and the eye. Microfilariae probably reach the eye by multiple routes:

- Direct invasion of the cornea from the conjunctiva
- Penetration of the sclera, both directly and through the vascular bundles
- Possibly by hematogenous spread

Live microfilariae are usually well tolerated, but dead microfilariae initiate a focal inflammatory response.

Anterior segment signs of onchocerciasis are common. Microfilariae can be observed swimming freely in the anterior chamber. Live microfilariae can be seen in the cornea; dead microfilariae cause a small stromal punctate inflammatory opacity that clears with time. Mild uveitis and limbitis are common, but severe anterior uveitis may occur and lead to synechiae, secondary glaucoma, and secondary cataract. Chorioretinal changes are common and vary widely in severity. Early disruption of the RPE is typical, with pigment dispersion and focal areas of atrophy. Later, severe chorioretinal atrophy occurs, predominantly in the posterior pole. Optic atrophy is common in advanced disease.

Diagnosis is based on clinical appearance and history of exposure in an endemic area. The diagnosis is confirmed by finding microfilariae in small skin biopsies or in the eye. Ivermectin, a macrolytic lactone, is the treatment of choice for onchocerciasis. Although not approved for sale in the United States, ivermectin is available on a compassionate basis for individual treatment. Ivermectin safely kills the microfilariae but does not have a permanent effect on the adult worms. A single oral dose of 150 µg/kg should be repeated annually, probably for 10 years. Topical corticosteroids can be used to control any anterior uveitis.

The former treatment, a course of diethylcarbamazine, was associated with many severe adverse reactions *(Mazzotti reaction)* caused by massive worm kill. This treatment has now been totally replaced by ivermectin. Although annual ivermectin treatment reduces anterior chamber microfilarial load and the development of new anterior chamber lesions, it does not reduce the macrofilarial load even at doses as high as 1600 µg/kg. Ivermectin does not appear to reduce the development of new chorioretinal lesions or to resolve existing lesions. It does appear to slow progression of visual field loss and optic atrophy, even in advanced disease. Nodules containing adult worms can be removed surgically, but this approach does not usually cure the disease because many nodules are deeply buried and cannot be found. Further research to develop more effective macrofilaricidal agents is needed to augment the beneficial effect of ivermectin in the control of onchocerciasis.

> Awadzi K, Attah SK, Addy ET, et al. The effects of high-dose ivermectin regimens on *Onchocerca volvulus* in onchocerciasis patients. *Trans R Soc Trop Med Hyg.* 1999;93:189–194.
> Chan CC, Nussenblatt RB, Kim MK, et al. Immunopathology of ocular onchocerciasis. 2. Anti-retinal autoantibodies in serum and ocular fluids. *Ophthalmology.* 1987;94:439–443.
> Cousens SN, Cassels-Brown A, Murdoch I, et al. Impact of annual dosing with ivermectin on progression of onchocercal visual field loss. *Bull WHO.* 1997;75:229–236.
> Ejere HY, Schwartz E, Wormald R. Ivermectin for onchocercal eye disease (river blindness). *Cochrane Database Syst Rev.* 2001;1:CD002219.
> Mabey D, Whitworth JA, Eckstein M, et al. The effects of multiple doses of ivermectin on ocular onchocerciasis. A six-year follow-up. *Ophthalmology.* 1996;103:1001–1008.

Immunologic and Granulomatous Diseases

Sarcoidosis

Sarcoidosis is a multisystem disease that primarily affects pulmonary function, although it is also capable of interfering with liver function and causing CNS disease. Sarcoidosis in the United States occurs 10 times more frequently among African Americans than among whites. Persons of all ages can be affected, but occurrence is most common between the ages of 20 and 50 years. Between 25% and 50% of patients with systemic sarcoidosis exhibit ocular inflammatory disease. Uveitis is the most frequent ocular manifestation. In most series, sarcoidosis accounts for 3%–10% of all uveitis.

The basic pathological lesion of sarcoidosis is the noncaseating epithelioid cell granuloma, or tubercle (Fig 10-14). The epithelioid cell is a polyhedral mononuclear histiocyte that is derived from the monocytes of the peripheral blood or the macrophage of the tissue. The tubercle of sarcoidosis is composed of

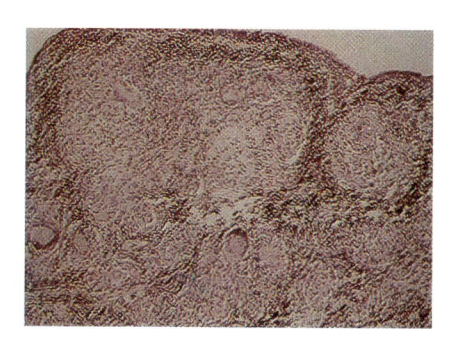

Figure 10-14 Sarcoidosis, histopathological view of conjunctival biopsy. Note giant cells and granulomatous inflammation.

- Epithelioid cells
- Multinucleated giant cells of the Langhans type, with nuclei at the periphery of the cell arranged in an arc or incomplete circle
- A thin rim of lymphocytes

Central areas of the tubercle seldom undergo fibrinoid degeneration or, in skin lesions (lupus pernio), micronecrosis. Various types of inclusion bodies may occur in the cytoplasm of the giant cells:

- *Schaumann's, or lamellar, bodies:* ovoid, basophilic, calcific bodies measuring up to 100 μm in diameter and also containing iron
- *Asteroid bodies:* star-shaped acidophilic bodies that measure up to 25 μm in diameter

A contagious etiologic agent has not been identified, although cell-wall–modified or cell-wall–deficient mycobacteria have been implicated.

Cutaneous involvement is frequent, and orbital and eyelid granulomas are common (Fig 10-15). Palpebral and bulbar conjunctival nodules also occur (Fig 10-16). Lacrimal gland infiltration may cause keratitis sicca. Symptoms of uveal involvement are variable and frequently include mild to moderate blurring of vision and aching about the eyes.

Sarcoidosis may involve all structures of the eye and present initially as a nongranulomatous process. A sizable proportion of patients develop chronic granulomatous iridocyclitis, accounting for two thirds of all cases of sarcoid uveitis. Typical findings are

- Mutton-fat keratic precipitates (Fig 10-17)
- Koeppe and Busacca iris nodules (Fig 10-18)
- White clumps of cells (snowballs) in the inferior anterior vitreous

Nummular corneal infiltrates, inferior corneal endothelial opacification, and large iris granulomas also occur. Posterior synechiae can be extensive and may lead to iris bombé and angle-closure glaucoma. Peripheral anterior synechiae may be extensive, encompassing the entire angle, for 360° in advanced cases. Secondary glaucoma can be severe, particularly when aggressive steroid therapy reverses ciliary body hyposecretion.

Posterior segment involvement is somewhat less frequent than anterior segment involvement. Nodular granulomas measuring ¼ to 1 disc diameter occur in both the

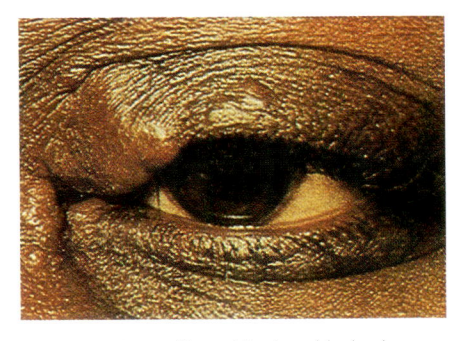

Figure 10-15 Sarcoidosis, skin lesions.

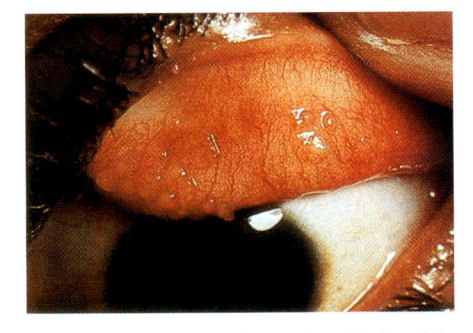

Figure 10-16 Sarcoidosis, conjunctival nodules.

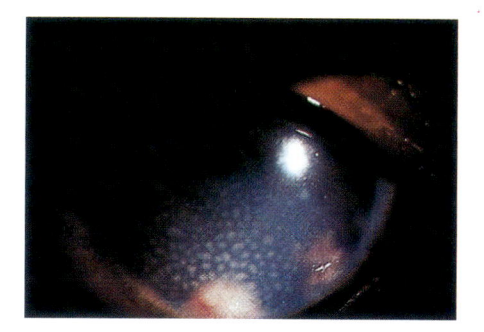

Figure 10-17 Sarcoidosis, keratic precipitates and iridocyclitis.

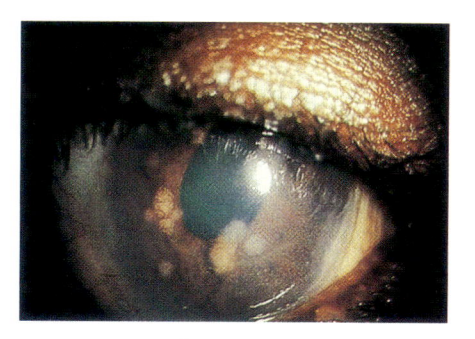

Figure 10-18 Sarcoidosis, iris nodules.

retina and the choroid. Rarely, large granulomas several disc diameters in size may occur. Irregular nodular granulomas along venules have been termed *candlewax drippings* or *taches de bougie*. Linear or patchy retinal periphlebitis presents as sheathing (Fig 10-19). Cystoid macular edema is common, and retinal neovascularization, disc edema, and optic nerve granulomas also occur.

Diagnosis and management

Because sarcoidosis is both variable in its presentation and known to be a frequent cause of uveitis, it must be considered as a possible cause in every patient with ocular inflammation. If sarcoidosis is suspected, serum lysozyme and angiotensin-converting enzyme (ACE) with chest radiography or chest CT are the most suitable tests. Frequently, a patient has a clinical picture compatible with sarcoidosis, yet laboratory data are inconclusive or negative. Additional testing may be useful, including a limited gallium scan of the head and neck. Gallium uptake is extremely sensitive to corticosteroids; a negative test result in patients taking even small doses of prednisone is unreliable. The combination of elevated ACE and positive gallium scans may be more specific for establishing the diagnosis of sarcoidosis in patients in whom chest radiographic results are negative or equivocal. Biopsy of suspicious skin or of conjunctival or lacrimal gland lesions may be considered (see Fig 10-14). Transconjunctival lacrimal gland biopsy may be diagnostic, especially when the lacrimal gland is enlarged or nodular. This procedure may obviate the need for a more invasive transbronchial biopsy.

Topical, periocular, and systemic corticosteroids are the mainstay of therapy. Cycloplegia is required for comfort and for prevention of synechiae. Systemic immunosuppressive therapy with methotrexate or azathioprine may be required in cases of corticosteroid intolerance or failure. When systemic disease is present, cooperation between the ophthalmologist and internist is required to devise an optimal therapeutic plan.

Aaberg TM. The role of the ophthalmologist in the management of sarcoidosis. *Am J Ophthalmol*. 1987;103:99–101.

Dana MR, Merayo-Lloves J, Schaumberg DA, et al. Prognosticators for visual outcome in sarcoid uveitis. *Ophthalmology*. 1996;103:1846–1853.

Jabs DA, Johns CJ. Ocular involvement in chronic sarcoidosis. *Am J Ophthalmol*. 1986;102:297–301.

Mayers M. Ocular sarcoidosis. *Int Ophthalmol Clin.* 1990;30:257–263.

Power WJ, Neves RA, Rodriguez A, et al. The value of combined serum angiotensin-converting enzyme and gallium scan in diagnosing ocular sarcoidosis. *Ophthalmology.* 1995;102:2007–2011.

Sympathetic Ophthalmia

Sympathetic ophthalmia (SO) is a rare bilateral, nonnecrotizing, granulomatous panuveitis that occurs after injury to one eye, the *exciting eye*, followed by a latent period and the development of uveitis in the uninjured globe, the *sympathizing eye* (Fig 10-20). Improved wound closure and early removal of severely damaged eyes have significantly reduced the incidence of SO. Because enucleation has supplanted evisceration as the operation of choice in the removal of ocular contents, another potential source for sympathetic disease has been largely eliminated. BCSC Section 7, *Orbit, Eyelids, and Lacrimal System*, discusses the advantages and disadvantages of enucleation and evisceration in greater detail.

The cause of SO is not known, but theories include

- Hypersensitivity to melanin and melanin-associated protein
- An infectious causal agent
- Sensitivity to retinal S antigen or other retinal or uveal proteins

Experimental animal studies suggest that these intraocular antigens require processing and presentation by the lymphatic system and that the antigens may gain access to the system through penetrating ocular injury.

Figure 10-19 Sarcoidosis, retinal vascular sheathing.

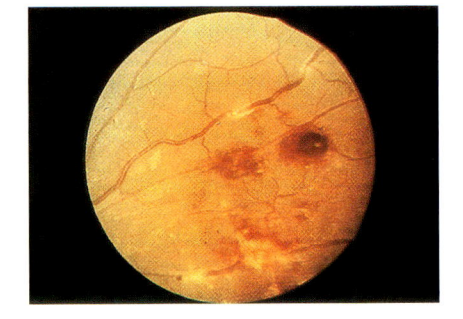

Figure 10-20 Sympathetic ophthalmia, sympathizing eye with synechiae.

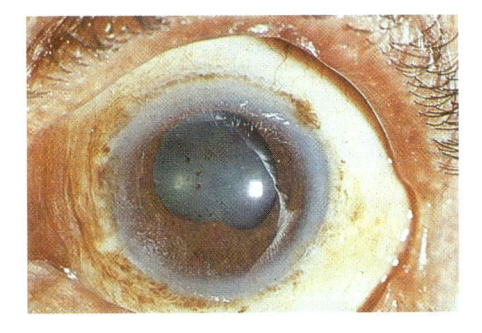

Histopathological features include the following, some of which are shown in Figures 10-21 and 10-22:

- Diffuse granulomatous uveal involvement, primarily with lymphocytes and epithelioid cells and occasionally with eosinophils
- Absence of reaction at the choriocapillaris
- Phagocytosis of uveal pigment by epithelioid cells

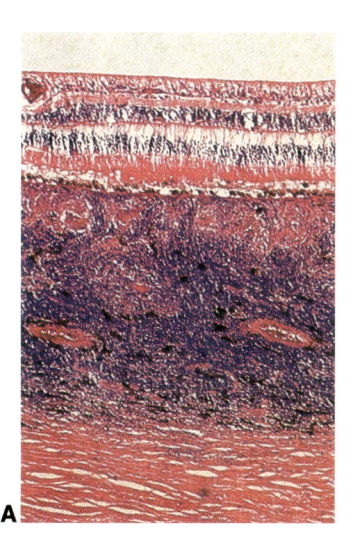

Figure 10-21 **A,** Diffuse granulomatous inflammation in sympathetic ophthalmia. **B,** Peripapillary and multifocal choroiditis (yellowish subretinal inflammatory infiltrates) with exudative retinal detachment in macula. **C,** Peripheral multifocal choroiditis and hazy view due to vitritis. *(Photographs B and C courtesy of Ramana S. Moorthy, MD.)*

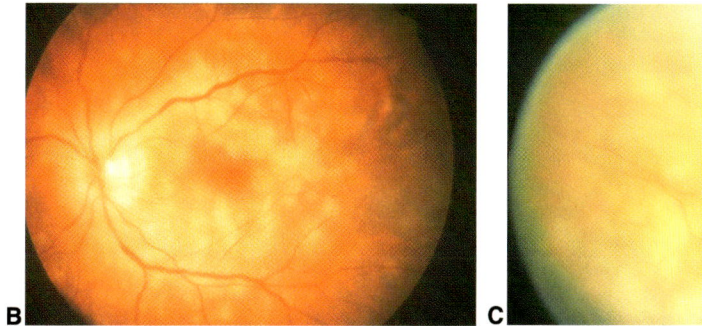

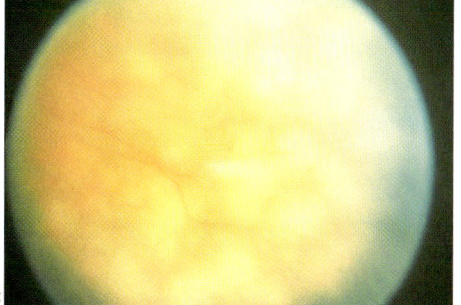

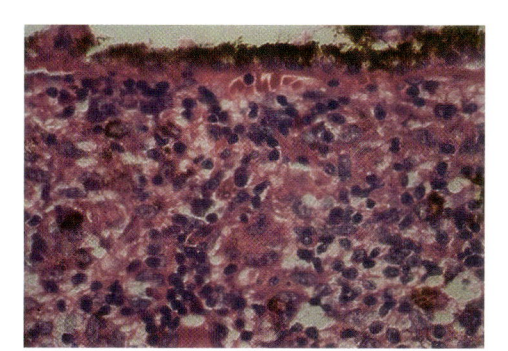

Figure 10-22 Sympathetic ophthalmia (histopathological view). Note giant cells in choroid.

- Presence of Dalen-Fuchs nodules
- Extension of the granulomatous process into scleral canals and the optic disc

Clinical features appear at least 10 days after injury or operation: minimal problems in near vision, mild photophobia, and slight redness in the previously unaffected eye. Because the patient is already receiving treatment for the initially affected eye, these symptoms usually are brought quickly to the attention of the ophthalmologist. Severe panuveitis is found in the injured or operated eye. Thickening of the uveal tract, large mutton-fat keratic precipitates, nodular infiltration in the iris, extensive peripheral anterior synechiae, and papillitis are seen in the sympathizing eye.

Diagnosis and management

Bilateral uveitis following any ocular trauma or surgery should suggest SO. The inflammation may occur as early as 10 days or as late as 50 years following the suspected triggering incident, but it usually occurs after 4–8 weeks. Table 10-1 lists surgical procedures and injuries known to have provoked SO.

The course of SO is chronic, with frequent exacerbations. Local, systemic, and periocular corticosteroids may be effective therapy. Topical cycloplegic/mydriatic agents are also indicated to relieve symptoms. Frequently, treatment with antimetabolites is effective when corticosteroids have failed to reduce the inflammation. Cyclosporine has also been shown to be an effective treatment for selected patients with SO. The advent of multiple routes of corticosteroid therapy and antimetabolite treatment has greatly improved the prognosis, with partial or full recovery of vision possible.

Some evidence suggests that once SO has developed, the clinical course can be moderated by removing the exciting eye within 2 weeks of disease onset. With advances in microsurgical techniques, however, an exciting eye that may have potentially useful vision may turn out to be the eye with the best acuity and should not be removed.

> Chan CC, Roberge RG, Whitcup SM, et al. 32 cases of sympathetic ophthalmia: a retrospective study at the National Eye Institute, Bethesda, Md., from 1982 to 1992. *Arch Ophthalmol.* 1995;113:597–600.

Table 10-1 Surgical Procedures and Injuries That May Lead to Sympathetic Ophthalmia

Surgical procedures associated with sympathetic ophthalmia
Vitrectomy
Secondary IOL placement
Trabeculectomy
Iridencleisis
Contact and noncontact YAG laser cyclodestruction
Cyclocryotherapy
Proton beam and helium ion irradiation for choroidal melanoma
Cataract extraction, particularly when the iris is entrapped within the wound

Injuries associated with sympathetic ophthalmia
Perforating ulcers
Severe contusion
Subconjunctival scleral rupture
Any perforating injury, with or without direct uveal involvement or uveal prolapse

Lam S, Tessler HH, Lam BL, et al. High incidence of sympathetic ophthalmia after contact and noncontact neodymium:YAG cyclotherapy. *Ophthalmology.* 1992;99:1818–1822.

Lubin JR, Albert DM, Weinstein M. Sixty-five years of sympathetic ophthalmia: a clinicopathologic review of 105 cases (1913–1978). *Ophthalmology.* 1980;87:109–121.

Marak GE Jr. Sympathetic ophthalmia. *Surv Ophthalmol.* 1982;89:1291–1292.

Rao NA, Robin J, Hartmann D, et al. The role of the penetrating wound in the development of sympathetic ophthalmia: experimental observations. *Arch Ophthalmol.* 1983;101:102–104.

Reynard M, Shulman IA, Azen SP, et al. Histocompatibility antigens in sympathetic ophthalmia. *Am J Ophthalmol.* 1983;95:216–221.

Sharp DC, Bell RA, Patterson E, et al. Sympathetic ophthalmia: histopathologic and fluorescein angiographic correlation. *Arch Ophthalmol.* 1984;102:232–235.

Sheppard JD. Sympathetic ophthalmia. *Semin Ophthalmol.* 1994;9:177–184.

Vogt-Koyanagi-Harada (VKH) Disease

VKH disease is a rare cause of posterior or diffuse uveitis, even within the most commonly affected group of patients: persons of Asian or American Indian ancestry between 30 and 50 years of age. However, any dark-skinned persons are considered to be at risk. An immune reaction to uveal melanin-associated protein, melanocytes, or pigment epithelium has been suggested as a mechanism, but the cause remains unknown. A chronic, diffuse granulomatous uveitis resembling that of SO is seen (Fig 10-23). Unlike with SO, however, patients with VKH disease do not have a history of antecedent ocular injury.

VKH disease may be clinically described in four phases—namely, the prodromal, uveitic, chronic, and recurrent phases. The prodromal phase is marked by flulike symptoms. Systemic symptoms include headache, stiff neck, loss of consciousness, paralysis, and seizures. CNS signs include fever, nuchal rigidity, coma, seizures, monoparesis, hemiparesis, and focal neurologic signs. Optic neuropathy is present. CSF examination may show an increased number of lymphocytes, but this pleocytosis is transient. Skin and hair signs include alopecia, vitiligo, or poliosis in about 30% of patients. Temporary deafness or tinnitus occurs in about 30% of patients early in the course of the disease.

Within 1–2 days after the onset of CNS signs, the patient may complain of photophobia, redness, blurry vision, and ocular pain. The uveitic phase is marked by bilateral anterior chamber cells, variable vitreous cells, and exudative retinal detachments (Fig 10-24A). Profound loss of vision may occur during this phase. Exudative retinal detachments are often shallow and have a cloverleaf pattern around the posterior pole. The optic disc is often edematous and hyperemic.

Several weeks later, the chronic (convalescent) phase begins. It is marked by resolution of exudative retinal detachments and gradual depigmentation of the choroid, resulting in the classic orange-red discoloration called the *sunset-glow fundus appearance* (Fig 10-24B). In addition, small, round, discrete depigmented lesions develop in the inferior peripheral fundus, representing resolved Dalen-Fuchs nodules (Fig 10-25). Peripapillary atrophy may also be seen (see Fig 10-24B). Perilimbal vitiligo (Sugiura's sign) develops in more than 75% of cases. Extraocular manifestations in the chronic phase include the development of vitiligo, alopecia, and poliosis in about 30% of patients (Figs 10-26, 10-27). Generally, these skin and hair signs occur several weeks to months after

204 • Intraocular Inflammation and Uveitis

Figure 10-23 Vogt-Koyanagi-Harada disease, choroiditis (histopathological view).

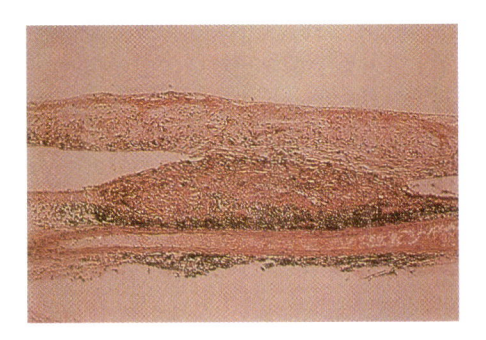

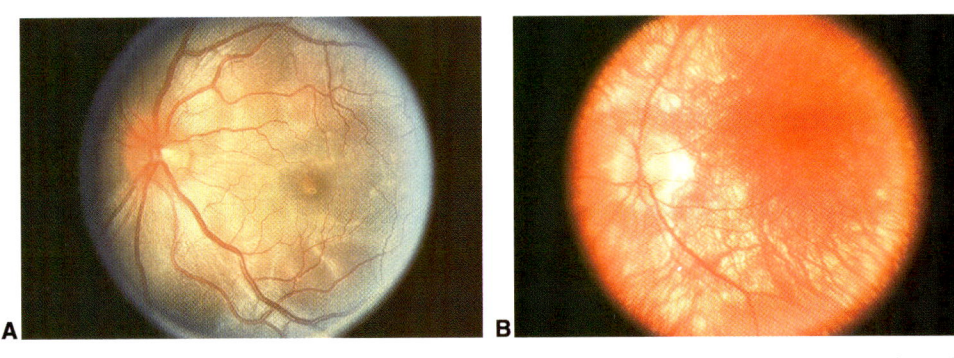

Figure 10-24 A, Disc hyperemia and multiple serous retinal detachments in the posterior pole of the left eye of a Hispanic patient in the acute phase of VKH disease. **B,** Sunset-glow fundus appearance in the chronic phase of VKH disease in a Hispanic patient. *(Reprinted with permission from Moorthy RS, Inomata H, Rao NA. Vogt-Koyanagi-Harada syndrome.* Surv Ophthalmol. *1995;39:271, 272.)*

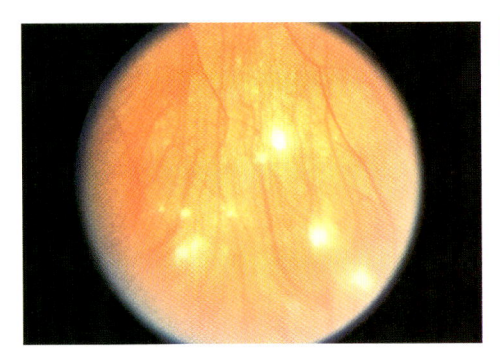

Figure 10-25 Multiple inferior peripheral punched-out chorioretinal lesions representing resolved Dalen-Fuchs nodules in the chronic phase of VKH disease. *(Photograph courtesy of Ramana S. Moorthy, MD.)*

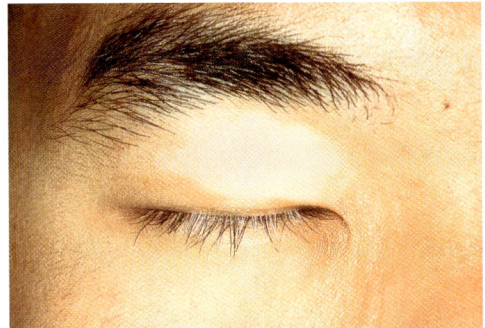

Figure 10-26 Vitiligo of the upper eyelid and marked poliosis in the chronic phase of VKH disease. *(Photograph courtesy of Ramana S. Moorthy, MD.)*

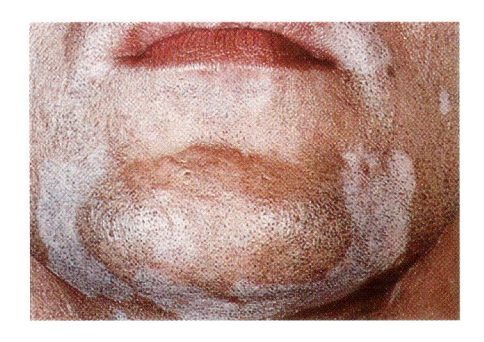

Figure 10-27 VKH disease, skin lesion.

the onset of ocular inflammation, but they may appear simultaneously. Perilimbal vitiligo, Sugiura's sign, occurs in more than 75% of cases.

If the uveitic and chronic phases are not adequately treated with systemic corticosteroids, the recurrent phase of the disease may ensue. This is marked by recurrent granulomatous anterior uveitis with development of keratic precipitates, posterior synechiae, iris nodules, iris depigmentation, and stromal atrophy. Visual loss occurs due to three main complications—namely, cataract (50%), glaucoma (33%), and choroidal neovascularization (10%).

Diagnosis and management

Diagnosis of VKH disease is suggested by the pathognomonic clinical picture. SO must be ruled out. Fluorescein angiography is helpful and may reveal multiple focal areas of subretinal leakage in the early phase of the angiogram (Fig 10-28). Ultrasonography has been useful in detecting diffuse choroidal thickening. Lumbar puncture showing lymphocytosis may be diagnostic in a patient with bilateral anterior and posterior segment inflammation. HLA-DR4 is strongly associated with VKH disease.

Treatment includes the vigorous use of systemic, local, and periocular corticosteroids as well as cycloplegic/mydriatic agents. Systemic corticosteroids should be tapered slowly over a minimum period of 3 months to reduce the risk of the recurrent phase. Many patients respond favorably to treatment, with some recovering nearly normal vision, but the recurrent phase may lead to peripheral anterior synechiae and secondary glaucoma, choroidal neovascularization, complicated cataract, and phthisis bulbi. Immunosuppressive therapy is considered mandatory in the treatment of VKH disease. In most cases, cyclosporine or another form of immunosuppressive therapy may be needed to control chronic recurrent inflammation and its associated complications.

> Beniz J, Forster DJ, Lean JS, et al. Variations in clinical features of the Vogt-Koyanagi-Harada syndrome. *Retina*. 1991;11:275–280.
> Davis JL, Mittal KK, Friedlin V, et al. HLA associations and ancestry in Vogt-Koyanagi-Harada disease and sympathetic ophthalmia. *Ophthalmology*. 1990;97:1137–1142.
> Moorthy RS, Inomata H, Rao NA. Vogt-Koyanagi-Harada syndrome. *Surv Ophthalmol*. 1995;39:265–292.
> Palestine AG. Medical therapy of uveitis. In: *Focal Points: Clinical Modules for Ophthalmologists*. San Francisco: American Academy of Ophthalmology; 1989;7:8.

206 • Intraocular Inflammation and Uveitis

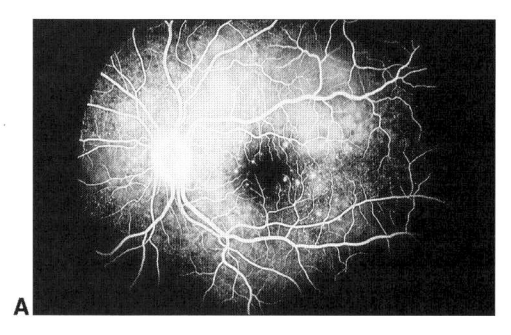

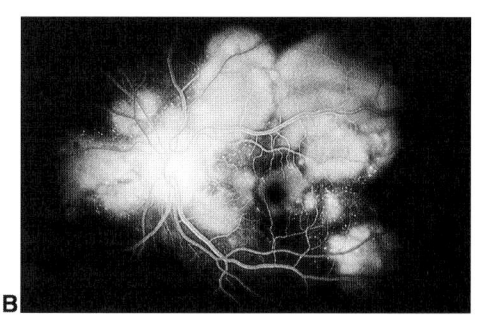

Figure 10-28 A, Early arteriovenous phase fluorescein angiogram showing multiple pinpoint foci of hyperfluorescence in the posterior pole of the left eye of a patient in the acute phase of VKH disease. **B,** Late arteriovenous phase fluorescein angiogram showing fluorescein pooling in multiple serous retinal detachments in the posterior pole in the same eye. *(Photographs courtesy of Ramana S. Moorthy, MD.)*

Smith RD, Nozik RA. *Uveitis: A Clinical Approach to Diagnosis and Management.* 2nd ed. Baltimore: Williams & Wilkins; 1989:144–146.

Zhang XY, Wang XM, Hu TS. Profiling human leukocyte antigens in Vogt-Koyanagi-Harada syndrome. *Am J Ophthalmol.* 1992;113:567–572.

CHAPTER 11

Endophthalmitis

The term *endophthalmitis* refers to intraocular inflammation predominantly involving the vitreous cavity and anterior chamber of the eye. Contiguous ocular structures such as the retina or the choroid may also be involved. *Infectious endophthalmitis,* inflammation associated with an infectious process, is the most common form and the focus of this chapter. Less often, a noninfectious stimulus such as retained lens material or a toxic substance introduced into the eye during trauma or intraocular surgery may be responsible for the inflammatory response, resulting in *sterile endophthalmitis.*

Signs and Symptoms

The most common signs of endophthalmitis are decreased vision, anterior chamber reaction (hypopyon), and vitritis. Immediate visual loss ranges from mild to more profound. Although patients may have endophthalmitis without significant pain, pain is often present. Conjunctival hyperemia and chemosis, eyelid edema, and corneal edema may also be observed.

Infectious Endophthalmitis

Infectious endophthalmitis can be classified according to the circumstances by which the infecting organism is introduced into the eye. *Exogenous endophthalmitis,* in which the organism enters the eye from the external environment, accounts for most cases, as in the following categories (Table 11-1):

- *Postoperative endophthalmitis:* through a surgical incision (Fig 11-1)
- *Posttraumatic endophthalmitis:* a traumatic laceration
- *Bleb-associated endophthalmitis:* a conjunctival filtering bleb

A miscellaneous category includes cases associated with suture removal, wound infection, microbial keratitis, wound leaks, and infectious scleritis. The organism may also gain access to the eye from the internal environment or hematogenously, a classification known as *endogenous endophthalmitis* (Fig 11-2).

Overall, the incidence of postoperative endophthalmitis for cataract surgery by extracapsular cataract extraction or phacoemulsification ranges between 0.07% and 0.12%; for penetrating keratoplasty, the incidence is 0.11%; and for pars plana vitrectomy, 0.05%.

Table 11-1 Characteristics of Exogenous Endophthalmitis

Category	Incidence	Most Common Organisms	Onset After Surgery or Trauma	Symptoms	Clinical Findings
Acute postoperative (cataract surgery)	0.07%–0.12%				
Mild		Staphylococcus epidermidis Sterile	1–14 days	Photophobia, floaters	Slow progression, vision >20/400, ± hypopyon, mild vitritis, fundus visible
Severe		Staphylococcus aureus Streptococcus species Gram-negative bacteria	1–4 days	Pain, decreased vision	Rapid progression, vision <20/400, ± hypopyon, marked vitritis, fundus not visible
Chronic postoperative	?	Propionibacterium acnes S epidermidis Fungus	2 weeks to 2 years	Photophobia, hazy vision	Sometimes appearing with granulomatous keratic precipitates, ± hypopyon, mild to moderate vitritis, capsular plaque
Posttraumatic	2.4%–8.0% (as high as 30.0% in rural settings)	S epidermidis Bacillus species	1–5 days (fungi 1–4 weeks)	± increasing pain, decreasing vision	Increasing inflammation, hypopyon, increasing vitritis
Associated with filtering bleb	0.2%–9.6%	Streptococcus species Haemophilus influenzae	Anytime	Red eye, discharge, pain, decreasing vision	Infected bleb, hypopyon, vitritis

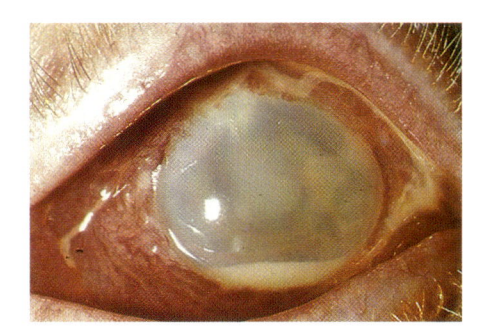

Figure 11-1 Exogenous postoperative endophthalmitis (bacterial).

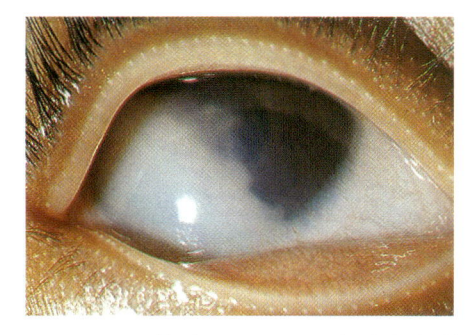

Figure 11-2 Endogenous endophthalmitis (meningococcal meningitis).

The cumulative incidence of bleb-related endophthalmitis after glaucoma filtering surgery has been reported to range from 0.2% to 9.6%.

High rates of endophthalmitis follow trauma. The incidence of posttraumatic endophthalmitis ranges between 2.4% and 8.0%. In rural settings or in cases with a retained intraocular foreign body, the incidence has been reported to be as high as 30%.

Postoperative Endophthalmitis

The eyelids and conjunctiva are the primary source of infection in postoperative endophthalmitis, and the organisms responsible may represent normal ocular surface flora such as *Staphylococcus* species and *Propionibacterium acnes*. The ocular microbiology of the eyelids and conjunctiva is discussed in detail in BCSC Section 8, *External Disease and Cornea*. Studies have demonstrated identical strains isolated from the ocular surface and from intraocular specimens taken from endophthalmitis cases. Other sources of contamination include

- Secondary infection from other sites such as the lacrimal system
- Blepharitis
- Contaminated eyedrops
- Contaminated surgical instruments, intraocular lenses, or irrigation fluids
- Other agents introduced into the eye
- Major breaches in sterile technique

In addition, IOLs may be the vector by which pathogens are introduced into the anterior chamber. Studies have suggested that bacteria bind to IOL components such as polypropylene.

In most cases of postoperative endophthalmitis, the causative organism is introduced into the eye at the time of surgery. A sutureless cataract operation occasionally allows postoperative entry of bacteria into the eye. Fortunately, the anterior chamber has a clearing capacity for bacteria, which may account for the small number of endophthalmitis cases despite possible contamination at the time of surgery.

Aaberg TM Jr, Flynn HW Jr, Schiffman J, et al. Nosocomial acute-onset postoperative endophthalmitis survey: a 10-year review of incidence and outcomes. *Ophthalmology*. 1998; 105:1004–1010.

Kattan HM, Flynn HW Jr, Pflugfelder SC, et al. Nosocomial endophthalmitis survey: current incidence of infection after intraocular surgery. *Ophthalmology*. 1991;98:227–238.

Speaker MG, Menikoff JA. Postoperative endophthalmitis: pathogenesis, prophylaxis, and management. In: Smolin G, Friedlaender MH, eds. *New and Evolving Ocular Infections. Int Ophthalmol Clin*. 1993;33:51–70.

Winward KE, Pflugfelder SC, Flynn HW Jr, et al. Postoperative *Propionibacterium* endophthalmitis. Treatment strategies and long-term results. *Ophthalmology*. 1993;100:447–451.

Acute-onset postoperative endophthalmitis

Acute-onset postoperative endophthalmitis develops within 1–14 days following intraocular surgery. In general, the more prolonged and complicated the surgery, the greater the risk. Endophthalmitis may occur following any surgical procedure in which the intraocular space is entered or inadvertently violated:

- Cataract surgery
- Secondary IOL implantation
- Glaucoma procedures
- Penetrating keratoplasty
- Keratorefractive surgery
- Pterygium excision
- Strabismus surgery
- Scleral buckling surgery
- Retinal/vitreous surgery
- Anterior chamber paracentesis
- Intravitreal administration of antiviral agents

For prognostic and therapeutic purposes, it is useful to distinguish between *mild* cases of acute endophthalmitis, with a slowly developing course, and *severe* cases, with a rapidly progressive course. The mild cases are less painful, involve a presenting visual acuity of 20/400 or better, and may present as late as 7–14 days postoperatively. *Staphylococcus epidermidis* and other coagulase-negative *Staphylococcus* species are the organisms most commonly recovered in culture (Fig 11-3). When intraocular cultures are negative,

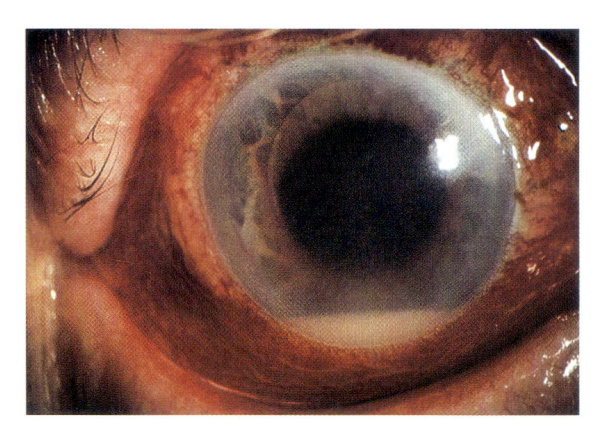

Figure 11-3 Mild acute postoperative endophthalmitis caused by *S epidermidis*.

the excessive intraocular inflammation is presumed to be caused by some unknown toxic or irritative factor or an infectious agent that cannot be cultured or identified.

Severe acute-onset postoperative endophthalmitis usually presents within 1–4 days after surgery. Vision is usually worse than 20/400, and patients report pain. Marked vitritis is common, and the fundus details are not visible. More virulent bacteria are often isolated in these cases, including *Staphylococcus aureus, Streptococcus* species, and gram-negative organisms such as *Serratia marcescens* (Fig 11-4), *Proteus,* and *Pseudomonas* species. Prompt recognition and treatment of severe acute-onset postoperative endophthalmitis are critical in limiting intraocular damage.

Chronic, or delayed-onset, postoperative endophthalmitis

Chronic postoperative endophthalmitis develops 4 weeks or more after surgery and can even be seen months to years later. The onset of signs and symptoms is gradual, with good vision, minimal pain, and mild vitritis. A hypopyon is less commonly present. Chronic postoperative endophthalmitis can be caused by bacteria or fungi, including *P acnes, S epidermidis,* or *Candida* species. *S epidermidis* infection presents within 6 weeks of surgery with nongranulomatous inflammation. Fungal endophthalmitis usually begins within 3 months after surgery and is most commonly caused by *Candida* species. *P acnes* endophthalmitis may develop from 2 months to 2 years following cataract surgery and is characterized by granulomatous keratic precipitates, a small hypopyon, vitritis, and a white plaque containing *P acnes* and residual lens material sequestered within the capsular bag (Fig 11-5).

Chronic postoperative endophthalmitis can rarely be precipitated by Nd:YAG laser capsulotomy. It is hypothesized that the laser allows the dissemination of sequestered pathogens from the capsular bag into the vitreous cavity and anterior chamber.

Posttraumatic Endophthalmitis

Posttraumatic endophthalmitis can occur following any penetrating ocular injury; however, the incidence appears to be higher in rural settings and when intraocular foreign bodies are retained. The most common organisms found are *S epidermidis, Bacillus* spe-

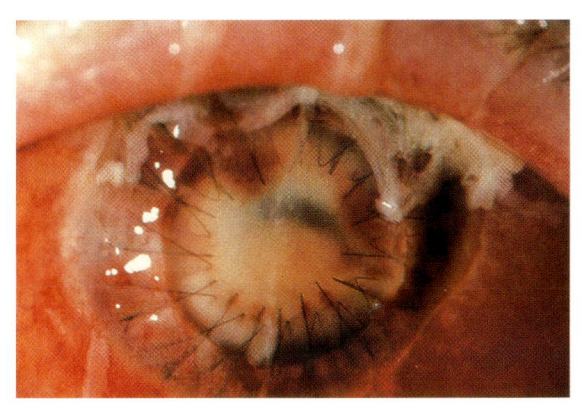

Figure 11-4 Severe acute postoperative endophthalmitis caused by *Serratia marcescens,* following penetrating keratoplasty.

212 • Intraocular Inflammation and Uveitis

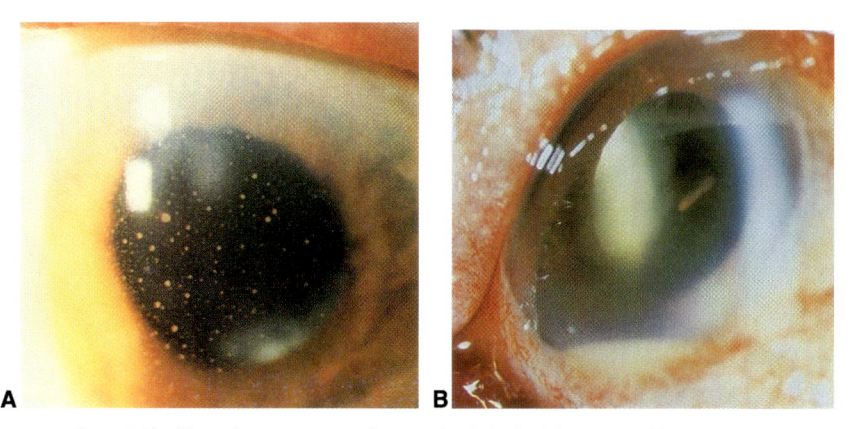

Figure 11-5 A and **B,** Chronic postoperative endophthalmitis caused by *P acnes*. Note granulomatous keratic precipitates and white plaque in the capsular bag. *(Photographs courtesy of David Meisler, MD.)*

cies, *Streptococcus* species, *S aureus*, and various fungi. *Bacillus* species such as *B cereus*, which are recovered in 25%–50% of culture-positive cases, cause a particularly fulminant endophthalmitis. In general, the larger and more contaminated the injury, the more likely endophthalmitis will develop. However, even small nonorganic materials such as a tiny hot metal shaving may occasionally cause endophthalmitis.

Removal of a retained intraocular foreign body within 24 hours of injury may reduce the risk of infectious endophthalmitis. Unfortunately, prompt recognition of the signs of possible endophthalmitis may be obscured by coexisting ocular injuries and the expected inflammatory response that normally follows a severe injury, resulting in treatment delay. Endophthalmitis should be suspected whenever a patient exhibits signs of increasing pain, intraocular inflammation (retinal periphlebitis), or a hypopyon after repair of a penetrating injury.

> Boldt HC, Pulido JS, Blodi CF, et al. Rural endophthalmitis. *Ophthalmology*. 1989;96: 1722–1726.
> Foster RE, Martinez JA, Murray TG, et al. Useful visual outcomes after treatment of *Bacillus cereus* endophthalmitis. *Ophthalmology*. 1996;103:390–397.
> Thompson JT, Parver LM, Enger CL, et al. Infectious endophthalmitis after penetrating injuries with retained intraocular foreign bodies. National Eye Trauma System. *Ophthalmology*. 1993;100:1468–1474.

Endophthalmitis Associated With Filtering Blebs

Bacteria may enter the eye through either intact or leaking conjunctival filtering blebs. Thin-walled blebs, as seen with mitomycin-C therapy, and inferiorly placed blebs may increase the risk of bacterial infection. BCSC Section 10, *Glaucoma*, discusses filtering blebs and their complications in more detail. Infection may occur months to years after filtering surgery. It is important to differentiate between low-grade bleb infection, or *blebitis*, and bleb-associated endophthalmitis.

In endophthalmitis, patients present with an infected bleb, marked intraocular inflammation with hypopyon, and vitritis. The organisms responsible include *Streptococcus* species, *S epidermidis, H influenzae, Moraxella* species, and *Enterococcus* species. The prognosis is usually poor, with profound visual loss.

In blebitis, the organisms are usually of low virulence, the bleb appears thin and cystic, and there is no evidence of vitreous inflammation. These cases may be treated conservatively with good visual outcomes. However, the physician must be aware (1) that bleb infection caused by more virulent organisms, such as *Streptococcus* species and *H influenzae*, may progress rapidly to endophthalmitis with pain and loss of vision and (2) that prompt intervention may be necessary.

>Brown RH, Yang LH, Walker SD, et al. Treatment of bleb infection after glaucoma surgery. *Arch Ophthalmol.* 1994;112:57–61.
>
>Ciulla TA, Beck AD, Topping MT, et al. Blebitis, early endophthalmitis, and late endophthalmitis after glaucoma-filtering surgery. *Ophthalmology.* 1997;104:986–995.
>
>Greenfield DS. Dysfunctional glaucoma filtration blebs. In: *Focal Points: Clinical Modules for Ophthalmologists.* San Francisco: American Academy of Ophthalmology; 2002;21:4.
>
>Higginbotham EJ, Stevens RK, Musch DC, et al. Bleb-related endophthalmitis after trabeculectomy with mitomycin C. *Ophthalmology.* 1996;103:650–656.
>
>Kangas TA, Greenfield DS, Flynn HW Jr, et al. Delayed-onset endophthalmitis associated with conjunctival filtering blebs. *Ophthalmology.* 1997;104:746–752.
>
>Mandelbaum S, Forster RK, Gelender H, et al. Late onset endophthalmitis associated with filtering blebs. *Ophthalmology.* 1985;92:964–972.

Endogenous Endophthalmitis

Endogenous endophthalmitis results from the bloodborne spread of bacteria or fungi during generalized septicemia. The source may be remote and nonocular, such as an infected intravenous line or an infected organ as in endocarditis, gastrointestinal disorders, pyelonephritis, meningitis, or osteomyelitis. Predisposed patients are chronically ill (ie, diabetes or chronic renal failure) or immunosuppressed, use intravenous drugs, have indwelling catheters, or are in the immediate postoperative or postpartum period.

Endogenous bacterial endophthalmitis is characterized by an acute onset with pain, decreased vision, hypopyon, and vitritis. Sometimes, both eyes are affected simultaneously. A wide variety of bacteria has been reported. The most common gram-positive organisms are *Streptococcus* species (endocarditis), *S aureus* (cutaneous infections), and *Bacillus* species (intravenous drug use). The most common gram-negative organisms are *Neisseria meningitidis* and *H influenzae* and enteric organisms such as *Escherichia coli* and *Klebsiella*.

Endogenous fungal endophthalmitis develops slowly as focal or multifocal areas of chorioretinitis. Granulomatous or nongranulomatous inflammation is observed with keratic precipitates, hypopyon, and vitritis with cellular aggregates. The infection usually begins in the choroid, appearing as yellow-white lesions with indistinct borders, ranging in size from small cotton-wool spots to several disc diameters (Fig 11-6). The infection subsequently can break through into the vitreous, producing localized cellular and fungal aggregates overlying the original site(s).

Candida is the most common causative organism (see Chapter 9, Figs 9-15 and 9-16); isolated cases of *Aspergillus* endophthalmitis have been reported. *Candida albicans* endophthalmitis occurs in association with hyperalimentation; indwelling intravascular

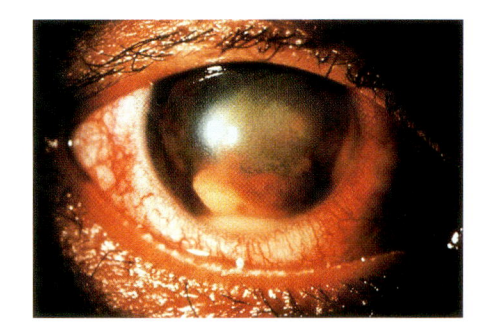

Figure 11-6 Fungal endophthalmitis.

lines; and IV drug use, recent major surgery, or immunosuppression. *Candida* endophthalmitis develops in a small percentage of patients with candidemia if not treated with antifungal therapies. In one study, patients treated with antifungal agents after a single positive fungal culture had an incidence of endogenous endophthalmitis of 2.8%, which appears to be lower than previous reports, in which 10%–37% of untreated patients developed endophthalmitis.

Accurate diagnosis of the agent causing endogenous endophthalmitis is crucial for proper antibiotic treatment of both ocular and systemic infections. Often, the cause may be presumed in light of existing positive cultures of blood or other suspected sites. If the agent is unknown, fungal and bacterial blood cultures should be obtained.

> Donahue SP, Greven CM, Zuravleff JJ, et al. Intraocular candidiasis in patients with candidemia. Clinical implications derived from a prospective multicenter study. *Ophthalmology*. 1994;101:1302–1309.
>
> Essman TF, Flynn HW Jr, Smiddy WE, et al. Treatment outcomes in a 10-year study of endogenous fungal endophthalmitis. *Ophthalmic Surg Lasers*. 1997;28:185–194.
>
> Okada AA, Johnson RP, Liles WC, et al. Endogenous bacterial endophthalmitis: report of a ten-year retrospective study. *Ophthalmology*. 1994;101:832–838.
>
> Scherer WJ, Lee K. Implications of early systemic therapy on the incidence of endogenous fungal endophthalmitis. *Ophthalmology*. 1997;104:1593–1598.

Prophylaxis

No study has established definitive standards for prophylaxis of endophthalmitis. Rather, an accumulation of data has led to trends, some of which remain controversial.

For cataract surgery, current literature strongly supports the use of preoperative povidone-iodine antisepsis. Preparation of the eyelids and conjunctiva with a 5% povidone-iodine solution just before surgery substantially reduces the bacterial load of the external structures.

Preoperative eyelid and conjunctival treatment with appropriate topical antibiotics may benefit patients who are at high risk for infection, such as those who have severe chronic blepharitis, lacrimal drainage abnormalities, cicatricial conjunctivitis, or a prosthesis in the other eye or who are diabetic or immunosuppressed. Preventive measures include preoperative topically applied broad-spectrum antibiotics, which can decrease the number of eyelid and conjunctival bacteria compared to no treatment. Isolation of the eyelids and lashes from the surgical field with careful draping is also important.

The use of intraocular antibiotics, either as a specific injection into the anterior chamber or as a concentration in irrigation fluids, has also been advocated. Subconjunctival antibiotics may be given at the end of intraocular surgery. The effectiveness of these methods in preventing endophthalmitis is uncertain. The efficacy of systemic administration of antibiotics in the prevention of endophthalmitis is also uncertain. Even so, some authors have advocated IV antibiotics for endophthalmitis prophylaxis in the setting of penetrating ocular injuries.

In general, the true effectiveness of any of these prophylactic strategies in the actual prevention of endophthalmitis is unknown. Moreover, routine antibiotic prophylaxis has raised concerns regarding costs, the risk of toxicity, and the emergence of resistant organisms.

Ciulla TA, Starr MB, Masket S. Bacterial endophthalmitis prophylaxis for cataract surgery. *Ophthalmology*. 2002;109:13–24.

Diagnosis

Differential Diagnosis

Infectious endophthalmitis caused by bacteria and fungi is often difficult to distinguish from other types of intraocular inflammation. Excessive inflammation without endophthalmitis is often encountered postoperatively in the setting of complicated surgery, preexisting uveitis and keratitis, diabetes, glaucoma therapy, and previous surgery. A vitreous and anterior chamber cellular reaction and a pseudohypopyon may be simulated by red blood cells, pigment, or debris. Retained lens material or other substances may cause sterile postoperative inflammation. Keratitis and postsurgical incision infections are often accompanied by a hypopyon without intraocular infection. It is important to avoid introducing a purely external infection (as in the case of bacterial keratitis) into the eye by performing an unnecessary paracentesis. Preexisting endogenous uveitis may flare up at any time following cataract surgery. Tumor cells from a lymphoma may accumulate in the vitreous, or retinoblastoma cells may accumulate in the anterior chamber, simulating intraocular inflammation.

The most helpful distinguishing characteristic of true infectious endophthalmitis is that the vitritis is progressive and out of proportion to other anterior segment findings. When in doubt, the clinician should manage the condition as an infectious process.

Obtaining Intraocular Specimens

Identification of an infective pathogen establishes diagnosis. Whenever possible, aqueous and vitreous specimens should be obtained for culture and microscopic study before antibiotic therapy is initiated. Obtaining vitreous specimens is important because postoperative infection might have disseminated to the vitreous without clinical evidence. Vitreous cultures are often positive, even when aqueous cultures in the same case are negative; the reverse may also be true.

Aqueous is obtained by passing a small-gauge needle through the limbus into the anterior chamber and withdrawing a 0.1 mL sample. Vitreous may be obtained by a vitreous tap using a needle or by a biopsy with an automated vitrector. For the tap, a 23-gauge 1-inch needle is passed through the pars plana 3.5 mm posterior to the limbus into the anterior vitreous cavity. If possible, the needle tip is visualized through the pupil to be in the proper position, and 0.2 mL of undiluted vitreous is withdrawn.

An alternative method is to perform the biopsy with a vitrector through the pars plana. Vitreous biopsy with a cutting instrument places less traction on a possibly inflamed and fragile retina as well as the vitreous base than does a vitreous tap performed with a needle.

Pars plana vitrectomy has been recommended for when fundus details are obscured by rapidly progressive cellular infiltration of the vitreous. The theoretical benefits of vitrectomy include

- Obtaining a larger sample of vitreous for culture and laboratory testing than is possible with a vitreous tap
- Removing potentially toxic bacterial by-products, endotoxins, and inflammatory cells
- Removing the vitreous scaffolding
- Reducing the bacterial load
- Clearing the ocular media

The disadvantages of vitrectomy are its technical difficulty and the delay it may create in therapeutic intervention while the patient is referred to an experienced vitreous surgeon. Thus, any benefits of a pars plana vitrectomy must be weighed against the potential risks of surgery.

Cultures and Laboratory Evaluation of Intraocular Specimens

Regardless of how the intraocular specimens are obtained, the aqueous and vitreous specimens should promptly be inoculated directly onto culture media. Drops of the sample should be placed onto blood agar, Sabouraud's agar, chocolate agar, thioglycollate broth, or similar media. In cases of chronic postoperative endophthalmitis, the laboratory should hold anaerobic cultures for 2 weeks because it may take that long for *P acnes* to grow out.

One drop each of the aqueous and vitreous specimens should be placed on clean slides for Gram and Giemsa stains for bacteria and fungi. Additional slides should be prepared and available for special stains (eg, calcofluor white) as indicated. If the responsible organism is definitively observed on these slides under the microscope, then treatment may be tailored accordingly before culture results are obtained. However, stains of aqueous and vitreous are often negative in spite of florid bacterial and fungal endophthalmitis and, thus, may be of limited value in the selection of appropriate therapy.

Barza M, Pavan PR, Doft BH, et al. Evaluation of microbiological diagnostic techniques in postoperative endophthalmitis in the Endophthalmitis Vitrectomy Study. *Arch Ophthalmol.* 1997;115:1142–1150.

Brod RD, Flynn HW Jr. Advances in the diagnosis and treatment of infectious endophthalmitis. *Curr Opin Ophthalmol.* 1991;2:306–314.

Treatment

Once infectious endophthalmitis is suspected, management should be tailored according to the course, severity, and extent of inflammation upon presentation. For example, mild cases of postoperative endophthalmitis may be treated by less aggressive means, whereas more severe cases often need vitrectomy.

Surgical Management

Vitrectomy is thought to debride the infected and inflamed vitreous cavity, allowing better antibiotic distribution in the vitreous cavity. It does not appear necessary to remove an IOL unless it hampers adequate visualization during vitrectomy. A national collaborative study, the Endophthalmitis Vitrectomy Study (EVS), investigated the management of postoperative endophthalmitis occurring within 6 weeks after cataract surgery with primary IOL or secondary IOL implantation. The study found that in eyes with vision better than light perception (defined as hand-motions acuity at 2 feet or more) at the time of presentation, visual results were not significantly different between eyes treated with immediate three-port pars plana vitrectomy and eyes treated with vitreous tap/biopsy in conjunction with intravitreal antibiotics (Table 11-2). However, in eyes with light perception–only vision, the vitrectomy group had significantly better outcomes than the vitreous tap/biopsy group. The EVS did not address the role of vitrectomy for other categories of endophthalmitis (ie, posttraumatic, filtering bleb–associated, endogenous, and chronic postoperative cases).

Medical Management

Antibacterial treatment of endophthalmitis should provide broad-spectrum coverage for both gram-positive and gram-negative organisms when the organism is not known (see Table 11-2). With the rising incidence of resistance to β-lactam antibiotics, many physicians have turned to vancomycin for gram-positive coverage. Aminoglycosides, including gentamicin, tobramycin, and amikacin, are usually effective treatment for gram-negative infection and may also be synergistic with vancomycin against certain gram-positive organisms. However, concern regarding aminoglycoside retinal toxicity (ie, macular infarction) has led many physicians to use third-generation cephalosporins such as ceftazidime to cover gram-negative bacilli. It has been suggested that fluoroquinolones be used since they can be given orally, penetrate the eye, and have a broad spectrum of activity. Unfortunately, they have limited effectiveness against anaerobic organisms, *Streptococcus* species, and other emerging resistant gram-positive bacteria.

Antibiotics may be administered by topical, subconjunctival, intraocular (usually intravitreal), and intravenous routes. The EVS employed intravitreal (vancomycin/amikacin), subconjunctival (vancomycin/ceftazidime), and topical (vancomycin/amikacin) antibiotics to treat acute postoperative endophthalmitis. The use of systemic antibiotics remains controversial. The EVS showed that IV antibiotics (amikacin/ceftazidime) made no difference in visual acuity outcomes comparing treated and untreated groups. The efficacy of IV antibiotics for the other categories of endophthalmitis mentioned above has not been established through the use of randomized controlled trials.

Table 11-2 Medications Used in Exogenous Endophthalmitis

	Topical	Subconjunctival	Route and Dose Intravitreal	Systemic
Antibiotic				
Gentamicin	9 mg/mL	20 mg/0.5 mL	01 mg/0.1 mL	1 mg/kg IV q8hr
Vancomycin	50 mg/mL	25 mg/0.5 mL	1.0 mg/0.1 mL	1.0 g IV q12hr
Amikacin	—	—	0.4 mg/0.1 mL	—
Chloramphenicol	—	—	1.0 mg/0.1 mL	—
Amphotericin B	—	—	5.0 µg/0.1 mL	1.0 mg/kg IV daily
Ceftazidime	—	—	2.0–2.25 mg/0.1 mL	1.0–2.0 g IV q8hr
Nafcillin	—	—	—	1.0 g IV q12hr
Ceftriaxone	—	—	—	1.0 g IV q12hr
Ketoconazole	—	—	—	400 mg PO daily
Fluconazole	—	—	—	200 mg PO daily
Itraconazole	—	—	—	100–200 mg (PO qd)
Ciprofloxacin	—	—	—	250–750 mg (PO bid)
Corticosteroid Preparations				
Prednisolone acetate 1% drops	Every hour	—	—	—
Dexamethasone 0.1% drops	Every hour	—	—	—
Dexamethasone injection 4 mg/mL	—	1.0 mL (4.0 mg)	0.1 mL (0.4 mg)	—
Prednisone tablets	—	—	—	1 mg/kg/day PO

Although corticosteroids may diminish the destructive intraocular inflammatory response to endophthalmitis, their timing and use is controversial. It has been suggested that corticosteroids should be withheld if a fungal pathogen is suspected.

General Considerations for Treatment

Mild acute-onset postoperative cases of infectious endophthalmitis are generally managed by injection of intraocular antibiotics alone, without vitrectomy, followed by topical antibiotics and steroids. In contrast, treatment of severe acute postoperative endophthalmitis includes

- Pars plana vitrectomy with vitreous and aqueous cultures
- Intravitreal, subconjunctival, and topical antibiotics
- Topical and periocular corticosteroids

The value of adjunctive intravitreal corticosteroids and systemic antibiotics is still debated. As in postoperative endophthalmitis, the treatment of posttraumatic endophthalmitis should be guided by the severity of the clinical course.

Chronic postoperative endophthalmitis therapy depends on the organism isolated. *S epidermidis* responds to intraocular vancomycin injection alone. In *P acnes* cases, intraocular vancomycin injection and local debridement or excision of the white intracapsular plaque and capsulectomy have been effective in eradicating the infection and reducing rates of recurrence.

Exogenous fungal endophthalmitis is treated by pars plana vitrectomy and intravitreal injection of amphotericin B. Topical, subconjunctival, and systemic antibiotics are given concomitantly, but their additional therapeutic value is unknown.

Treatment of endogenous bacterial and fungal endophthalmitis usually includes systemic antibiotic administration to treat not only the intraocular infection but also the systemic source of the pathogen. Treatment of endogenous bacterial endophthalmitis also usually includes intravitreal antibiotics. Systemic treatment of *Candida* chorioretinitis includes 5-flucytosine or oral fluconazole or, in more severe cases, IV amphotericin B. Intravenous amphotericin is nephrotoxic, and serum creatinine should be closely monitored during the course of treatment. When intravitreal involvement is present, intravitreal amphotericin B is usually used in combination with vitrectomy.

Blebitis usually responds to topical and subconjunctival antibiotic therapy. Infection in filtering blebs, however, may progress rapidly to endophthalmitis with pain and loss of vision. Vitreous inflammation dictates prompt intervention with vitreous cultures followed by intravitreal antibiotic injection, similar to the treatment of acute-onset postoperative cases.

Outcomes of Treatment

Visual loss in endophthalmitis results from the damage caused both by the toxins and proteases produced by the infectious organism and by the host's inflammatory response to the infection. The retina and anterior segment structures may be directly injured, which may lead to tractional or rhegmatogenous retinal detachments, ciliary body damage, hypotony, and phthisis bulbi.

In general, more virulent organisms capable of producing exotoxins, endotoxins, or proteases, such as *S aureus, Streptococcus* species, *Bacillus* species, and gram-negative organisms *(Pseudomonas, Serratia marcescens, Proteus),* cause the most rapidly progressive and fulminant disease and have the worst visual acuity outcomes. The less virulent organisms, such as *S epidermidis* and *P acnes,* are associated with more indolent clinical courses and better visual acuity outcomes.

The EVS reported the following findings:

- *At 3 months:* 41% of patients achieved 20/40 or better visual acuity; 69% had 20/100 or better acuity
- *At 9–12 months:* 53% of patients achieved visual acuity of 20/40 or better; 74% achieved 20/100 or better; 15% had worse than 5/200 vision
- *At the final follow-up visit:* 5% of patients had no light perception

Chronic endophthalmitis usually carries a favorable visual prognosis, with one study showing visual acuity of 20/40 or better in 80% of cases. The incidence for achieving 20/400 or better visual acuity in endophthalmitis associated with infected filtering blebs was 47% in one study. Only 10% of patients who develop bacterial endophthalmitis after trauma obtain a visual acuity of 20/400 or better.

> Aaberg TM Jr, Flynn HW Jr, Murray TG. Intraocular ceftazidime as an alternative to the aminoglycosides in the treatment of endophthalmitis. *Arch Ophthalmol.* 1994;112:18–19.
>
> Campochiaro PA, Lim JI. Aminoglycoside toxicity in the treatment of endophthalmitis. The Aminoglycoside Toxicity Study Group. *Arch Ophthalmol.* 1994;112:48–53.
>
> Doft BH. The Endophthalmitis Vitrectomy Study. *Arch Ophthalmol.* 1991;109:487–489.
>
> Doft BH, Barza M. Ceftazidime or amikacin: choice of intravitreal antimicrobials in the treatment of postoperative endophthalmitis [letter]. *Arch Ophthalmol.* 1994;112:17–18.
>
> Endophthalmitis Vitrectomy Study Group. Results of the Endophthalmitis Vitrectomy Study: a randomized trial of immediate vitrectomy and of intravenous antibiotics for the treatment of postoperative bacterial endophthalmitis. *Arch Ophthalmol.* 1995;113:1479–1496.

This chapter was prepared with the assistance of Dennis P. Han, MD, and Peter K. Kaiser, MD. The author also wishes to acknowledge the contribution of Harry W. Flynn, Jr, MD.

CHAPTER 12

Masquerade Syndromes

Masquerade syndromes are classically defined as those conditions that include, as part of their clinical findings, the presence of intraocular cells but are not due to immune-mediated uveitis entities. These may be divided into nonneoplastic conditions and neoplastic conditions.

Nonneoplastic Masquerade Syndromes

The nonneoplastic masquerade syndromes classically include retinitis pigmentosa (RP), ocular ischemic syndrome, and chronic peripheral retinal detachment. Endogenous fungal endophthalmitis and *Nocardia* endophthalmitis also are included in this group since they can be confused with other uveitic entities.

Retinitis Pigmentosa

Patients with RP often have variable numbers of vitreous cells. In addition, to confuse matters further, patients with RP can also develop cystoid macular edema. Classically, cystoid macular edema is seen angiographically as leakage from the retinal pigment epithelium. Unlike the case with most uveitic entities, patients with RP uniformly complain of nyctalopia. RP is usually a bilateral disease with a positive family history. In addition, fundus examination demonstrates waxy disc pallor, attenuation of arterioles, and a bone spiculing pattern of pigmentary changes in the midperiphery. The electroretinogram of patients with RP often appears severely depressed or extinguished, even early in the course of the disease process. These criteria can be used to differentiate RP from true uveitis.

Ocular Ischemic Syndrome

Ocular ischemic syndrome is defined by a generalized hypoperfusion of the entire eye and sometimes the orbit, usually due to carotid artery obstruction. Patients with ocular ischemic syndrome present with decreased vision and mild ocular pain. Examination may demonstrate corneal edema, a variable number of anterior chamber cells, and moderate flare. The flare often is greater and out of proportion to the number of cells in the anterior chamber. Rubeosis may be present on the iris, and neovascularization may be present in the angle on gonioscopy. The cataract may be more prominent on the side of the ocular ischemia. The vitreous is usually clear. Dilated fundus examination may show mild disc edema associated with dilated tortuous retinal venules, narrowed arterioles, and scattered blot intraretinal hemorrhages of medium to large size in the midperiphery and far periphery of the eye. Neovascularization may be present in the disc or elsewhere in the retina.

Fluorescein angiography shows delayed arteriolar filling, diffuse leakage in the posterior pole as well as from the optic disc, and signs of capillary nonperfusion in the posterior pole of the midperiphery. Retinal vascular staining may be present in the absence of any physical vascular sheathing on examination.

Patients with ocular ischemic syndrome should undergo carotid Doppler studies to determine whether there is ipsilateral carotid stenosis of greater than 75%, which often supports the diagnosis.

Treatment involves carotid endarterectomy of the ipsilateral site, if indicated, along with a local ocular treatment with both topical corticosteroid agents and cycloplegics as well as panretinal photocoagulation treatment, especially if rubeosis or retinal neovascularization is present. The 5-year mortality rate of patients with ocular ischemic syndrome is 40%. The visual prognosis is guarded, and many patients transiently improve with treatment but eventually worsen.

Differentiating ocular ischemia from true uveitis can be difficult. The combination of ischemic signs in the iris and in the posterior pole along with the age of the patient, usually over 65 years, and ipsilateral carotid stenosis can be very useful in differentiating ocular ischemic syndrome from uveitis.

Sivalingam A, Brown GC, Magargal LE, et al. The ocular ischemic syndrome. II. Mortality and systemic morbidity. *Int Ophthalmol.* 1990;13:187–191.

Sivalingam A, Brown GC, Magargal LE. The ocular ischemic syndrome. III. Visual prognosis and the effect of treatment. *Int Ophthalmol.* 1991;15:15–20.

Chronic Peripheral Rhegmatogenous Retinal Detachment

Chronic peripheral rhegmatogenous retinal detachment can be associated with anterior segment cell and flare and vitreous inflammatory and pigment cells. Patients often have good vision but can sometimes develop decreased vision due to cystoid macular edema. The key to the diagnosis of peripheral retinal detachment is the dilated fundus examination with scleral depression. Peripheral pigment demarcation lines, subretinal fluid, retinal breaks, subretinal fibrosis, and peripheral retinal cysts may be present. In some cases, the anterior segment cells may not represent true inflammation but rather the presence of photoreceptor outer segments that have been liberated from the subretinal space. In these situations, IOP can be elevated. Photoreceptor outer segments are phagocytosed by the endothelial cells in the trabecular meshwork and result in secondary open-angle glaucoma. This condition is called *Schwartz syndrome*.

Matsuo N, Takabatake M, Ueno H, et al. Photoreceptor outer segments in the aqueous humor and rhegmatogenous retinal detachment. *Am J Ophthalmol.* 1986;101:673–679.

Schwartz A. Chronic open angle glaucoma secondary to rhegmatogenous retinal detachment. *Am J Ophthalmol.* 1973;75:205–211.

Endogenous Nocardial Endophthalmitis

Nocardia asteroides *disease*

Although ocular involvement with *Nocardia asteroides* is rare, ocular disease may be the presenting complaint in this potentially lethal but treatable systemic disease characterized by pneumonia and disseminated abscesses. Ocular involvement occurs by hematogenous spread. Choroidal abscess has been described in heart transplant recipients. The responsible organism is commonly found in soil, and initial infection occurs by ingestion or inhalation. Symptoms of ocular infection caused by *N asteroides* may vary from the mild pain and redness of iridocyclitis to the severe pain and decreased vision of panophthalmitis. Findings range from an isolated, unilateral chorioretinal mass with minimal vitritis to diffuse iridocyclitis with cell and flare, vitritis, and multiple choroidal abscesses with overlying retinal detachment (Fig 12-1).

Diagnosis can be established with a culture of the organism taken from tissue or fluid, by vitreous aspiration for Gram stain and culture, or occasionally by enucleation and microscopic identification of organisms. Treatment of systemic *N asteroides* infection is systemic sulfonamide for 6 weeks in immunologically competent patients and up to 1 year in immunosuppressed patients.

Davitt B, Gehrs K, Bowers T. Endogenous *Nocardia* endophthalmitis. *Retina*. 1998;18:71–73.

Endogenous Fungal Endophthalmitis

Endogenous fungal endophthalmitis due to *Candida*, *Aspergillus*, and *Coccidioides* can all be considered nonneoplastic masquerade syndromes since, in many patients, the condition can be mistaken for noninfectious uveitis and treated with corticosteroids alone. This usually worsens the clinical course of the disease, necessitating further investigation to establish the correct diagnosis. These conditions often require aggressive systemic and local therapy as well as surgical intervention.

Candida *endophthalmitis (ocular candidiasis)*—Candida albicans

Ocular inflammatory disease caused by *Candida albicans*, although still uncommon, has increased notably as a result of the widespread use of immunosuppressive therapy, hyperalimentation, and intravenous drugs. Rarely, *Candida* retinitis is seen in AIDS patients following intravenous drug use (Figs 12-2, 12-3). Endogenous *Candida* endophthalmitis occurs in 10%–37% of patients with candidemia if they are not receiving antifungal

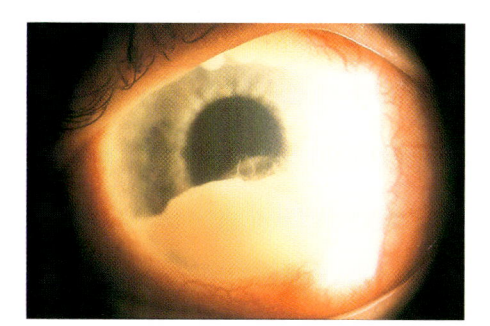

Figure 12-1 Hypopyon due to *Nocardia* endophthalmitis in a patient with rheumatoid arthritis. *(Photograph courtesy of Ramana S. Moorthy, MD.)*

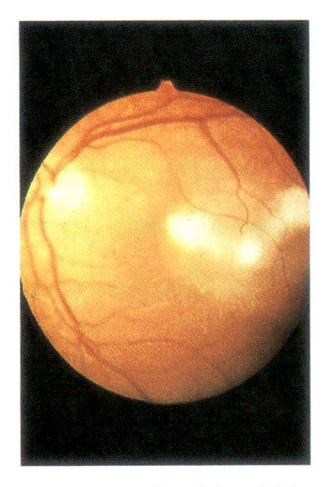

Figure 12-2 *Candida* retinitis.

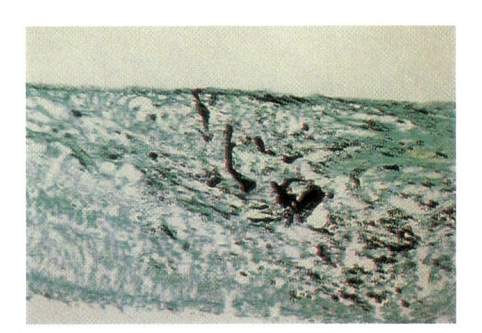

Figure 12-3 Pathological specimen of *Candida* retinitis. Note fungi *(black)* in the Gomori methenamine silver stain of the retina.

therapy. Ocular involvement drops to 3% in patients who are receiving treatment for their disease.

The organism spreads through metastasis to the choroid. Fungal replication results in secondary retinal and vitreous involvement. Symptoms of endogenous *Candida* endophthalmitis include decreased vision or perception of floaters, depending on the location of the lesions. Mimicking toxoplasmic choroiditis, posterior pole lesions appear yellow white with fluffy borders, ranging in size from small cotton-wool spots to several disc diameters wide. The lesions originate in the retina and result in exudation into the vitreous. Peripheral lesions may resemble pars planitis.

Diagnosis of endogenous *Candida* endophthalmitis can be confirmed by positive blood cultures obtained during candidemia. Recent advances in polymerase chain reaction assays allow detection of *C albicans* DNA in intraocular fluid. This method can be used to evaluate vitreous specimens obtained from pars plana vitrectomy in suspected cases. The physician should be alert to the possible diagnosis of candidiasis in hospitalized patients with indwelling intravenous catheters or those receiving hyperalimentation or systemic therapy with antibiotics, steroids, and antimetabolites. Symptomatic or newly diagnosed, untreated cases of candidemia should prompt examination for ocular involvement. These patients should undergo two dilated fundus examinations 1–2 weeks apart to detect metastatic ocular disease.

Treatment of endogenous *Candida* endophthalmitis includes intravenous, periocular, and intraocular administration of antifungal agents such as amphotericin B and ketoconazole. Oral flucytosine, fluconazole, or rifampin may be administered in addition to intravenous amphotericin B. If the infectious process breaks through the retina into the vitreous cavity, intravitreal antifungal agents and vitrectomy should be considered. Prompt treatment of peripherally located lesions promotes a favorable prognosis. However, early treatment of central lesions seldom salvages useful vision because of damage to central photoreceptors. Consultation with an infectious disease specialist may be extremely helpful.

> Brooks RG. Prospective study of *Candida* endophthalmitis in hospitalized patients with candidemia. *Arch Intern Med.* 1989;149:2226–2228.
> Essman TF, Flynn HW, Smiddy WE, et al. Treatment outcomes in a 10-year study of endogenous fungal endophthalmitis. *Ophthal Surg Lasers.* 1997;28:185–194.
> Hidalgo JA, Alangaden GJ, Eliot D, et al. Fungal endophthalmitis diagnosis by detection of *Candida albicans* DNA in intraocular fluid by use of species-specific polymerase chain reaction assay. *J Infect Dis.* 2000;181:1198–1201.
> Menezes AV, Sigesmund DA, Demajo WA, et al. Mortality of hospitalized patients with *Candida* endophthalmitis. *Arch Intern Med.* 1994;154:2093–2097.
> Rao NA, Hidayat AA. Endogenous mycotic endophthalmitis: variations in clinical and histopathologic changes in candidiasis compared with aspergillosis. *Am J Ophthalmol.* 2001;132:244–251.

Aspergillus flavus *and* fumigatus *endophthalmitis*

Endogenous *Aspergillus* endophthalmitis is a rare disorder associated with disseminated aspergillosis among patients with severe chronic pulmonary diseases or severe immunocompromise and with intravenous drug abuse. It is particularly common among patients following orthotopic liver transplantation. Rarely, *Aspergillus* endophthalmitis may occur in immunocompetent patients with no apparent predisposing factors.

Aspergillus species are found in soils and decaying vegetation. The spores of these ubiquitous saprophytic spore-forming molds become airborne and seed the lungs and paranasal sinuses of humans. Human exposure is very common, but infection is rare and depends on the virulence of the fungal pathogen and immunocompetence of the host. Ocular disease occurs via hematogenous dissemination of *Aspergillus* to the choroid.

Endogenous *Aspergillus* endophthalmitis results in rapid onset of pain and visual loss. A confluent yellowish infiltrate is seen in the macula beginning in the choroid and subretinal space. A hypopyon develops in the subretinal or subhyaloidal space (Fig 12-4A). Retinal hemorrhages, retinal vascular occlusions, and full-thickness retinal necrosis occur. The infection can spread to produce a dense vitritis and variable degrees of cells, flare,

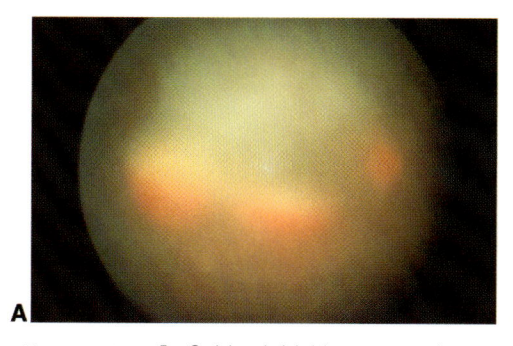

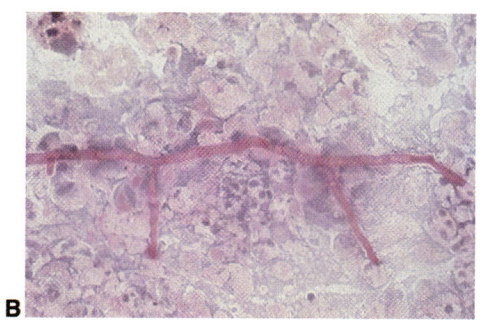

Figure 12-4 **A,** Subhyaloidal hypopyon due to endogenous *Aspergillus* endophthalmitis in an immunocompetent patient. **B,** Light micrograph shows branching hyphae of *Aspergillus fumigatus* (periodic acid–Schiff × 220). *(Reprinted with permission from Valluri S, Moorthy RS, Liggett PE, et al. Endogenous* Aspergillus *endophthalmitis in an immunocompetent individual.* Int Ophthalmol. *1993;17:131–135.)*

and hypopyon in the anterior chamber. The macular lesions heal to form a central atrophic scar.

The diagnosis of endogenous *Aspergillus* endophthalmitis is based on clinical findings combined with pars plana vitreous biopsy and cultures and Gram and Giemsa stains. Coexisting systemic aspergillosis can be a strong clue, especially among high-risk patients.

The differential diagnosis of endogenous *Aspergillus* endophthalmitis includes *Candida* endophthalmitis, cytomegalovirus retinitis, *Toxoplasma* retinochoroiditis, coccidioidomycotic choroiditis/endophthalmitis, and bacterial endophthalmitis.

Aspergillus endophthalmitis lesions are histologically angiocentric. Mixed acute (polymorphonuclear leukocytes) and chronic (lymphocytes and plasma cells) inflammatory cells infiltrate the infected areas of the choroid and retina. Hemorrhage is present in all retinal layers. Granulomas contain rare giant cells. Fungal hyphae may be seen spreading on the surface of Bruch's membrane without penetrating it. Polymorphonuclear leukocytes are present in the vitreous. Fungal hyphae are often surrounded by macrophages and lymphocytes, which form small vitreous abscesses (Fig 12-4B). In candidal endophthalmitis, the vitreous is the primary focus of infection, but in *Aspergillus* endophthalmitis, retinal and choroidal vessel invasion and subretinal/sub-RPE infection primarily occur.

Endogenous *Aspergillus* endophthalmitis must be treated aggressively with diagnostic and therapeutic pars plana vitrectomy combined with intravitreal injection of amphotericin B. Intravitreal corticosteroids may be used in conjunction with amphotericin B. Since most patients with endogenous *Aspergillus* endophthalmitis have disseminated aspergillosis, systemic treatment with intravenous amphotericin B is often required. Other systemic antifungals such as itraconazole, miconazole, fluconazole, and ketoconazole may also be used. Systemic aspergillosis is best managed by an infectious disease specialist.

Despite aggressive treatment, the visual prognosis is poor because of macular involvement. Final visual acuity is usually less than 20/200.

Ocular coccidioidomycosis

Coccidioides immitis is a dimorphic fungus that causes pulmonary and rarely disseminated visceral disease that sometimes involves the CNS. Ocular disease is extremely rare. Disseminated disease more commonly results in adnexal and phlyctenular conjunctival inflammation. Uveal involvement is still rarer, with fewer than 20 pathologically verified cases having been reported. Coccidioidal uveitis should be considered in the differential diagnosis of any patient with apparent idiopathic iritis who has lived or traveled through endemic areas of the American Southwest, specifically southern California and the San Joaquin Valley, northern Mexico, or Argentina.

Intraocular manifestations of coccidioidomycosis consist of iridocyclitis, iris granuloma (Fig 12-5), choroiditis, or chorioretinitis. One half of patients with ocular involvement have systemic disease, and complement fixation titers are often elevated (>1:32). The anterior segment and posterior segment are equally involved. With isolated anterior segment involvement, an anterior chamber tap may be useful. Culturing for the organism may delay diagnosis. The material from the anterior chamber tap may also be directly examined for coccidioidal organisms using the Papanicolaou stain. The differential diagnosis of coccidioidal uveitis includes *Candida, Aspergillus,* and *Histoplasma* endophthalmitis and tuberculous uveitis.

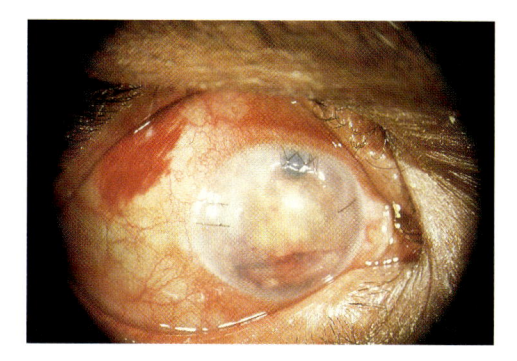

Figure 12-5 Coccidioidal iris granuloma in the pupil. This granuloma was biopsied and a peripheral iridectomy had just been performed because it was causing pupillary block and angle-closure glaucoma. *(Photograph courtesy of Ramana S. Moorthy, MD.)*

Histopathologically, *C immitis* evokes pyogenic, granulomatous, and mixed reactions. Intraocular lesions from the anterior segment usually demonstrate zonal granulomatous inflammation that involves the uvea and angle structure, and *Coccidioides* organisms are usually seen.

Intravenous amphotericin is the mainstay of treatment for intraocular coccidioidomycosis. Surgical debulking of anterior chamber granulomas, pars plana vitrectomy, and intraocular injections of amphotericin may be required. With systemic disease, much higher doses and a longer duration of intravenous amphotericin therapy may be needed. An infectious disease specialist is essential in the management of coccidioidomycosis. Despite aggressive treatment, ocular coccidioidomycosis carries a poor visual prognosis, with most eyes requiring enucleation because of pain and blindness.

Endogenous fungal endophthalmitis due to *Cryptococcus neoformans*, *Sporothrix schenckii*, and *Blastomyces dermatitidis* is less common than that due to *Candida* and *Aspergillus*.

Crump JR, Elner SG, Elner VM, et al. Cryptococcal endophthalmitis: case report and review. *Clin Infect Dis.* 1992;14:1069–1073.

Hunt KE, Glasgow BJ. *Aspergillus* endophthalmitis: an unrecognized endemic disease in orthotopic liver transplantation. *Ophthalmology.* 1996;103:757–767.

Moorthy RS, Sidikaro Y, Foos RY, et al. Coccidioidomycosis iridocyclitis. *Ophthalmology.* 1994;101:1923–1928.

Rodenbiker HT, Ganley JP. Ocular coccidioidomycosis. *Surv Ophthalmol.* 1980;24:263–290.

Safneck JR, Hogg GR, Napier LB. Endophthalmitis due to *Blastomyces dermatitidis*. Case report and review of the literature. *Ophthalmology.* 1990;97:212–216.

Valluri S, Moorthy RS, Liggett PE, et al. Endogenous *Aspergillus* endophthalmitis in an immunocompetent individual. *Int Ophthalmol.* 1993;17:131–135.

Weishaar PD, Flynn HW Jr, Murray TG, et al. Endogenous *Aspergillus* endophthalmitis: clinical features and treatment outcomes. *Ophthalmology.* 1998;105:57–65.

Witherspoon CD, Kuhn F, Owens SD, et al. Endophthalmitis due to *Sporothrix schenckii* after penetrating ocular injury. *Ann Ophthalmol.* 1990;22:385–388.

Neoplastic Masquerade Syndromes

Neoplastic masquerade syndromes may account for 2%–3% of all patients seen in the tertiary uveitis referral clinic. The vast majority of these are patients with intraocular involvement from primary CNS lymphoma.

Primary Central Nervous System Lymphoma

Nearly all (98%) primary CNS lymphomas (PCNSLs) are non-Hodgkin B-cell lymphomas. Approximately 2% are T-cell lymphomas. PCNSL mainly affects patients in their sixth to seventh decade of life, although PCNSL rarely occurs in children and adolescents. The incidence of PCNSL appears to be increasing and is projected to occur in 51 of 10 million immunocompetent patients.

Clinical features and findings

Approximately 25% of patients with PCNSL have ocular involvement. Approximately 15% may have ocular involvement alone. Fifteen percent may have ocular and visceral involvement. Approximately 60% have ocular and CNS involvement, and 4% have ocular, CNS, and visceral involvement. Sites of ocular involvement include the vitreous, retina, sub-RPE, or any combination thereof. The most common complaints of presenting patients are decreased vision and floaters.

Examination reveals spillover anterior chamber cells and a variable degree of vitritis, often severe. Retinal examination shows the characteristic retinal lesions. These often appear as creamy yellow subretinal infiltrates with overlying retinal pigment epithelial detachments (Fig 12-6). They can look like discrete white lesions from acute retinal necrosis, toxoplasmosis, frosted branch angiitis, or retinal arteriolar obstruction with coexisting multifocal chorioretinal scars and retinal vasculitis. These lesions vary in thickness from about 1 mm to 2 mm.

Many of these patients are mistakenly treated with systemic corticosteroids. This can improve the vitreous cellular infiltration, but the effect is not long-lasting and the uveitis often becomes resistant to steroid therapy. Immunosuppressive agents are then added in these situations. These immunosuppressive agents also reduce vitreous cells temporarily. This therapy also eventually meets with failure. Subsequently, a vitrectomy is often performed; the vitrectomy specimens are nondiagnostic because of the previous intensive

Figure 12-6 Primary CNS lymphoma. Fundus photograph of multifocal, subretinal pigment epithelial lesions. *(Photograph courtesy of E. Mitchel Opremcak, MD.)*

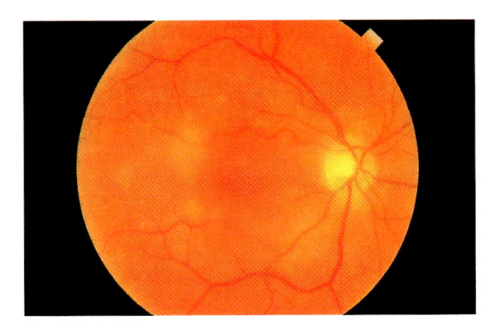

treatment. Diagnosis is much easier to make when retinal lesions are present because the lesions have a characteristic appearance (see Fig 12-6).

CNS signs may vary. Behavioral changes appear to be the single most frequent symptom reported, often at the time these patients are admitted for hospitalization. These behavioral changes occur because of the periventricular location of many of the CNS lesions in PCNSL. Other neurologic signs include heavy paresis, cerebellar signs, epileptic seizures, and cranial nerve palsies. Cerebrospinal fluid seeding of lymphoma cells occurs in 42% of patients with PCNSL. A new syndrome can also occur in which glaucoma, uveitis, and neurologic symptoms *(GUN syndrome)* are all associated together in PCNSL.

Ancillary tests

Ultrasonography shows choroidal thickening, vitreous debris, elevated chorioretinal lesions, and serous retinal detachment. Fluorescein angiography shows hypofluorescent areas due to blockage from sub-RPE tumor mass or from RPE clumping. Hyperfluorescent window defects may also be present from RPE atrophy from spontaneously resolved RPE infiltration. An unusual leopard spot pattern of alternating hyper- and hypofluorescence may also be noted.

MRI studies of the brain show isointense lesions on T1 and iso- to hyperintense lesions on T2. Computed tomography shows multiple diffuse periventricular lesions when no contrast is present. If intravenous contrast is used, these periventricular lesions may enhance.

Results of cerebrospinal fluid analysis are positive in one third of patients with PCNSL and show lymphoma cells.

Diagnostic testing

Tissue diagnosis is the most effective and accurate method of determining whether a patient has PCNSL. If lymphoma cells are found in the cerebrospinal fluid from a lumbar puncture, or if MRI demonstrates characteristic intracranial lesions, pars plana vitreous biopsy may not be necessary. However, the presence of vitreous cells of unidentifiable cause, especially in a patient over the age of 65, necessitates a vitreous biopsy. Usually this is performed via a pars plana vitrectomy. Ideally, 1 mL of undiluted vitreous sample should be obtained in a syringe that contains 3 mL of tissue culture medium to maximize cellular viability. In addition, a retinal biopsy, an aspirate of sub-RPE material, or both may also be obtained during vitrectomy. This approach may improve diagnostic yield when previous vitreous biopsies have been negative. The vitreous specimen should be fixed in an equal volume of 95% alcohol immediately after its removal from the eye. Samples stored in balanced salt solution will result in cellular degradation and loss of detail. Proper diagnosis requires an expert cytopathologist with experience in interpreting lymphomas.

Histopathology

Cyologic specimens obtained from the vitreous or subretinal space often show pleomorphic cells with hyperchromatic nuclei and an elevated nuclear/cytoplasmic ratio (Fig 12-7). The cytoplasm is very scant, and multiple irregular nucleoli may be seen. Necrotic cellular debris is present in the background. Equivocal vitreous biopsies may require

Figure 12-7 Vitreous aspirate showing mitotic figure and cellular atypia in large-cell lymphoma. *(Photograph courtesy of E. Mitchel Opremcak, MD.)*

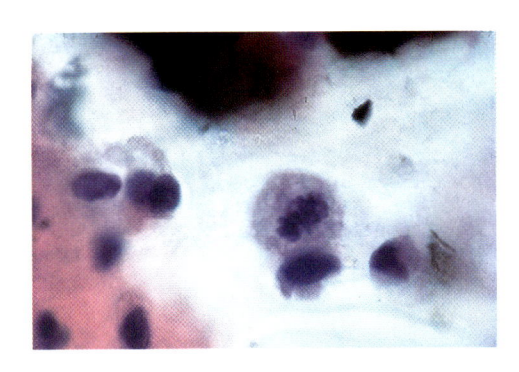

immunophenotypic or genetic testing. Immunophenotyping is used to establish clonality of B lymphocytes by demonstrating the presence of abnormal immunoglobulin κ or λ light chain predominance. This is performed by flow cytometry and immunohistochemistry. Monoclonal populations of cells are likely to be present in cases of PCNSL. Molecular diagnosis using genetic techniques relies on the fact that cancers such as PCNSL are clonal growths. As a result, gene translocations or oncogene translocations or gene rearrangements are often repeated in all of the cells in a given PCNSL. Polymerase chain reaction (PCR) techniques are invaluable in the detection of these oncogene translocations or gene rearrangements.

If diagnosis by vitreous aspiration or subretinal aspiration cannot be performed, either internal or external chorioretinal biopsy techniques may be used to aid in the diagnosis of PCNSL.

Treatment

Without treatment and supportive care, the prognosis of PCNSL is dismal. Median survival is 2–3 months with supportive care alone. However, the patient does not fare much better with surgical removal of CNS lesions. Median survival still remains in the range of 1–5 months with surgery alone. Even with disease isolated to the eye, prophylactic CNS treatment is warranted since approximately 56% of patients with ocular involvement eventually develop CNS involvement with PCNSL. Currently, a combination of chemotherapy and coned-down radiotherapy is advocated.

Investigators from the Memorial Sloan-Kettering Cancer Center have reported some success using high-dose methotrexate delivered intravenously along with intrathecal administration via Ommaya reservoir in combination with radiation therapy and intravenous cytarabine. In addition, local ocular treatment with repeated biweekly or weekly intravitreal methotrexate injections of 400 μg can also be used in conjunction with systemic treatment. The role of this treatment alone in isolated ocular disease has been studied and may be effective in controlling local disease. The regimen's effect on median survival compared to systemic treatment is not known. Based on the available information, chemotherapy alone is indicated for patients 60 years and older because of potential CNS toxicity from radiation; for patients younger than 60, combination radiation therapy and chemotherapy is preferred.

Prognosis

Despite the availability of multiple treatment modalities and regimens, the long-term prognosis for PCNSL remains poor. The longest median survival in various reports approaches 40 months with treatment. Factors that can influence outcome include age; neurologic functional classification level; single versus multiple lesions in the CNS; superficial cerebral, cerebellar hemispheric lesions versus deep nuclei/periventricular lesions; and Karnofsky performance status.

> Read RW, Zamir E, Rao NA. Neoplastic masquerade syndromes. *Surv Ophthalmol.* 2002; 47:81–124.
>
> Valluri S, Moorthy RS, Khan A, et al. Combination treatment of intraocular lymphoma. *Retina.* 1995;15:125–129.
>
> Whitcup SM, de Smet MD, Rubin BI, et al. Intraocular lymphoma. Clinical and histopathologic diagnosis. *Ophthalmology.* 1993;100:1399–1406.

Neoplastic Masquerade Syndromes Secondary to Systemic Lymphoma

Systemic lymphomas hematogenously spread to the choroid, to the subretinal space, into the vitreous, and occasionally into the anterior chamber. These entities often present with vitritis and creamy subretinal infiltrates of variable size, number, and extent. Retinal vasculitis, necrotizing retinitis, and diffuse choroiditis or uveal masses may also be present. All T-cell lymphomas (including mycosis fungoides, HTLV-1 lymphoma, systemic B-cell lymphoma, and Ki-1 lymphoma), Hodgkin disease, and primary intravascular lymphoma can present in this fashion. Reports of these entities are rare and scattered throughout the literature.

Neoplastic Masquerade Syndromes Secondary to Leukemia

Patients with leukemia may have retinal findings, including intraretinal hemorrhages, cotton-wool spots, white-centered hemorrhages, microaneurysms, and peripheral neovascularization. Rarely, leukemic cells may invade the vitreous cavity in the simulated vitritis. If the choroid is involved, exudative retinal detachment may be present and is angiographically similar to Vogt-Koyanagi-Harada disease. Leukemia may also present with a hypopyon/hyphema, iris heterochromia, or a pseudohypopyon, which can be gray-yellow.

> Kincaid MC, Green WR. Ocular and orbital involvement in leukemia. *Surv Ophthalmol.* 1983;27:211–232.

Neoplastic Masquerade Syndromes Secondary to Uveal Lymphoid Proliferations

The uveal tract may also be a site for lymphoid proliferations that can mimic chronic uveitis. These can range from benign reactive uveal lymphoid proliferations to frank lymphomas that may or may not be associated with systemic lymphomas. Patients with these conditions clinically may present with gradual painless unilateral or bilateral vision loss. Early stages show multifocal creamy choroidal lesions that may mimic inflammatory entities, including sarcoid uveitis or birdshot choroidopathy. Cystoid macular edema may be present. Anterior uveitis with acute symptoms of pain, redness, and photophobia may also be present. Glaucoma and elevated IOP are common. Angle structures may be infiltrated by lymphocytes resulting in elevation of IOP.

Clinical appearances may seem malignant even though these processes may be benign histopathologically. These intraocular processes may extend to the epibulbar area and may manifest as fleshy episcleral or conjunctival masses. These may be salmon pink. Unlike subconjunctival lymphomas, they are not mobile and are attached firmly to the sclera. These conditions should be differentiated from posterior scleritis as well as from uveal effusion syndrome. Needle aspiration biopsy and biopsy of extrascleral portions of the tumors can aid diagnosis. Biopsy specimens demonstrate mature lymphocytes and plasma cells that are quite different from those seen with PCNSL. Therapy with corticosteroids, radiation, or both has been used with variable results. Systemic and periocular corticosteroid therapy can result in rapid regression of the lesions, as can external beam radiation.

Jakobiec FA, Sacks E, Kronish JW, et al. Multifocal static creamy choroidal infiltrates. An early sign of lymphoid neoplasia. *Ophthalmology*. 1987;94:397–406.

Nonlymphoid Malignancies

Uveal melanoma

Approximately 5% of patients with uveal melanoma may present with ocular inflammation, including episcleritis, anterior or posterior uveitis, endophthalmitis, or panophthalmitis. Most of the tumors that present in this fashion are epithelioid cell or mixed cell choroidal melanoma. Ultrasonography can be very useful in the diagnosis of atypical cases because of the characteristic low internal reflectivity of these lesions. The management of uveal melanomas is discussed in BCSC Section 4, *Ophthalmic Pathology and Intraocular Tumors*.

Fraser DJ Jr, Font RL. Ocular inflammation and hemorrhage as initial manifestations of uveal malignant melanoma. Incidence and prognosis. *Arch Ophthalmol*. 1979;97:1311–1314.

Retinoblastoma

Approximately 1%–3% of retinoblastomas may present with inflammation. Patients are usually between 4 and 6 years of age at presentation. Most cases that present with inflammation are due to the relatively rare variant of diffuse infiltrating retinoblastoma. These cases can be diagnostically confusing because of the limited visibility of the fundus and the lack of calcification on radiography or ultrasonography. Patients may have conjunctival chemosis, pseudohypopyon, and vitritis. The pseudohypopyon typically shifts with changes in head position. The pseudohypopyon of retinoblastoma is usually white. Diagnostic aspiration of the aqueous humor may be required, but there is a significant risk of tumor spread through the needle tract. Histopathological examination shows round cells with hyperchromatic nuclei and scanty cytoplasm.

Bhatnagar R, Vine AK. Diffuse infiltrating retinoblastoma. *Ophthalmology*. 1991;98:1657–1661.

Juvenile xanthogranuloma

Juvenile xanthogranuloma is a histiocytic process affecting mainly the skin and eyes, and, rarely, viscera. Patients usually present before the age of 1 with characteristic skin lesions that are reddish yellow. Histopathological investigation shows large histiocytes with foamy cytoplasm and Touton giant cells containing fat. Ocular lesions can involve the iris, from which spontaneous hyphema may occur. Iris biopsy shows fewer foamy histiocytes and fewer Touton giant cells than a skin biopsy. Other ocular structures may be involved, but this is rare. If the skin of the eyelids is involved, the globe is usually spared. Intraocular lesions may respond to topical, periocular, or systemic corticosteroid therapy. Resistant cases may require local resection, radiation, or immunosuppressive therapy.

Zamir E, Rao NA, Krishnakumar S, et al. Juvenile xanthogranuloma masquerading as pediatric chronic uveitis: a clinicopathologic study. *Surv Ophthalmol.* 2001;46:164–171.

Metastatic Tumors

The most common intraocular malignancies in adults are metastatic tumors. The most common primaries include lung and breast cancer. Choroidal metastasis may be marked by vitritis, serous retinal detachment, and occasionally cystoid macular edema. These lesions are often bilateral and multifocal. Vitritis may be very mild.

Anterior uveal metastasis may present with cells in the aqueous humor, iris nodules, rubeosis iridis, and elevated IOP. Anterior chamber paracentesis may aid the diagnosis.

Retinal metastases are extremely rare. The most common primary cancers metastatic to the retina include cutaneous melanoma (the most common), followed by lung cancer, gastrointestinal cancer, and breast cancer. Metastatic tumors to the retina can present with vitreous cells. Metastatic melanoma often produces brown spherules in the retina, whereas other metastatic cancers are white to yellow and result in perivascular sheathing, simulating a retinal vasculitis or necrotizing retinitis. Vitreous biopsy and aspiration may be diagnostic if vitreous cells are present.

Bilateral Diffuse Uveal Melanocytic Proliferation

Bilateral diffuse uveal melanocytic tumors have been associated with systemic malignancy. Such tumors can be associated with rapid vision loss; cataracts; multiple pigmented and nonpigmented, placoid iris and choroidal nodules; and serous retinal detachments. This condition can mimic Vogt-Koyanagi-Harada disease. Histopathological investigation shows diffuse infiltration of the uveal tract by benign nevoid or spindle-shaped cells. Necrosis within the tumors may be present, and scleral involvement is common. The cause of this entity is unknown.

Treatment should be directed at finding and treating the underlying primary lesion.

Barr CC, Zimmerman LE, Curtin VT, et al. Bilateral diffuse melanocytic uveal tumors associated with systemic malignant neoplasms. A recently recognized syndrome. *Arch Ophthalmol.* 1982;100:249–255.

CHAPTER 13

Complications of Uveitis

Cataracts

Any eye with chronic or recurrent uveitis may develop cataract due to both the inflammation itself and the corticosteroids used to treat it. Cataract surgery should be considered whenever functional benefit is likely. See also BCSC Section 11, *Lens and Cataract*, for more information on many of the issues covered in this discussion.

Careful evaluation is necessary to ascertain how much the cataract is actually contributing to visual dysfunction, since visual loss in uveitis may stem from a variety of other ocular problems such as macular edema or vitritis. Sometimes a cataract precludes an adequate view of the posterior segment of the eye, and surgery can be justified to permit examination, diagnosis, and treatment of posterior segment abnormalities.

Studies have shown that extracapsular cataract extraction or phacoemulsification with posterior chamber IOL implantation effectively improves vision and is well tolerated in many eyes with uveitis, even over long periods. For example, excellent surgical and visual results have been reported for eyes with Fuchs heterochromic cyclitis. Cataract surgery in other types of uveitis—including idiopathic uveitis, pars planitis, and uveitis associated with sarcoidosis, herpes simplex virus, herpes zoster, syphilis, toxoplasmosis, and spondyloarthropathies—can be more problematic, although such surgery may also yield very good results.

Pars plana lensectomy/vitrectomy has been advocated for uveitis associated with JRA, although acceptable results have also been reported with combined phacoemulsification and vitrectomy. IOL implantation is in general contraindicated in children with JRA-associated iridocyclitis, but IOLs may be successful in selected adults with JRA whose inflammation has been adequately controlled.

Extracapsular cataract extraction and phacoemulsification may be more challenging in uveitic eyes than in noninflamed eyes, and intraocular inflammation should be controlled before surgery is performed. It is imperative to eliminate anterior chamber cells and to have the eye quiet without flare-ups of inflammation for at least 3 months prior to cataract surgery. Approximately 1 week before surgery, oral corticosteroids (0.5–1.0 mg/kg per day) and hourly topical corticosteroids should be administered. These may be tapered after surgery, depending on the postoperative inflammatory response. Cataract surgery in the uveitic eye may be more challenging than in the nonuveitic eye. Extensive posterior synechiae and pupillary miosis may require pupil stretching, sphincterotomies, or use of iris retractors. A fibrotic anterior capsule may be more difficult to open with a capsulorrhexis. The zonules may be inherently weak, which may make phacoemulsification and lens implantation challenging or impossible.

Nucleus extraction is performed in the usual manner. If logistically possible, phacoemulsification may be the preferred alternative for nucleus removal. Capsulorrhexis in conjunction with phacoemulsification may minimize the risk of postoperative posterior synechiae and may facilitate implantation of the IOL haptics in the capsular bag. Cortical cleanup should be meticulous. Extracapsular cataract extraction or phacoemulsification can be done in conjunction with pars plana vitrectomy if clinical or ultrasonic examination suggests the presence of substantial vision-limiting vitreous debris. Perioperative immunosuppressive agents (eg, topical, subconjunctival, and oral corticosteroids), other immunosuppressives, or both should be administered.

Visual compromise following extracapsular cataract extraction with posterior chamber lens implantation in patients with uveitis is usually attributed to posterior segment abnormalities, most commonly cystoid macular edema. The postoperative course may also be complicated by recurrence or exacerbation of uveitis. The incidence of posterior capsule opacification is higher in uveitic eyes, leading to earlier use of Nd:YAG laser capsulotomy. In some uveitic conditions such as pars planitis, inflammatory debris may accumulate and membranes may form on the surface of the IOL, necessitating frequent Nd:YAG laser procedures. On occasion, posterior chamber IOLs have been removed from these eyes. The use of surface-modified IOLs has also been advocated to minimize deposit formation on the optics. Heparin-surface-modified intraocular lenses have been shown to have fewer surface deposits than polymethylmethacrylate (PMMA) lenses for up to 1 year after cataract extraction. Among patients with uveitis, the frequency of postoperative posterior synechiae formation and cystoid macular edema appears similar with both PMMA and heparin-surface-modified lenses. Frequent follow-up, a high index of suspicion, and aggressive immunosuppressive treatment of these complications optimize short- and long-term visual results.

> Flynn HW Jr, Davis JL, Culbertson WW. Pars plana lensectomy and vitrectomy for complicated cataracts in juvenile rheumatoid arthritis. *Ophthalmology.* 1988;95:1114–1119.
>
> Foster CS. Cataract surgery in the patient with uveitis. In: *Focal Points: Clinical Modules for Ophthalmologists* San Francisco: American Academy of Ophthalmology; 1994;12:4.
>
> Foster CS, Barrett F. Cataract development and cataract surgery in patients with juvenile rheumatoid arthritis–associated iridocyclitis. *Ophthalmology.* 1993;100:809–817.
>
> Foster CS, Fong LP, Singh G. Cataract surgery and intraocular lens implantation in patients with uveitis. *Ophthalmology.* 1989;96:281–288.
>
> Foster RE, Lowder CY, Meisler DM, et al. Combined extracapsular cataract extraction, posterior chamber intraocular lens implantation, and pars plana vitrectomy. *Ophthalmic Surg.* 1993;24:446–452.
>
> Foster RE, Lowder CY, Meisler DM, et al. Extracapsular cataract extraction and posterior chamber intraocular lens implantation in uveitis patients. *Ophthalmology.* 1992;99:1234–1241.
>
> Kaufman AH, Foster CS. Cataract extraction in patients with pars planitis. *Ophthalmology.* 1993;100:1210–1217.
>
> Krishna R, Meisler DM, Lowder CY, et al. Long-term follow-up of extracapsular cataract extraction and posterior chamber intraocular lens implantation in patients with uveitis. *Ophthalmology.* 1998;105:1765–1769.

Probst LE, Holland EJ. Intraocular lens implantation in patients with juvenile rheumatoid arthritis. *Am J Ophthalmol.* 1996;122:161–170.

Tabbara KF, Al-Kaff AS, Al-Rajhi AA, et al. Heparin surface-modified intraocular lenses in patients with inactive uveitis or diabetes. *Ophthalmology.* 1998;105:843–845.

Trocme SD, Li H. Effect of heparin-surface-modified intraocular lenses on postoperative inflammation after phacoemulsification: a randomized trial in a United States patient population. Heparin-Surface-Modified Lens Study Group. *Ophthalmology.* 2000;107:1031–1037.

Glaucoma

Secondary glaucoma is a well-recognized complication of uveitis. Elevated IOP may be acute, chronic, or recurrent. In eyes with long-term ciliary body inflammation, the IOP may fluctuate between abnormally high and low values. Numerous morphologic, cellular, and biochemical alterations occur in the uveitic eye that cause uveitic glaucoma and ocular hypertension (Table 13-1). Successful management of uveitic glaucoma requires the identification and treatment of each of these contributing factors. See also BCSC Section 10, *Glaucoma.*

Inflammatory open-angle glaucoma occurs when the trabecular meshwork is inflamed or blocked by inflammatory cells and debris as commonly occurs with infectious causes of uveitis, such as *Toxoplasma* retinitis, acute retinal necrosis, and herpes simplex and varicella-zoster iridocyclitis. This type of glaucoma usually responds to topical cycloplegics, corticosteroids, and specific treatment of the infectious agent.

Chronic outflow obstruction in anterior chamber inflammation may be caused by peripheral anterior synechiae as well as by direct damage to the trabecular meshwork. Common examples of these mechanisms are chronic iridocyclitis associated with JRA, sarcoidosis, and Fuchs heterochromic iridocyclitis. Initial treatment is with topical and oral glaucoma medications such as carbonic anhydrase inhibitors, β-blockers, and α-agonists. However, parasympathomimetic medications should be avoided. The β-blocker metipranolol (OptiPranolol) has been associated with granulomatous intraocular inflammation, and it is possible that the new agent latanoprost (Xalatan) may also provoke inflammation, especially in eyes with a history of anterior uveitis.

When medical management fails, glaucoma filtering surgery is indicated, although standard trabeculectomy may have a greater risk of failure in these eyes. Results may be improved by using 5-fluorouracil or mitomycin-C with intensive topical corticosteroids. Trabeculodialysis, a modified goniotomy, and laser sclerostomy have also been suggested for treatment of uveitic glaucomas. Some eyes require aqueous drainage devices. Cyclodestructive procedures may worsen ocular inflammation and lead to hypotony and phthisis bulbi. Laser trabeculoplasty should be avoided in eyes with active intraocular inflammation or iris neovascularization.

Formation of posterior synechiae may result in pupillary block and iris bombé with acute secondary peripheral angle closure. This condition occasionally occurs in patients with chronic granulomatous iridocyclitis associated with sarcoidosis or Vogt-Koyanagi-Harada disease and in those with acute recurrent nongranulomatous iridocyclitis, as is seen with ankylosing spondylitis. Peripheral iridotomy with the Nd:YAG or argon laser results in resolution of the bombé and angle closure if performed before permanent peripheral synechiae form. Iridotomies should be multiple and as large as possible. Con-

Table 13-1 Pathogenesis of Uveitic Glaucoma

I. Cellular and biochemical alterations of aqueous in uveitis
   A. Inflammatory cells
   B. Protein
   C. Prostaglandins
   D. Inflammatory mediators (cytokines) and toxic agents (oxygen free radicals)
II. Morphologic changes in anterior chamber angle
   A. Closed angle
      1. Primary angle-closure glaucoma
      2. Secondary angle-closure glaucoma
         a. Posterior synechiae and pupillary block
         b. Peripheral anterior synechiae (PAS)
            i. PAS secondary to inflammation
            ii. PAS secondary to iris neovascularization
            iii. PAS secondary to prolonged iris bombé
         c. Forward rotation of ciliary body (due to inflammation)
   B. Open angle
      1. Primary open-angle glaucoma
      2. Secondary open-angle glaucoma
         a. Aqueous misdirection
         b. Mechanical blockage of trabecular meshwork
            i. Serum components (proteins)
            ii. Precipitates (cells, cellular debris)
         c. Trabeculitis (trabecular dysfunction)
         d. Damage to trabeculum and endothelium from chronic inflammation
         e. Corticosteroid-induced glaucoma
   C. Combined-mechanism glaucoma

siderable inflammation can be anticipated following laser iridotomy procedures in these eyes. Intensive topical corticosteroid and cycloplegic therapy is given following the procedure. Surgical iridotomy may be indicated if laser iridotomy is not successful.

Topical periocular and oral corticosteroid therapy for uveitis may produce a steroid-induced elevation in IOP, which may be difficult to distinguish from other causes of glaucoma in uveitis. This IOP rise may be avoided with a less potent steroid preparation, a less frequent administration schedule, or both. Fluorometholone or rimexolone may be less likely to cause a corticosteroid-induced IOP elevation but may also be less effective in controlling intraocular inflammation than other topical ocular corticosteroid preparations. If these measures do not reduce intraocular pressure and further optic nervehead damage, medical and possibly surgical treatment of the glaucoma may be required.

In many cases of uveitic glaucoma, multiple mechanisms may be responsible. Treatment should be aimed at controlling the inflammation and IOP through a multimodal approach of both medical and surgical therapy aimed at each of the responsible mechanisms.

Hill RA, Nguyen QH, Baerveldt G, et al. Trabeculectomy and Molteno implantation for glaucomas associated with uveitis. *Ophthalmology.* 1993;100:903–908.

Moorthy RS, Mermoud A, Baerveldt G, et al. Glaucoma associated with uveitis. *Surv Ophthalmol.* 1997;41:361–394.

Panek WC, Holland GN, Lee DA, et al. Glaucoma in patients with uveitis. *Br J Ophthalmol.* 1990;74:223–227.

Patel NP, Patel KH, Moster MR. Metipranolol-associated nongranulomatous anterior uveitis. *Am J Ophthalmol.* 1997;123:843–844.

Patitsas CJ, Rockwood EJ, Meisler DM, et al. Glaucoma filtering surgery with postoperative 5-fluorouracil in patients with intraocular inflammatory disease. *Ophthalmology.* 1992; 99:594–599.

Watanabe TM, Hodes BL. Bilateral anterior uveitis associated with a brand of metipranolol. *Arch Ophthalmol.* 1997;115:421–422.

Hypotony

Hypotony in uveitis is usually caused by decreased aqueous production from the ciliary body and may follow intraocular surgery in patients with uveitis. Acute inflammation of the ciliary body may cause temporary hyposecretion, whereas chronic ciliary body damage results in permanent hypotony. Serous choroidal detachment often accompanies hypotony and complicates management.

Hypotony usually responds to intensive corticosteroid and cycloplegic therapy, although prolonged choroidal effusions may require surgical drainage. In eyes with ciliary body traction from a cyclitic membrane, pars plana membranectomy may restore normal pressure. In select cases, vitrectomy and intraocular silicone oil may help maintain ocular anatomy and IOP.

Cystoid Macular Edema

Cystoid macular edema is a common cause of visual loss in eyes with uveitis. Therapy that reduces intraocular inflammation in general often has beneficial effects. Nonspecific therapy includes topical, periocular, and oral corticosteroids as well as oral and topical NSAIDs. Oral acetazolamide, 500 mg daily, has been effective in some patients. Eyes with chronic vitritis occasionally respond to pars plana vitrectomy or other systemic immunosuppressive therapy. See also BCSC Section 12, *Retina and Vitreous*.

Farber MD, Lam S, Tessler HH, et al. Reduction of macular oedema by acetazolamide in patients with chronic iridocyclitis: a randomised prospective crossover study. *Br J Ophthalmol.* 1994;78:4–7.

Jennings T, Rusin MM, Tessler HH, et al. Posterior sub-Tenon's injections of corticosteroids in uveitis patients with cystoid macular edema. *Jpn J Ophthalmol.* 1988;32:385–391.

Vitreous Opacification and Vitritis

Permanent vitreous opacification affecting vision occasionally occurs in uveitis, particularly in eyes with toxoplasma retinitis and pars planitis. In other cases of vitritis, the diagnosis is uncertain. Pars plana vitrectomy may be therapeutic or diagnostic in eyes with vitritis. This procedure can be used both to debride vitreous and to obtain a vitreous sample that may be studied by culture, stains, and cytology to determine the cause of the vitritis.

Retinal Detachment

Pars planitis and posterior uveitis occasionally cause a rhegmatogenous or tractional retinal detachment. Repair is often complicated by vitreous organization and poor visualization. Scleral buckling with cryoretinopexy is still useful in cases of retinal detachment associated with pars planitis. Acute retinal necrosis and cytomegalovirus retinitis frequently lead to retinal detachments that are difficult to repair because of multiple, large, and posterior retinal breaks. Pars plana vitrectomy and endolaser treatment with internal gas or silicone oil tamponade may be required to repair the detachment, remove epiretinal membranes, or both.

> Freeman WR, Friedberg DN, Berry C, et al. Risk factors for development of rhegmatogenous retinal detachment in patients with cytomegalovirus retinitis. *Am J Ophthalmol.* 1993; 116:713–720.
>
> Kuppermann BD, Flores-Aguilar M, Quiceno JI, et al. A masked prospective evaluation of outcome parameters for cytomegalovirus-related retinal detachment surgery in patients with acquired immune deficiency syndrome. *Ophthalmology.* 1994;101:46–55.
>
> Nussenblatt RB, Whitcup SM, Palestine AG. *Uveitis: Fundamentals and Clinical Practice.* 2nd ed. St Louis: Mosby; 1996.
>
> Sternberg P Jr, Han DP, Yeo JH, et al. Photocoagulation to prevent retinal detachment in acute retinal necrosis. *Ophthalmology.* 1988;95:1389–1393.

Retinal and Choroidal Neovascularization

Retinal neovascularization may develop in any chronic uveitic condition but is particularly common in pars planitis, sarcoid panuveitis, and retinal vasculitis of various causes, including Eales disease. Any condition that results in retinal capillary nonperfusion and ischemia can lead to retinal neovascularization on the disc or elsewhere. Treatment is directed first toward reduction of inflammation with corticosteroids and/or immunosuppressive agents and then scatter laser photocoagulation in the ischemic areas and associated watershed zones.

Choroidal neovascularization (CNV) can develop in posterior uveitis and panuveitis. A disruption of Bruch's membrane from choroidal inflammation and the presence of inflammatory cytokines that promote angiogenesis results in CNV in such cases. The prevalence of CNV varies among different entities. It can occur in up to 10% of patients with Vogt-Koyanagi-Harada disease. Patients present with metamorphopsia and scotoma of rapid onset. Diagnosis is based on clinical and angiographic findings. Treatment should be directed toward reducing inflammation as well as on anatomical ablation of the CNV. Focal laser photocoagulation of peripapillary and extrafoveal CNV may be performed. The treatment of subfoveal CNV is controversial. Corticosteroids and immunosuppressives alone may be used in an attempt to cause involution of CNV. If these agents alone do not work, pars plana vitrectomy and subfoveal CNV extraction may be considered.

> Kuo IC, Cunningham ET. Ocular neovascularization in patients with uveitis. *Int Ophthalmol Clin.* 2000;40:111–126.
>
> Moorthy RS, Chong LP, Smith RE, et al. Subretinal neovascular membranes in Vogt-Koyanagi-Harada syndrome. *Am J Ophthalmol.* 1993;116:164–170.

CHAPTER 14

Ocular Involvement in AIDS

Acquired immunodeficiency syndrome (AIDS) is the first pandemic since the first half of the 20th century. This syndrome, first described in 1981 in Los Angeles, is now thought to be a new infection of humans that originated in central Africa, perhaps in the 1950s. From there, it probably spread to the Caribbean and then to the United States, Europe, and other parts of the world. This syndrome is caused by a retrovirus commonly known as *human immunodeficiency virus (HIV)*.

The HIV epidemic has now entered its third decade, with new cases steadily being reported around the world. Although the infection was recognized initially in the United States, its spread continues to increase at an alarming rate, particularly in countries with large populations and areas of poverty such as India and Thailand and in many countries of sub-Saharan Africa. It is estimated that more than 40 million people are known to be infected with HIV worldwide. Most people with HIV/AIDS live in impoverished countries, particularly in those countries with high rates of sexually transmitted diseases, which are known to be important cofactors in the transmission of HIV. The proportion of new cases involving homosexual and bisexual men is dropping, whereas the proportion of new HIV infections in intravenous drug users, women, minorities, and children is rising. The World Health Organization estimates that 3 million children under the age of 15 and 11.8 million young adults 15–24 years old are now infected worldwide.

During the first decade of the HIV epidemic, it became clear that aggressive educational programs could reduce the transmission of HIV. This mass education had a positive influence on changing high-risk sexual behavior in the United States and other parts of the industrialized world. HIV-infected persons now live significantly longer, and the quality of their lives has also been improved by the introduction of various antiviral agents and drugs that reduce morbidity and mortality from the myriad opportunistic infections that occur so frequently in the late stages of HIV infection. However, a cure for this deadly disease is nowhere near. But although HIV infection is not yet curable, it is now recognized to be a manageable, albeit chronic and severe, medical condition. Moreover, if HIV infection is detected prior to the development of symptoms, prophylactic administration of the newer anti-HIV agents can have a significant beneficial effect on the overall course of the disease.

Cunningham ET Jr, Belfort R. *HIV/AIDS and the Eye: A Global Perspective.* Ophthalmology Monograph 15. San Francisco: American Academy of Ophthalmology; 2002.

Virology of HIV

HIV is a retrovirus that is a member of the *Lentivirinae* subfamily. Currently, two lentiviruses are known to infect humans:

- HIV-1, the more prevalent, is seen worldwide
- HIV-2 is identified primarily in western Africa

HIV-2 virus shares roughly 40% homology in nucleotide sequence with HIV-1 and about 75% homology with simian immunodeficiency virus.

HIV-1 and HIV-2 viruses are each approximately 100 nm in diameter. The virion has a cylindrical nucleocapsid. This capsid contains the single-stranded RNA and viral enzymes, including proteinase, integrase, and reverse transcriptase. Surrounding the capsid is a lipid envelope, which is derived from the infected host cell. This envelope contains virus-encoded glycoproteins. The viral genome contains three structural genes: *gag, pol,* and *env*. HIV-1 and HIV-2 are genetically similar in the *gag* and *pol* regions; the *env* regions, however, are different, resulting in differences in the envelope glycoproteins of these viruses. Such heterogeneity among these viruses leads to specific immune responses and necessitates different HIV-1 and HIV-2 immune assays or Western blot procedures for serologic diagnosis. In addition to the three structural genes, HIV contains six regulatory genes: *tat, rev, nef, vif, vpr,* and *vpu*. Two of these regulatory genes *(tat* and *rev)* are essential for virus replication. HIV isolates show marked heterogeneity in the *env* and the *nef* genes, with the following results:

- Differing tissue and cell tropisms
- Variations in pathogenesis
- Disparate responses to therapy
- Potential challenges in developing a broadly cross-reactive protective vaccine

This viral heterogeneity exists from continent to continent, from one infected individual to another, and even within the same infected host. Causes of this heterogeneity may include spontaneous mutation of the virus, the frequent error rate of the reverse transcriptase enzyme, and possibly antiviral therapy. See also BCSC Section 2, *Fundamentals and Principles of Ophthalmology,* Part III, Genetics.

Pathogenesis

Initial events in HIV infection include attachment of the virus to a distinct group of T cells and monocytes/macrophages that display a membrane antigen complex known as *CD4*. However, other molecules on these cells may also play a role in the attachment of HIV, particularly chemokine receptors such as CCR5 and CXCR4. After attachment, the lipid membrane of the virus fuses with the target cell, allowing entry of the viral core into host cell cytoplasm. This viral core is subsequently uncoated and transcribed by reverse transcriptase enzyme, resulting in a complementary strand of DNA. The action of cellular enzymes transforms this DNA into the typical double-stranded form that subsequently enters the cell nucleus.

Once intranuclear, the proviral DNA integrates into the genome of the host cell by means of a viral endonuclease. This host cell can be either latently or actively infected. If latently infected, no viral RNA is produced, and a productive infection may not develop. If actively infected, however, the cell may produce mature virions by transcription of proviral DNA. This transcription also generates messenger RNA (mRNA). In the cytoplasm, mRNA is translated into HIV-specific structural proteins that are integrated with the viral core particles.

These assembled virus particles then migrate to the plasma membrane of the infected cell. The virus undergoes final maturation by a process of reverse endocytosis (budding) at the plasma membrane. Subsequent dissemination of the virus occurs either through free infectious particles that are released by the budding process or, more likely, by cell-to-cell transfer.

The initial target cells of HIV—namely, $CD4^+$ helper T cells and macrophages—show different cytopathic effects. The T cells gradually become fewer as the virus replicates. Helper T cells are known to play a pivotal role in immunologic response, and their decrease in number leads to immune deficiency and subsequent secondary opportunistic infections (see Part I, Immunology, of this volume). In contrast, the infected macrophages rarely undergo lysis or decrease in number. These circulating infected cells harbor the HIV and may disseminate it throughout the body. HIV alters the immune-related functions of these infected monocytes/macrophages in the following ways:

- Decreased migration response to chemoattractants
- Defective intracellular killing of various microorganisms such as *Toxoplasma gondii* and *Candida* spp
- Reduced expression of class II MHC molecules, which impairs the processing and presentation of antigen to helper T cells
- Excessive production by the macrophages of tumor necrosis factor–α, which leads to dementia, wasting syndrome, and unexplained fever

Weiss RA. How does HIV cause AIDS? *Science.* 1993;260:1273–1279.

Natural History

Although the illness that results from HIV infection differs from one individual to another, various predictable stages ultimately lead to death. In general, infected persons initially experience an acute primary infection followed by a relatively asymptomatic infection that can include generalized lymphadenopathy. This progresses to symptomatic disease associated with progressive decline in helper T cells and eventually to advanced HIV disease, with the development of opportunistic infections, malignancies, or both. This advanced stage is what was first recognized as AIDS. These AIDS-defining illnesses are summarized in Table 14-1, which represents the 1993 Centers for Disease Control and Prevention (CDC) revised classification system for HIV infection and AIDS.

The acute HIV infection usually lasts for about 1–2 weeks and is characterized by symptoms typical of a nonspecific viral illness. Patients then enter an asymptomatic phase of variable duration, from 2 to more than 10 years. During this phase, the CD4 lym-

Table 14-1 1993 Revised Classification System for HIV Infection and AIDS-Defining Illnesses

CD4+ T Lymphocyte Categories

Category 1: >500 cells/mm^3
Category 2: 200–499 cells/mm^3
Category 3: <200 cells/mm^3

Clinical Categories of HIV Infection

Category A: One or more of the following conditions, but no conditions in category B or C:
  Asymptomatic HIV infection
  Persistent generalized lymphadenopathy
  Acute (primary) HIV infection

Category B: Symptomatic conditions in an HIV-infected adolescent or adult that are not included in category C (AIDS-defining illnesses) and that meet at least one of the following criteria:
  (1) the conditions are attributed to HIV infection or are indicative of a defect in cell-mediated immunity or
  (2) the conditions are considered by physicians to have a clinical course or to require management that is complicated by HIV infection

  Examples of conditions in category B include, but are not limited to
    Bacillary angiomatosis *(Bartonella henselae, B quintana)*
    Candidiasis, oropharyngeal (thrush)
    Candidiasis, vulvovaginal; persistent, frequent, or poorly responsive to therapy
    Cervical dysplasia (moderate or severe)/cervical carcinoma in situ
    Constitutional symptoms, such as fever (38.5°C) or diarrhea lasting >1 month
    Hairy leukoplakia, oral
    Herpes zoster (shingles), involving at least two distinct episodes or more than one dermatome
    Idiopathic thrombocytopenic purpura
    Listeriosis
    Pelvic inflammatory disease, particularly if complicated by tubo-ovarian abscess
    Peripheral neuropathy

Category C (AIDS): Includes the clinical conditions listed below *(AIDS-defining illnesses):*
  Candidiasis of bronchi, trachea, or lungs
  Candidiasis, esophageal
  Cervical cancer, invasive*
  Coccidioidomycosis, disseminated or extrapulmonary
  Cryptococcosis, extrapulmonary
  Cryptosporidiosis, chronic intestinal (>1 month's duration)
  Cytomegalovirus disease (other than liver, spleen, or nodes)
  Cytomegalovirus retinitis (with loss of vision)
  Encephalopathy, HIV-related
  Herpes simplex: chronic ulcer(s) (>1 month's duration), or bronchitis, pneumonitis, or esophagitis
  Histoplasmosis, disseminated or extrapulmonary
  Isosporiasis, chronic intestinal (>1 month's duration)
  Kaposi sarcoma
  Lymphoma, Burkitt (or equivalent term)
  Lymphoma, immunoblastic (or equivalent term)
  Lymphoma, primary, of brain
  Mycobacterium avium complex or *M kansasii,* disseminated or extrapulmonary
  Mycobacterium tuberculosis, any site (pulmonary* or extrapulmonary)
  Mycobacterium, other species or unidentified species, disseminated or extrapulmonary
  Pneumocystis carinii pneumonia

(Continues)

Table 14-1 **1993 Revised Classification System for HIV Infection and AIDS-Defining Illnesses (Continued)**

Category C (continued)
  Pneumonia, recurrent*
  Progressive multifocal leukoencephalopathy
  Salmonella septicemia, recurrent
  Toxoplasmosis of brain
  Wasting syndrome due to HIV

* Added in the 1993 expansion of the AIDS surveillance case definition. In addition, a CD4+ T lymphocyte count of <200/mm³ or a CD4+ T lymphocyte percentage of total lymphocytes <14 is now considered an AIDS-defining condition.

(Data from the Centers for Disease Control. 1993 revised classification system for HIV infection and expanded surveillance case definition for AIDS among adolescents and adults. *MMWR*. 1992;41:1–19. Reproduced with permission from Gold JWM. The diagnosis and management of HIV infection. In: *Med Clin North Am*. Philadelphia: Saunders; 1996;80:1286.)

phocyte count varies from about 200 to 750 cells/mm³ (CD4 counts in immunocompetent adults vary from 600 to 1500 cells/mm³). Advanced HIV disease may last for up to 3 years; during this stage, the CD4 cells decrease to less than 200 cells/mm³.

Transmission

Transmission of HIV occurs predominantly by sexual contact, by parenteral (IV drug use) or mucous membrane exposure to contaminated blood or blood products, and perinatally. HIV has been isolated from blood, semen, saliva, cerebrospinal fluid, tears, breast milk, amniotic fluid, vaginal secretions, cervical cells, and bronchoalveolar lavage fluid. A 1997 study broke down the transmission of HIV:

- Sexual intercourse accounted for 70% of cases
- Intravenous drug use accounted for 27% of cases
- Blood transfusions accounted for 2%–3% of cases
- Perinatal transmission accounted for about 1% of cases

There are rare instances in which HIV has been transmitted through transplantation of organs such as the heart, liver, kidney, bone, or pancreas. No cases of HIV transmission have been reported from corneal transplantation.

Diagnosis

Laboratory investigations are essential to establish the diagnosis of HIV infection, which depends on demonstration of virus-specific antibodies by enzyme-linked immunosorbent assay (ELISA) and Western blot, viral antigen by enzyme immunoassay, direct isolation of HIV from the blood by culture, or detection of HIV nucleic acid by polymerase chain reaction (PCR). Enzyme immunoassays such as ELISA are the most widely used method for screening individuals for antibody to HIV or for direct detection of HIV antigen. The specificity and sensitivity of the commercially available HIV antibody kits (ELISA) are generally in excess of 95%. However, even though ELISA is a highly sensitive and specific test, false-positive results do occur. Mainly to minimize the reporting of false-positive results, Western blot analysis is used to confirm the results of ELISA. The Western blot assay has the advantage of direct visualization of the antibodies directed to specific major proteins of HIV. The additional investigations such as PCR and viral P24 antigen detection are usually employed only when the immunoassays do not provide clearly positive results or in testing seronegative persons who are at high risk.

Management of HIV Infection

Systemic Conditions

As the number of HIV-infected persons increases throughout the world, particularly in impoverished countries, it is important that physicians in these countries learn how to manage the viral infection and prevent the complications associated with this deadly disease. The prevention of complications involves not only antiretroviral therapy and prophylactic antimicrobial agents but also immunization (eg, hepatitis B, influenza, and other vaccines) and early disease detection. Progression of the infection leads to deterioration of the protective immune function, and symptoms such as fatigue, night sweats, malaise, fever, and weight loss will develop. Although thorough clinical examination provides some clues as to the stage of HIV infection, measurement of T lymphocyte subsets, particularly absolute CD4 counts, has become a fundamental aspect of staging HIV infection:

- CD4 counts between 200 and 500 cells/mm^3 are associated with oral candidiasis, Kaposi sarcoma, lymphoma, and herpes zoster ophthalmicus
- Counts between 150 and 200 cells/mm^3 are associated with disseminated tuberculosis, pneumocystosis, and toxoplasmosis
- Counts less than 100 cells/mm^3 are associated with cytomegalovirus (CMV) infection and *Mycobacterium avium* complex

Cunningham ET Jr, Margolis TP. Ocular manifestations of HIV infection. *N Engl J Med.* 1998;339:236–244.

Medical therapy

Three broad classes of anti-HIV agents have been approved by the Food and Drug Administration (FDA): nucleoside analogues, nonnucleoside reverse-transcriptase inhibitors, and protease inhibitors (Table 14-2). All of these are nucleoside analogues that work through inhibition of the reverse transcriptase enzyme. These agents are all associated with toxic side effects, including severe bone marrow suppression, peripheral neuropathy, and gastrointestinal irritation. The combined use of three or more of these agents is referred to as *highly active antiretroviral therapy (HAART)*.

Havlir DV, Lange JM. New antiretrovirals and new combinations. *AIDS.* 1998;12:S165–S174.

Table 14-2	Antiretroviral Agents

Nucleoside analogues
  Zidovudine (ZDV, AZT, Retrovir)
  Didanosine (ddl, Videx)
  Zalcitabine (ddC, Hivid)
  Stavudine (d4T, Zerit)
  Lamivudine (3TC, Epivir)
  Abacavir (ABC, Ziagen)

Nonnucleoside reverse-transcriptase inhibitors
  Nevirapine (Viramune)
  Delavirdine (Rescriptor)
  Efavirenz (Sustiva)

Protease inhibitors
  Amprenavir (Agenerase)
  Indinavir (Crixivan)
  Nelfinavir (Viracept)
  Ritonavir (Norvir)
  Saquinavir (Invirase)
  Lopinovir, which is available in combination with ritonavir (Kaletra)

Management of each HIV-infected individual requires an in-depth clinical and laboratory evaluation, including

- CD4 T-cell counts
- Determination of plasma HIV RNA level by reverse transcriptase polymerase chain reaction (RT-PCR) or by signal amplification assays such as branched DNA (bDNA)
- Detection of AIDS-defining illnesses (see Table 14-1)

Even though treatment of HIV infection is continually changing as a result of the introduction of new antiretroviral agents and the information gathered from various clinical trials, recent guidelines (1997) have emerged from recommendations by the International AIDS Society–USA. Treatment is indicated for any person with acute HIV infection or who is within 6 months of seroconversion and for any chronically infected patient when HIV RNA levels are above 10,000 copies/mL or when the CD4 count falls below 500 cells/mm^3. Initial treatment often includes a combination of three agents: two reverse transcriptase enzyme inhibitors and a protease inhibitor. Specific recommendations need to be tailored to each patient, however.

When the CD4 count falls below 200 cells/mm^3, the patient requires prophylaxis against *Pneumocystis* pneumonia by trimethoprim/sulfamethoxazole (TMP/SMX). During this stage, it is also important to rule out tuberculosis, which is a common complication of HIV infection and 500 times more common in HIV-infected persons than in the general population. HIV-infected patients with positive PPD results require prophylaxis with isoniazid and pyridoxine for at least 12 months. The physician must remember that the PPD is notoriously unreliable in HIV-infected patients because of their altered cellular immune function. Because the skin test reaction is decreased in HIV-infected patients, any skin test result that measures greater than 2 mm may be considered positive in some patients at high risk for tuberculosis.

HIV-infected patients with low CD4 counts also require prophylaxis against recurrent opportunistic infections such as cerebral toxoplasmosis, cryptococcosis, *Mycobacterium avium–intracellulare* complex (MAI), oroesophageal or vulvovaginal candidiasis, and histoplasmosis. Rifabutin is commonly used for prophylaxis against MAI, and fluconazole is used for mycotic infections.

All HIV-infected patients should be tested for syphilis.

Carpenter CC, Fischl MA, Hammer SM, et al. Antiretroviral therapy for HIV infection in 1996: recommendations of an international panel. International AIDS Study–USA. *JAMA*. 1996;276:146–154.

Ophthalmic Complications

Ocular manifestations have been reported in up to 70% of persons infected with HIV, and it has become apparent that the ocular manifestations almost invariably reflect systemic disease and may be the first sign of disseminated systemic infection. The ophthalmologist thus has the opportunity to make not only a sight-saving, but indeed a life-prolonging, diagnosis in some patients with AIDS. These ocular manifestations include

- HIV-related microangiopathy of the retina
- Various opportunistic viral, bacterial, and fungal infections
- Kaposi sarcoma
- Lymphomas involving the retina (primary intraocular lymphoma), adnexal structures, and orbit
- Squamous cell carcinoma of conjunctiva

Reports also suggest that HIV itself may cause anterior uveitis or an inflammatory reaction in the vitreous that is not responsive to corticosteroids but improves with antiretroviral therapy.

Cunningham ET Jr. Uveitis in HIV positive patients. *Br J Ophthalmol*. 2000;84:233–235.

HIV retinopathy is the most common ocular finding in patients with AIDS, occurring in about 50%–70% of cases. It is characterized by retinal hemorrhages, microaneurysms, and cotton-wool spots (Fig 14-1). The cotton-wool spots are usually oriented along vascular arcades and represent focal areas of ischemia in the nerve fiber layer. HIV has been isolated from human retina, and its antigen has been detected in retinal endothelial cells by immunohistochemistry. It is thought that such HIV endothelial infection and/or hematologic alterations may play a role in the development of cotton-wool spots and other vascular alterations. The microaneurysms and hemorrhages that characterize HIV retinopathy are also distributed along the nerve fiber layer and in the inner retinal layers. Cotton-wool spots, retinal hemorrhages, and microaneurysms are probably the result of both an underlying microvasculopathy and hematologic abnormalities such as increased leukocyte activation and rigidity.

Goldenberg DT, Holland GN, Cumberland WG, et al. An assessment of polymorphonuclear leukocyte rigidity in HIV-infected individuals after immune recovery. *Invest Ophthalmol Vis Sci*. 2002;43:1857–1861.

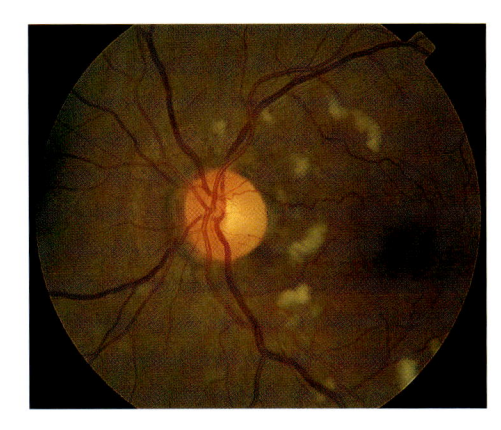

Figure 14-1 HIV retinopathy with numerous cotton-wool spots. *(Reprinted with permission from Cunningham ET Jr, Belfort R Jr. HIV/AIDS and the Eye: A Global Perspective. Ophthalmology Monograph 15. San Francisco: American Academy of Ophthalmology; 2002:55.)*

Other infectious agents that can affect the eye in patients with AIDS include CMV, herpes zoster virus, *T gondii*, *Mycobacterium tuberculosis*, MAI, *Cryptococcus neoformans*, *P carinii*, *Histoplasma capsulatum*, *Candid* spp, molluscum contagiosum, *Microsporida*, and others. These agents can infect the ocular adnexa, anterior segment, or posterior segment. Visual morbidity, however, occurs primarily with posterior segment involvement, particularly retinitis caused by CMV, herpes zoster virus, or *T gondii*.

Cytomegalovirus retinitis

CMV retinitis is the most common opportunistic ocular infection in patients with AIDS and can occasionally be the initial manifestation of AIDS. CMV is a double-stranded DNA virus that belongs to the Herpesviridae family, which also includes the herpes simplex, varicella-zoster, and Epstein-Barr viruses. Before the administration of HAART came into use against HIV, CMV disease occurring in the retina, colon, lung, and other sites was the most common opportunistic infection in AIDS. Even today, CMV disease could be the most common opportunistic infection in AIDS. Among the various affected organs, the retina most commonly presents with clinical manifestations.

Prior to HAART, CMV retinitis was known to occur in 15%–40% of patients with AIDS, and the median elapsed time between diagnosis of AIDS and the development of CMV retinitis was about 9 months. However, more recent studies have shown that this infection can occur as long as 3–5 years after the diagnosis of AIDS and usually develops when CD4 cell counts are below 50 cells/mm^3.

The modes of transmission for CMV are not completely understood, although epidemiologic and virologic studies implicate close or intimate contact with infected persons who are shedding virus in their urine, saliva, or other secretions. CMV infection in otherwise healthy adults and children is usually asymptomatic but occasionally is associated with a mononucleosis-like syndrome. In contrast to the generally benign course of CMV infection in healthy persons, CMV is a major cause of morbidity and mortality in immunocompromised patients. The high incidence of anti-CMV antibodies in the general population is evidence of widespread exposure to this virus. It is possible that CMV retinitis represents a dissemination of systemic infection or a reactivation of CMV that was already present in a latent form.

Well-established CMV retinitis is easily recognized as a full-thickness retinal opacification associated with hard exudates and hemorrhages (Fig 14-2). The infection may begin anywhere in the retina, including the far periphery. Because of severe immunosuppression in patients with AIDS, the amount of overlying vitreous inflammation is minimal. CMV infection may show granular white opacification of the retina with minimal or no retinal hemorrhage or may display a more edematous retinitis with hard exudates and hemorrhages. Occasionally, CMV retinitis may present with periphlebitis (frosted-branch angiitis) with some retinal necrosis. Very early CMV retinitis lesions may resemble cotton-wool spots.

Diagnosis The diagnosis of CMV retinitis is based on its characteristic clinical appearance. Serologic investigation and viral culture are of limited value, because many persons show evidence of previous exposure to CMV on serologic testing. In addition, the serologic diagnosis of CMV in patients with AIDS can be equivocal because of their profound immunosuppression. Although culture-confirmed presence of CMV in the throat, urine, and blood may be more reliable, immunosuppressed patients are often chronic carriers of this virus, so the mere presence of CMV does not necessarily indicate significant infection.

Because of these confounding factors and the fact that CMV infection involving the retina can be diagnosed easily and reliably, the ophthalmic examination has taken on great importance. Rarely, molecular techniques such as PCR for CMV DNA are used for diagnosis; however, these investigations are employed primarily for research purposes in predicting individual susceptibility to CMV retinitis.

Management In the United States, five medications are currently approved for treatment of CMV retinitis: ganciclovir, foscarnet, cidofovir, fomivirsen, and valganciclovir. Both ganciclovir and foscarnet show an initial response rate of 80%–100%. Moreover, treatment of CMV retinitis may prolong the survival of patients with AIDS. Prior to the introduction of HAART, the median survival time following the diagnosis of CMV retinitis was 6 weeks in patients receiving no treatment. Anti-CMV treatment increased the survival time to 10 months in patients who responded completely to ganciclovir treatment and to 3.1 months for those who responded partially. Recent studies show longer survival as a result of improved treatment of HIV infection with antiretroviral agents and management of various opportunistic infections and neoplasms.

Three forms of *ganciclovir* are currently approved for clinical use:

- Intravenous
- Oral
- Intravitreal in the form of an injection or implant

Ganciclovir is usually administered intravenously. The initial 2-week, high-dose induction therapy (5 mg/kg twice daily for 2 weeks) is aimed at controlling the infection and is followed by long-term maintenance therapy (5 mg/kg once daily 7 days a week or 6 mg/kg once daily 5 days a week). The primary side effect of ganciclovir is myelosuppression. Concomitant use of granulocyte-macrophage colony-stimulating factor can reduce or reverse neutropenia, the most serious component of myelosuppression, and may allow

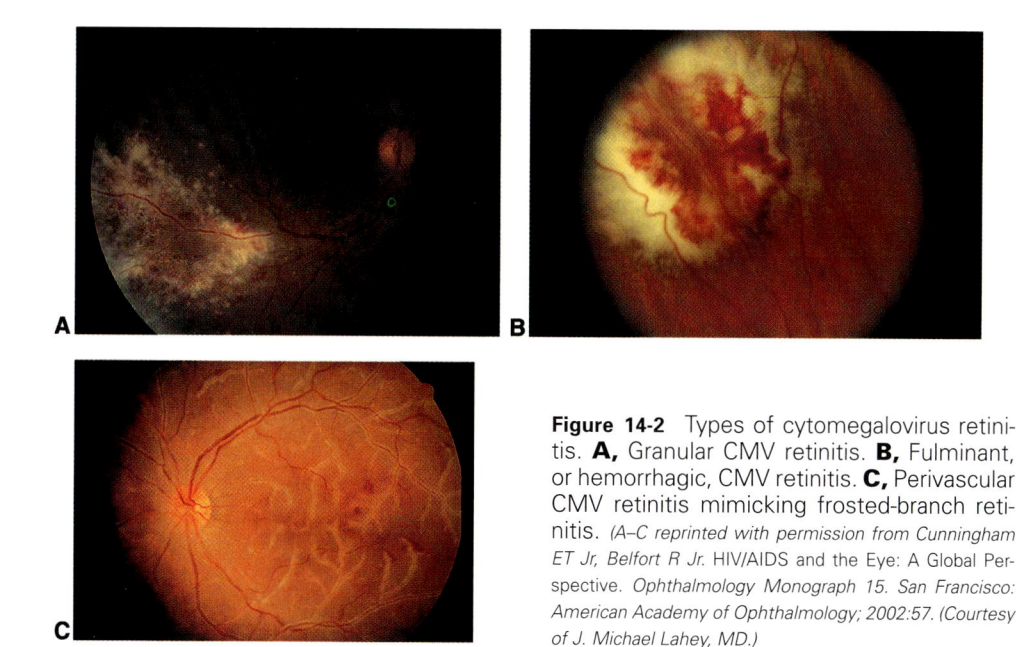

Figure 14-2 Types of cytomegalovirus retinitis. **A,** Granular CMV retinitis. **B,** Fulminant, or hemorrhagic, CMV retinitis. **C,** Perivascular CMV retinitis mimicking frosted-branch retinitis. *(A–C reprinted with permission from Cunningham ET Jr, Belfort R Jr. HIV/AIDS and the Eye: A Global Perspective.* Ophthalmology Monograph 15. *San Francisco: American Academy of Ophthalmology; 2002:57. (Courtesy of J. Michael Lahey, MD.)*

continuation of ganciclovir therapy. Neutropenia is usually reversible but may also necessitate interruption of the drug therapy. Thrombocytopenia has been reported to occur in 5%–10% of patients treated with ganciclovir. When CMV retinitis is diagnosed, patients may already be undergoing treatment with zidovudine (ZDV). Because ZDV also has toxic effects on the bone marrow, the dosage is usually decreased when used concomitantly with ganciclovir.

Ganciclovir is also available for oral administration, and this route of administration can be used as a maintenance therapy for patients with CMV retinitis who respond well to IV induction therapy with this agent. Drug toxicity is lower in patients maintained on oral administration. However, median time to progression of retinitis on oral ganciclovir (29 days) is less than with IV maintenance therapy (49 days). Moreover, the risk of CMV in the fellow eye is greater in patients receiving oral ganciclovir compared to those on IV maintenance.

Foscarnet is administered IV and, like ganciclovir, requires an initial 2-week, high-dose induction therapy (60 mg/kg every 8 hours for 2 or 3 weeks) followed by long-term maintenance therapy (90–120 mg/kg daily 5 or 7 days a week). Although foscarnet does not have a toxic effect on the bone marrow and can be used concurrently with full-dose ZDV therapy, it is toxic to the kidneys. Renal dysfunction and metabolic abnormalities of calcium and magnesium have been reported in up to 30% of patients who are receiving foscarnet, and seizures have been reported in approximately 10%.

Although the FDA has approved ganciclovir and foscarnet for IV use and ganciclovir for oral administration, patients who cannot tolerate these systemic anti-CMV drugs may receive them through intravitreal injection. Intravitreal ganciclovir or foscarnet can also be considered for patients who have shown progression of retinitis despite high-dose systemic therapy with ganciclovir, foscarnet, or both.

Under topical anesthesia, an intravitreal injection of 2.0 mg in 0.1 mL of ganciclovir is given once a week. Foscarnet, 2.4 mg in 0.1 mL, can be given instead of ganciclovir. Initial success rates are very high, with almost all patients showing early resolution of retinitis. As with IV forms of therapy, a substantial proportion of patients experience relapse. The risks associated with repeated intravitreal injections include cataract formation, vitreous hemorrhage, retinal detachment, and infectious endophthalmitis. Perhaps the most serious drawback of the intravitreal route of administration is that it does not provide the benefits of systemic anti-CMV treatment to the other eye and to extraocular sites of CMV infection.

A second proven method of intravitreal administration of ganciclovir is through an intravitreal device, which is surgically implanted and delivers the drug in effective concentrations over 4–8 months. The intravitreal device is also a useful alternative for patients who cannot tolerate IV therapy or do not respond well to it.

The FDA has also approved the antiviral *cidofovir* for the treatment of CMV disease including retinitis. This agent is administered intravenously with efficacy similar to IV ganciclovir. Cidofovir has a prolonged intracellular half-life and is administered at a dose of 5 mg/kg once a week for 2 weeks for induction, and 5 mg/kg every 2 weeks for maintenance therapy. During the administration of this agent, the patient requires IV hydration and probenecid to avoid severe renal toxicity. Up to 50% of patients may develop hypotony, anterior uveitis, or both while on cidofovir.

Another newly approved agent is an antisense compound *fomivirsen* (Vitravene, ISIS 2922), which is composed of 21 nucleotides. This agent inhibits the virus replication and is administered intravitreally. The agent is recommended at a dosage of 330 µg for the patient whose retinitis has failed to respond to other anti-CMV agents. Fomivirsen has been shown to be effective in controlling early or advanced CMV retinitis for up to 1 year when given as an intravitreal dose of 330 µg. In a study, fomivirsen was given weekly for three doses, then once every 2 weeks for maintenance therapy. Side effects of fomivirsen include anterior uveitis, vitritis, elevation of IOP, and cataract formation.

The most recent anti-CMV agent to be approved by the FDA is *valganciclovir*, which is taken orally. Valganciclovir is a prodrug of ganciclovir and achieves blood levels comparable to IV ganciclovir. Induction therapy involves 450 mg twice daily for 21 days, followed by 450 mg once daily as maintenance therapy. The systemic side effects and toxicities are similar to IV ganciclovir, but the oral agent is much more convenient for the patient and eliminates complications associated with placement of an indwelling catheter or repeated IV administration.

When assessing response to treatment, the most important clinical characteristic to evaluate is the size of the lesion. Careful attention to the border of the lesion, not the central area, is essential. The clinical appearance of the lesion can be compared against earlier clinical photographs to detect enlargement or stabilization of its size. The second most important clinical parameter is the degree of activity of the lesion, which is determined by the presence of retinal whitening and hemorrhage at the border of the lesion. Lesions in recurrent disease usually demonstrate fluffy white areas of active retinitis at the border of the original CMV lesion. In some cases of recurrence, lesions may enlarge despite minimal signs of retinal whitening or hemorrhage. As with the primary disease, it is the border of the lesion that reflects disease activity. In chronic stages of the disease, large atrophic holes may develop that can lead to retinal detachment.

Despite the impressive initial response to treatment with the agents described, without HAART, active retinitis recurs in 20%–50% of patients on maintenance therapy and in virtually all patients who discontinue anti-CMV therapy. Most investigators think that, given enough time, all patients eventually suffer a relapse, although they generally respond to a second course of induction (reinduction) therapy. If a patient experiences recurrence while receiving ganciclovir, foscarnet, or cidofovir, the following choices must be considered:

- Reinduction with the current medication
- New induction using the second or third medication
- Concomitant use of two medications

Concomitant use is found to be synergistic against CMV in vitro and beneficial in preventing progression of CMV retinitis that fails to respond to either agent administered alone.

In patients on HAART, the CD4 cell count may increase sufficiently to allow a decrease or discontinuation of anti-CMV therapy. Such patients need to be monitored closely every 6–12 months, however, for two reasons: CMV retinitis may recur even with CD4 counts over 100 cells/mm^3, and partial viral resistance, intolerance, or both occur in a sizable proportion of patients on HAART. More frequent follow-up may be warranted if CD4 counts drop.

Retinal detachment An additional complication of CMV retinitis is retinal detachment, which occurs in up to 50% of patients. It may occur either when the retinitis is active or when it is quiescent during successful treatment. In almost all patients with retinal detachment, the CMV lesions extend anteriorly to the pars plana, and the retinitis generally involves more than 50% of the retina. Myopia is an additional risk factor for the development of retinal detachment in patients with CMV retinitis.

Retinal detachments in patients with CMV retinitis are among the most difficult to repair because of extensive retinal necrosis and multiple, often posterior, hole formation. Most investigators agree that these detachments are not amenable to repair by scleral buckling alone; the procedure of choice is pars plana vitrectomy with long-term silicone oil tamponade. Anatomical reattachment can be achieved in 90% of these patients. Functional success, however, depends on the condition of the macula and the extent of affected retina.

Progressive outer retinal necrosis (PORN)

A rare infection in HIV-infected patients, PORN may be caused by the herpes zoster virus or herpes simplex virus. It may occur in the absence of, at the same time as, or subsequent to a cutaneous zoster infection (Fig 14-3).

In its early stages, PORN may be difficult to differentiate from peripheral CMV retinitis. However, PORN's characteristic rapid progression and relative absence of vitreous inflammation usually allow this entity to be distinguished from CMV retinitis and the acute retinal necrosis syndrome (ARN), respectively. There is a high incidence of

254 • Intraocular Inflammation and Uveitis

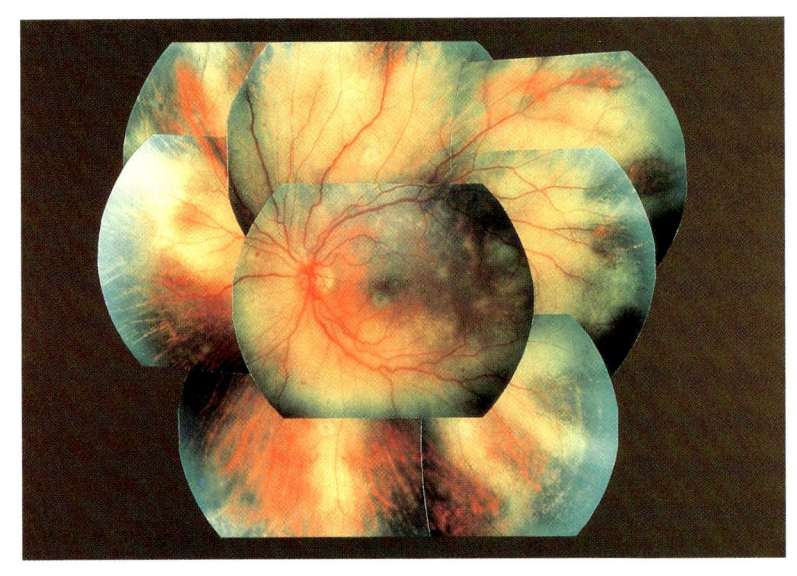

Figure 14-3 Retinal necrosis with preservation of vessels in a patient with progressive outer retinal necrosis. *(Photograph courtesy of Narsing A. Rao, MD.)*

retinal detachment, and bilateral involvement is common. Although no current therapy is adequate, intravitreal ganciclovir or foscarnet in combination with IV acyclovir may be more effective than IV acyclovir alone in stabilizing the infection.

Toxoplasma *retinochoroiditis*

A number of reports of toxoplasmosis in patients with AIDS have revealed important clinical differences from immunocompetent persons. In general, the size of the retinochoroiditic lesions is larger in patients with AIDS, with up to one third of lesions greater than 5 disc diameters. Bilateral disease is seen in 18%–38% of these cases. Solitary, multifocal, and miliary patterns of retinitis have been observed (Fig 14-4). A vitreous inflammatory reaction usually appears overlying the area of active retinochoroiditis, but the degree of vitreous reaction may be less than that observed in immunocompetent patients.

The diagnosis of ocular toxoplasmosis may be more difficult in patients with AIDS. Although this diagnosis in immunocompetent patients is frequently aided by the presence of old retinochoroiditic scars, patients with AIDS rarely demonstrate preexisting scars, which are present in only 4%–6% of such patients with ocular toxoplasmosis. Because the clinical manifestations in this population are so varied and may be more severe than in immunocompetent persons, ocular toxoplasmosis in patients with AIDS may be difficult to distinguish from ARN, necrotizing herpetic retinitis, or syphilitic retinitis.

The histologic features of ocular specimens from patients with AIDS reflect the immunologic abnormalities of the host. In general, the inflammatory reaction in the choroid, retina, and vitreous is less prominent than in patients with an intact immune system. Trophozoites and cysts can be observed in greater numbers within areas of retinitis, and *T gondii* organisms can occasionally be seen invading the choroid, which is not the case in immunocompetent persons.

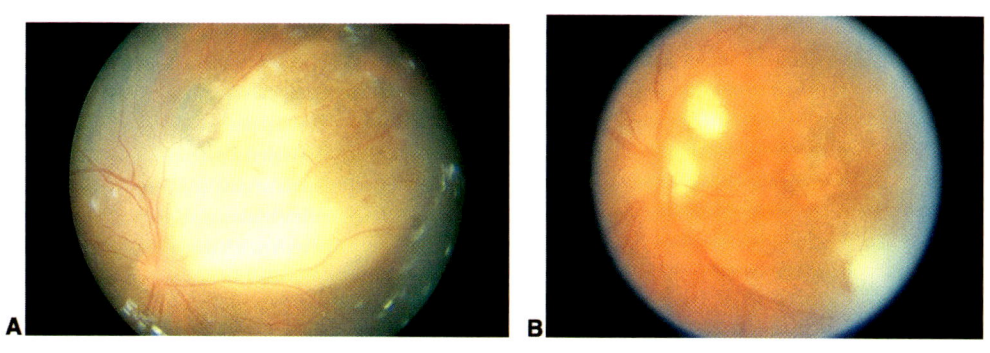

Figure 14-4 A, A large area of macular toxoplasmic retinochoroiditis in an HIV-infected patient. **B,** Multifocal toxoplasmic retinochoroiditis in another HIV-infected patient. *(Photographs courtesy of Emmett T. Cunningham, Jr, MD.)*

Ocular toxoplasmosis in immunocompetent patients is usually the result of reactivation of a congenital infection. In contrast, newly acquired infection or dissemination from a nonocular site of infection is most likely among patients with AIDS. These conclusions are drawn from the observations that preexisting retinochoroiditic scars are rarely present and *Toxoplasma*-specific IgM titers are found in 6%–12% of patients.

The prompt diagnosis of ocular toxoplasmosis is especially important in patients with immunosuppression because this condition inevitably progresses if left untreated, in contrast to the self-limited disease of immunocompetent patients. In addition, ocular toxoplasmosis in immunocompromised patients may be associated with cerebral or disseminated toxoplasmosis, an important cause of morbidity and mortality in patients with AIDS. HIV-infected patients with active ocular toxoplasmosis should therefore undergo MRI of the brain to rule out CNS involvement.

Antitoxoplasmic therapy with various combinations of pyrimethamine, sulfadiazine, and clindamycin is required. Corticosteroids should be used with caution and only in the presence of appropriate antimicrobial cover because of the risk of further immunosuppression in this population. In selecting the therapeutic regimen, the physician should consider the possibility of coexisting cerebral or disseminated toxoplasmosis and the toxic effects of pyrimethamine and sulfadiazine on the bone marrow. Even after the active retinitis has resolved, antitoxoplasmic therapy must be continued for the life of the patient in order to prevent recurrence.

Syphilitic chorioretinitis

The clinical presentations of syphilitic chorioretinitis include uveitis, optic neuritis, and retinitis. Patients may also experience dermatologic and CNS manifestations. Patients with AIDS who have syphilitic chorioretinitis may present with vitritis associated with large, bilateral, pale-yellow subretinal lesions that are solitary and placoid. Most of these lesions show evidence of central fading and a pattern of stippled hyperpigmentation of the RPE *(syphilitic posterior placoid chorioretinitis)*. Some HIV-positive patients with syphilis may present with dense vitritis without clinical evidence of chorioretinitis. In these patients, vitritis can be the first manifestation of syphilis.

256 • Intraocular Inflammation and Uveitis

The course of syphilis may be more aggressive in patients with AIDS. These patients require treatment with 12–24 million units of intravenous penicillin G administered daily for 10–14 days, followed by 2.4 million units of intramuscular benzathine penicillin G administered weekly for 3 weeks.

Aldave AJ, King JA, Cunningham ET Jr. *Curr Opin Ophthalmol.* 2001;12:433–441.

Pneumocystis carinii *choroiditis*

Patients with AIDS are at much greater risk for *P carinii* pneumonia, and this infection can be the opportunistic disease initially seen in these patients. Rarely, this infection can disseminate, and patients with such disseminated infection may present with choroidal infiltrates containing the responsible microorganisms.

Fundus changes characteristic of *P carinii* choroiditis consist of slightly elevated, plaquelike, yellow-white lesions located in the choroid with minimal vitritis (Figs 14-5, 14-6, 14-7). On fluorescein angiography, these lesions tend to be hypofluorescent in the

Figure 14-5 *Pneumocystis carinii* choroiditis. The fellow eye revealed similar findings. *(Reprinted with permission from Cunningham ET, Jr, Belfort R Jr. HIV/AIDS and the Eye: A Global Perspective. Ophthalmology Monograph 15. San Francisco: American Academy of Ophthalmology; 2002:67.)*

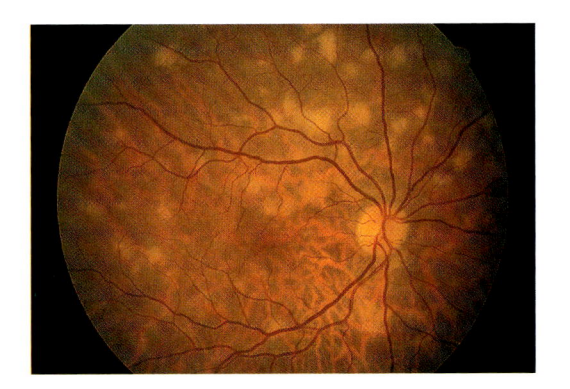

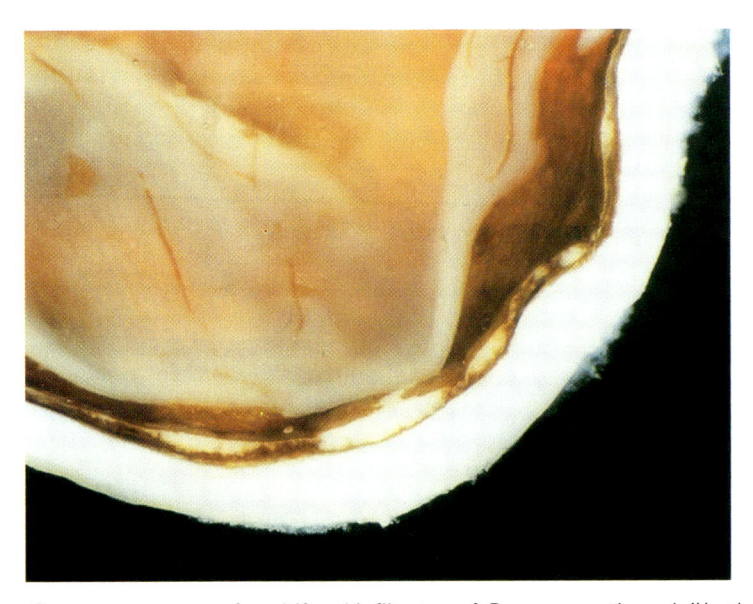

Figure 14-6 Gross appearance of multifocal infiltrates of *Pneumocystis carinii* in the choroid.

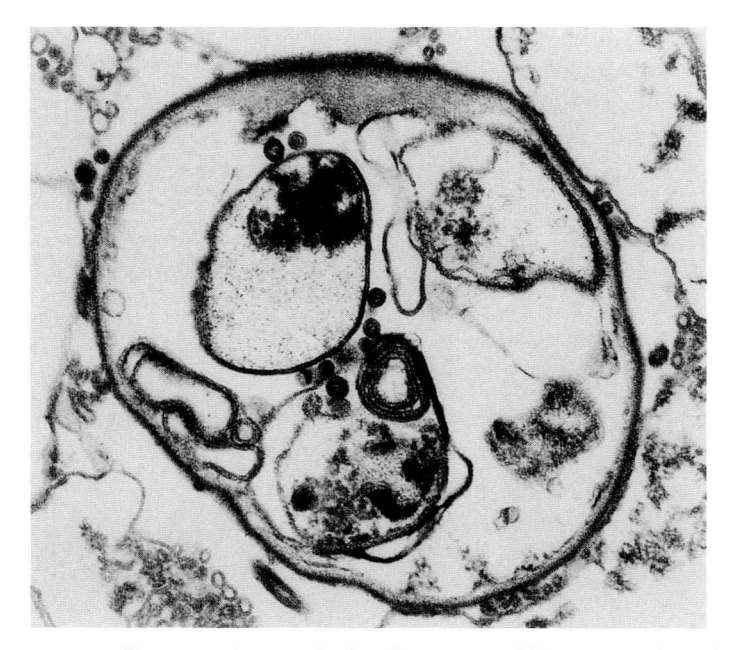

Figure 14-7 Electron micrograph showing a cyst of *Pneumocystis carinii.*

early phase and hyperfluorescent in the later phases. If disseminated *P carinii* is suspected, an extensive examination is required, including

- Chest radiography
- Arterial blood gas analysis
- Liver function testing
- Abdominal CT

Treatment of *P carinii* choroiditis requires hospitalization for a 3-week regimen of IV trimethoprim (20 mg/kg per day) and sulfamethoxazole (100 mg/kg per day) or pentamidine (4 mg/kg per day). Within 3–12 weeks, most of the yellow-white lesions disappear, leaving mild overlying pigmentary changes.

Cryptococcus neoformans *choroiditis*

The dissemination of *C neoformans* in patients with AIDS may result in a multifocal choroiditis similar to that seen in *P carinii* choroiditis. Some patients with *C neoformans* choroiditis show choroidal lesions before they develop clinical evidence of dissemination. Ocular manifestations may presage specific clinical systemic manifestations such as CNS disease. The alert clinician may use ophthalmic findings to reach an early diagnosis of disseminated cryptococcosis.

Multifocal choroiditis and systemic dissemination

Multifocal choroidal lesions from a variety of infectious agents, including those discussed above, are seen in about 5%–10% of patients with AIDS. Most of these lesions are caused by *C neoformans, P carinii, M tuberculosis,* or atypical mycobacteria. Although multifocal choroiditis caused by any one of these infectious organisms is seen in many patients with AIDS, occasionally two or more of them in combination can be responsible.

Because it is so often the site of opportunistic disseminated infections, the choroid is a critical structure that needs to be carefully examined in patients with AIDS. Although nonspecific, multifocal choroiditis is alarming and should prompt an exhaustive workup for disseminated infection. Because multifocal choroiditis frequently represents disseminated infection, the ophthalmologist may have a life-prolonging role in the diagnosis and treatment of these patients.

External Eye Manifestations

Other ophthalmic manifestations of AIDS include Kaposi sarcoma; molluscum contagiosum; herpes zoster ophthalmicus; and keratitis caused by various viruses, protozoa, conjunctival infections, and microvascular abnormalities. All of these conditions affect mainly the anterior segment of the globe and the ocular adnexa. These conditions are also discussed in BCSC Section 8, *External Disease and Cornea*.

Ocular adnexal Kaposi sarcoma

Since the initial description of Kaposi sarcoma in 1872, two more-aggressive variants of this tumor have been described. An endemic variety was described in 1959 in Africa; it is especially prevalent in Kenya and Nigeria, where it accounts for nearly 20% of all malignancies. The second variant, *epidemic Kaposi sarcoma*, was first noted in renal transplant recipients and currently occurs in 30% of all patients with AIDS. AIDS-associated Kaposi sarcoma is particularly aggressive, disseminating to visceral organs (gastrointestinal tract, lung, and liver) in 20%–50% of patients. Prior to 1981, fewer than 25 patients with ocular adnexal Kaposi sarcoma had been reported, but this condition is now noted to occur in approximately 20% of patients with AIDS-associated systemic Kaposi sarcoma.

Histopathologic investigation shows spindle cells mixed with vascular structures (Fig 14-8). Recent evidence suggests that AIDS-related Kaposi sarcoma may have an infectious origin. Human herpesvirus 8 has been isolated from patients with Kaposi sarcoma. That HIV may play a role in the pathogenesis of Kaposi sarcoma is evident from studies of transgenic mice bearing the HIV-1 transactivator *(tat)* gene under the control of the virus regulatory region (HIV-LTR). The HIV-*tat* protein has been shown to be a potent mi-

Figure 14-8 Histopathologically, Kaposi sarcoma is made up of large spindle cells forming slitlike spaces. These spaces contain erythrocytes.

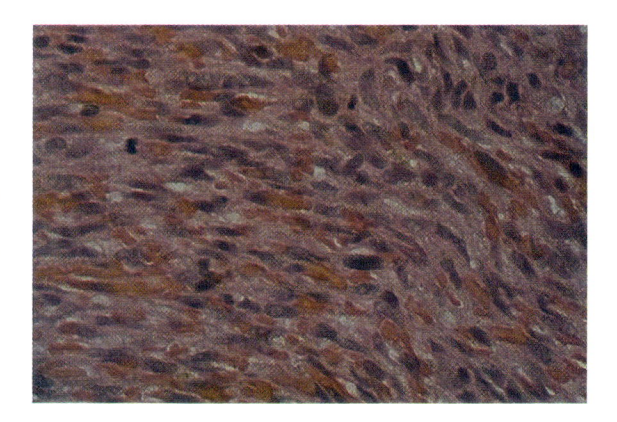

togen for human Kaposi sarcoma–derived cell lines. As in humans, these lesions in mice occur predominantly in males, which suggests that their development may be hormonally controlled.

Three clinical stages of ocular adnexal Kaposi sarcoma have been described:

- Stage I and stage II tumors are patchy, flat (<3 mm in height), and of less than 4 months' duration
- Stage III tumors are nodular, elevated (>3 mm in height), and of greater than 4 months' duration (Fig 14-9)

The treatment of Kaposi sarcoma is based on the clinical stage of the tumor as well as its location and the presence or absence of disseminated lesions. If the lesion is confined to the ocular adnexa, local treatment is appropriate. If the tumor is confined to the bulbar conjunctiva and is stage I or stage II, an excisional biopsy with 1–2 mm tumor-free margins should be considered only if the lesion is symptomatic. Stage III Kaposi sarcoma of the bulbar conjunctiva should be surgically excised, preferably after delineation by fluorescein angiography. Stage I and stage II Kaposi sarcoma involving the eyelid may be treated with cryotherapy. Stage III Kaposi sarcoma of the eyelid may be treated with either radiation or cryotherapy, although radiation is preferred because of a lower recurrence rate. In order to avoid radiation-related complications, however, lesions may be treated with cryotherapy if the patient is aware that recurrence is more likely and may necessitate retreatment.

When evaluating a patient with AIDS who has ocular adnexal Kaposi sarcoma, the physician should perform a full systemic examination for tumor dissemination. If chemotherapy is administered for systemic Kaposi sarcoma, the ophthalmologist should wait at least 4–6 weeks to observe response to treatment before deciding whether further therapy is warranted.

Molluscum contagiosum

Molluscum contagiosum is caused by a DNA virus of the poxvirus family. The characteristic skin lesions show a small elevation with central umbilication. Molluscum lesions in healthy persons are few, are unilateral, and involve the eyelids. In patients with AIDS, however, these lesions may be numerous and bilateral. If molluscum lesions in patients with AIDS are symptomatic or cause conjunctivitis, surgical excision may be necessary. However, surgery and cryotherapy sometimes fail to treat these viral lesions.

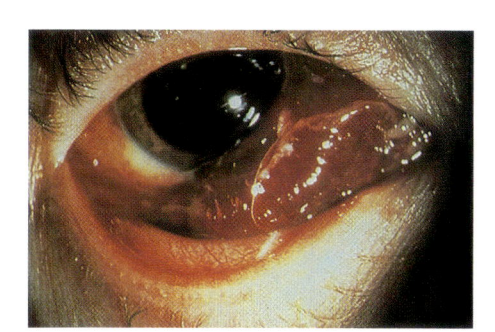

Figure 14-9 Conjunctival involvement in Kaposi sarcoma; hemorrhagic conjunctival tumor (stage III). *(Photograph courtesy of John D. Sheppard Jr, MD.)*

Herpes zoster

Apparently healthy young people who present with herpes zoster lesions of the face or eyelids should be suspected of having AIDS and tested for HIV. Corneal involvement can cause a persistent, chronic epithelial keratitis, and treatment consists of IV and topical acyclovir. See the discussion of PORN earlier in this chapter. Although PORN is rare, these patients should be followed periodically with retinal examination.

Other infections

HIV infection does not appear to predispose patients to bacterial keratitis. However, infections appear to be more severe and are more likely to cause perforation in patients with AIDS than in immunocompetent patients. Bacterial and fungal keratitis can occur in patients with AIDS with no obvious predisposing factors such as trauma or topical corticosteroid use. Although herpes simplex keratitis does not appear to have a higher incidence in patients with AIDS, it may have a prolonged course or multiple recurrences and involve the limbus in these patients (Fig 14-10). *Microsporida* organisms have been shown to cause a coarse, superficial punctate keratitis with a minimal conjunctival reaction in patients with AIDS (Fig 14-11). Electron microscopy of the epithelial scrapings has revealed the organism, which is an obligate, intracellular, protozoal parasite.

Solitary granulomatous conjunctivitis from cryptococcal infection, tuberculosis, or other mycotic infections can occur in HIV-infected persons. As with all other infections in AIDS, the possibility of dissemination must be considered and aggressively sought. Orbital lymphomas and intraocular lymphomas have been described in patients with AIDS. These neoplasms are mostly large B-cell lymphomas. Conjunctival squamous cell carcinomas have been reported, and in some patients these neoplasms show spindle cells with frequent abnormal mitotic figures.

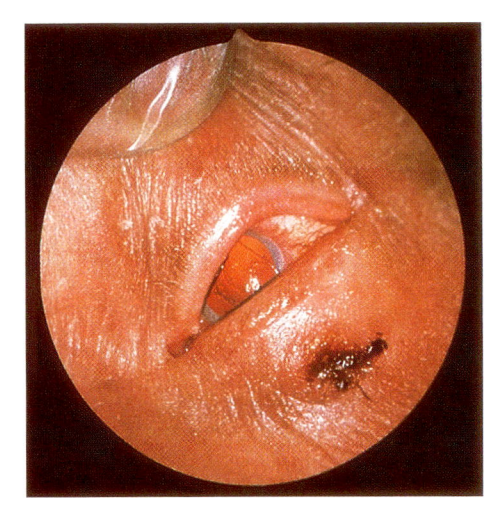

Figure 14-10 Lesions of the eyelid and cornea in a patient with AIDS and disseminated herpes simplex.

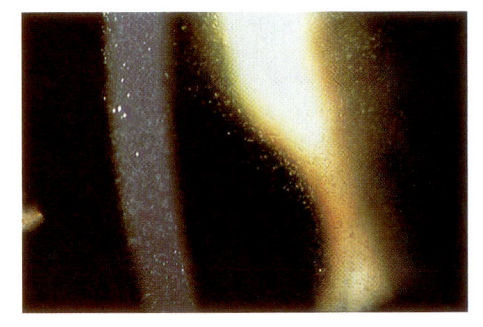

Figure 14-11 Superficial punctate keratitis caused by *Microsporida*.

The Ophthalmologist's Role

The role of the ophthalmologist in the diagnosis and management of patients with AIDS is becoming increasingly important. Not only does the eye reflect systemic disease, but ocular involvement may often precede systemic manifestations. The ophthalmologist treating a patient with AIDS truly has an opportunity to make not only a sight-saving, but also a life-sustaining, diagnosis. Therefore, it is the responsibility of the ophthalmologist to provide not only a thorough and accurate ophthalmologic examination but also a careful and pertinent systemic evaluation, timely referrals, and periodic follow-up care.

HIV infection is a major public health problem with almost 100% mortality. It is likely that new drugs to combat HIV infection, and other agents to suppress the opportunistic infections that accompany HIV, will continue to be developed. In the future, an anti-HIV vaccine may be introduced. However, at present, the most productive approach to combating HIV remains prevention of its transmission.

Precautions in the Health Care Setting

Specific precautionary measures against HIV infection have been advocated in the United States by the CDC and other governmental agencies, including the Occupational Safety and Health Administration (OSHA). These agencies insist on adoption of bloodborne pathogen standards, commonly referred to as *universal precautions*. These precautions should be followed whether or not a patient is known to be HIV-positive and include the following:

- Taking measures to prevent accidental needle-stick injury
- Routine wearing of gloves when collecting and handling specimens
- Disposing of contaminated sharp objects in puncture-resistant (sharps) containers
- Proper shielding of eyes and mouth for clinical and laboratory workers
- Thoroughly disinfecting examination equipment that touches mucosal surfaces after each use
- Prompt cleaning by a gloved person using 10% chlorine bleach solution of all blood spills in the examining rooms or waiting area
- Making hepatitis B vaccine available to all personnel who come in contact with patient blood

Precautions in Ophthalmic Practice

While it appears that ophthalmology presents a lower level of risk than some other, more hazardous specialties, the American Academy of Ophthalmology has advocated following precautionary measures against HIV infection in ophthalmic practice. These measures are meant to provide protection to patients, ancillary health care personnel, and ophthalmologists.

Even though there are no published reports of HIV transmission in ophthalmic health care settings, hand washing with soap and water and thorough drying with fresh or disposable towels is recommended between various tests on an individual and between patients. If an open wound or weeping lesion is present, disposable gloves should be worn and discarded appropriately.

Tonometers and diagnostic contact lenses should be wiped with an alcohol sponge. Similarly, the Schiøtz tonometer can be disassembled and cleaned with an alcohol sponge. However, the CDC recommends household chlorine bleach (1:10 dilution) to clean such instruments. These items must be carefully rinsed after use of either alcohol or chlorine. BCSC Section 10, *Glaucoma*, gives more specific instructions for infection control in tonometry.

Contact lens trial sets need to be disinfected between patients. For hard contact lenses and rigid gas-permeable contact lenses, hydrogen peroxide disinfection or a chlorhexidine-containing disinfectant system should be employed. For soft contact lenses, hydrogen peroxide or a heat disinfection system should be used.

Barrier precautions, such as disposable gloves, should be used during diagnostic procedures such as injection of dye for fluorescein angiographic studies. During surgical procedures, particularly when contact with blood or blood-contaminated fluids is likely, all health care personnel in attendance should wear disposable gloves, masks, and protective eye wear.

Corneal and scleral tissue used for transplantations should be screened for HIV and hepatitis B virus, in accordance with the guidelines provided by the Eye Bank Association of America, which are spelled out in BCSC Section 8, *External Disease and Cornea*.

> Minimizing transmission of bloodborne pathogens and surface infectious agents in ophthalmic offices and operating rooms. *Information Statement.* San Francisco: American Academy of Ophthalmology; 2002.

Basic Texts

Intraocular Inflammation and Uveitis

Giles CL. Uveitis in childhood. In: Tasman W, Jaeger EA, eds. *Duane's Clinical Ophthalmology.* Philadelphia: Lippincott; 2001.

Michelson JB. *Color Atlas of Uveitis Diagnosis.* 2nd ed. St Louis: Mosby; 1992.

Nussenblatt RB, Whitcup SM, Palestine AG. *Uveitis: Fundamentals and Clinical Practice.* 2nd ed. St Louis: Mosby; 1996.

Opremcak EM. *Uveitis: A Clinical Manual for Ocular Inflammation.* New York: Springer-Verlag; 1995.

Pepose JS, Holland GN, Wilhelmus KR, eds. *Ocular Infection and Immunity.* St Louis: Mosby; 1996.

Rao NA, Augsburger JJ, Forster DJ. *The Uvea: Uveitis and Intraocular Neoplasms.* New York: Gower; 1992.

Roitt IM. *Essential Immunology.* 10th ed. Malden, MA: Blackwell Science; 2001.

Smith RE, Nozik RA. *Uveitis: A Clinical Approach to Diagnosis and Management.* 2nd ed. Baltimore: Williams & Wilkins; 1989.

Related Academy Materials

Focal Points: Clinical Modules for Ophthalmologists

Cunningham ET. Diagnosis and management of anterior uveitis (Module 1, 2002).
Dinning WJ. Uveitis and juvenile chronic arthritis (Module 5, 1990).
Dodds EM. Ocular toxoplasmosis: clinical presentations, diagnosis, and therapy (Module 10, 1999).
Doft BH. Managing infectious endophthalmitis: results of the Endophthalmitis Vitrectomy Study (Module 3, 1997).
Dunn JP. Uveitis in children (Module 4, 1995).
Folk JC, Pulido JS, Wolf MD. White dot and chorioretinal inflammatory syndromes (Module 11, 1990).
Holland GN. An update on AIDS-related cytomegalovirus retinitis (Module 5, 1991).
Hooper PL. Pars planitis (Module 11, 1993).
Jaffe GJ. Cystoid macular edema (Module 11, 1994).
Jampol LM. Nonsteroidal anti-inflammatory drugs (Module 6, 1997).
Margo CE. Nonpigmented lesions of the ocular surface (Module 9, 1996).
Meisler DM. Intraocular inflammation and extracapsular cataract surgery (Module 7, 1990).
Moshfeghi DM, Muccioli C, Belfort R Jr. Laboratory evaluation of patients with uveitis (Module 12, 2001).
Opremcak EM. Topical therapy for iritis (Module 7, 1991).
Palestine AG. Medical therapy of uveitis (Module 8, 1989).
Rosenbaum JT. Practical diagnostic evaluation of uveitis (Module 6, 1993).
Rosenbaum JT, Smith JR. Immune–mediated systemic diseases associated with uveitis (Module 10, 2003).
Samples JR. Management of glaucoma secondary to uveitis (Module 5, 1995).
Tessler HH, Goldstein DA. Update on systemic immunosuppressive agents (Module 11, 2000).

Publications

Cunningham ET Jr, Belfort R Jr. *HIV/AIDS and the Eye: A Global Perspective.* Ophthalmology Monograph 15. San Francisco: American Academy of Ophthalmology; 2002:57.
Lane SS, Skuta GL, eds. *ProVision: Preferred Responses in Ophthalmology,* Series 3 (Self-Assessment Program, 1999).
Schwab L. *Eye Care in Developing Nations.* 3rd ed. (1999).

Skuta GL, ed. *ProVision: Preferred Responses in Ophthalmology,* Series 2 (Self-Assessment Program, 1996).

Wilson FM II, ed. *Practical Ophthalmology: A Manual for Beginning Residents.* 4th ed. (1996).

Slide Script

Tang RA. *Ocular Manifestations of Systemic Disease* (Eye Care Skills for the Primary Care Physician Series, 1996).

Multimedia

Eye Care Skills on CD-ROM (all seven titles from the Eye Care Skills for the Primary Care Physician Series) (1999).

Whitcup SM, Foster CS, Nussenblatt RB, et al. *LEO Clinical Update Course on Uveitis* (CD-ROM, 1999).

Continuing Ophthalmic Video Education

Kelly MP. *Basic Techniques of Fluorescein Angiography* (1994).
Osher RH. *More Challenging Cases in Cataract Surgery* (2001).

To order any of these materials, please call the Academy's Customer Service number at (415) 561-8540, or order online at www.aao.org.

Credit Reporting Form

Basic and Clinical Science Course, 2004–2005
Section 9

The American Academy of Ophthalmology is accredited by the Accreditation Council for Continuing Medical Education to provide continuing medical education for physicians.

The American Academy of Ophthalmology designates this educational activity for a maximum of 30 category 1 credits toward the AMA Physician's Recognition Award. Each physician should claim only those hours of credit that he/she actually spent in the activity.

The American Medical Association has determined that non-US licensed physicians who participate in this CME activity are eligible for AMA PRA category 1 credit.

If you wish to claim continuing medical education credit for your study of this section, you may claim your credit online or fill in the required forms and mail or fax them to the Academy.

To use the forms:

1. Complete the study questions and mark your answers on the Section Completion Form.
2. Complete the Section Evaluation.
3. Fill in and sign the statement below.
4. Return this page and the required forms by mail or fax to the CME Registrar (see below).

To claim credit online:

1. Log on to the Academy website (www.aao.org).
2. Go to Education Resource Center; click on CME Central.
3. Follow the instructions.

Important: These completed forms or the online claim must be received at the Academy within 3 years of purchase.

I hereby certify that I have spent _____ (up to 30) hours of study on the curriculum of this section and that I have completed the Study Questions.

Signature: _____

                                                                                                 Date

Name: _____

Address: _____

City and State: _____ Zip: _____

Telephone: (_____) _____ Academy Member ID# _____
              area code

Please return completed forms to: **Or you may fax them to:** 415-561-8557
American Academy of Ophthalmology
P.O. Box 7424
San Francisco, CA 94120-7424
Attn: CME Registrar, Clinical Education

2004–2005
Section Completion Form

Basic and Clinical Science Course

Answer Sheet for Section 9

Question	Answer	Question	Answer	Question	Answer
1	a b c d	18	a b c d	35	a b c d
2	a b c d	19	a b c d	36	a b c d
3	a b c d	20	a b c d	37	a b c d
4	a b c d	21	a b c d	38	a b c d
5	a b c d	22	a b c d	39	a b c d
6	a b c d	23	a b c d	40	a b c d
7	a b c d	24	a b c d	41	a b c d
8	a b c d	25	a b c d	42	a b c d
9	a b c d	26	a b c d	43	a b c d
10	a b c d	27	a b c d	44	a b c d
11	a b c d	28	a b c d	45	a b c d
12	a b c d	29	a b c d	46	a b c d
13	a b c d	30	a b c d	47	a b c d
14	a b c d	31	a b c d	48	a b c d
15	a b c d	32	a b c d	49	a b c d
16	a b c d	33	a b c d	50	a b c d
17	a b c d	34	a b c d		

Section Evaluation

Please complete this CME questionnaire.

1. To what degree will you use knowledge from BCSC Section 9 in your practice?
    - ☐ Regularly
    - ☐ Sometimes
    - ☐ Rarely

2. Please review the stated objectives for BCSC Section 9. How effective was the material at meeting those objectives?
    - ☐ All objectives were met.
    - ☐ Most objectives were met.
    - ☐ Some objectives were met.
    - ☐ Few or no objectives were met.

3. To what degree is BCSC Section 9 likely to have a positive impact on health outcomes of your patients?
    - ☐ Extremely likely
    - ☐ Highly likely
    - ☐ Somewhat likely
    - ☐ Not at all likely

4. After you review the stated objectives for BCSC Section 9, please let us know of any additional knowledge, skills, or information useful to your practice that were acquired but were not included in the objectives. [Optional]

5. Was BCSC Section 9 free of commercial bias?
    - ☐ Yes
    - ☐ No

6. If you selected "No" in the previous question, please comment. [Optional]

7. Please tell us what might improve the applicability of BCSC to your practice. [Optional]

Study Questions

Although a concerted effort has been made to avoid ambiguity and redundancy in these questions, the authors recognize that differences of opinion may occur regarding the "best" answer. The discussions are provided to demonstrate the rationale used to derive the answer. They may also be helpful in confirming that your approach to the problem was correct or, if necessary, in fixing the principle in your memory. Where relevant, additional references are given.

1. Which of the following statements about innate immunity is correct?
   a. It comprises recognition, processing, and effector phases.
   b. It is triggered by bacterial toxins and cell debris.
   c. It demonstrates specificity for each unique offending antigen.
   d. It demonstrates memory, with an accelerated and more vigorous response to a second antigenic exposure.

2. Which of the following is commonly associated with host defenses against parasitic infections?
   a. neutrophils
   b. basophils
   c. eosinophils
   d. macrophages

3. Which of the following blood cell types is a major effector of IgE-mediated hypersensitivity?
   a. neutrophils
   b. basophils
   c. eosinophils
   d. monocytes

4. Which antibody is produced in the effector phase of the primary immune response to antigens?
   a. IgM
   b. IgG
   c. IgD
   d. IgE

5. Which of the following disorders is associated with the least amount of inflammation?
   a. *Propionibacterium acnes* endophthalmitis
   b. sympathetic ophthalmia
   c. phacoantigenic endophthalmitis
   d. phacolytic glaucoma

6. HLA-B27–associated acute anterior uveitis is associated with all *except* which of the following systemic disorders?
   a. Behçet syndrome
   b. Reiter syndrome
   c. psoriatic arthritis
   d. ankylosing spondylitis

7. Patients with which of the following are most likely to present with granulomatous uveitis?

   a. sarcoidosis
   b. Behçet syndrome
   c. juvenile rheumatoid arthritis
   d. Reiter syndrome

8. Hypopyon is most likely to be seen in which of the following uveitic syndromes?

   a. sarcoidosis
   b. Behçet syndrome
   c. rheumatoid arthritis
   d. Reiter syndrome

9. Which of the following topical agents is most effective in controlling intraocular inflammation in uveitis?

   a. loteprednol (Lotemax)
   b. fluorometholone 0.25% (FML Forte)
   c. dexamethasone 0.1% (Decadron)
   d. prednisolone 1% (Pred Forte, Inflammase Forte)

10. Which of the following uveitic syndromes is least likely to require topical corticosteroid management?

    a. sarcoidosis
    b. juvenile rheumatoid arthritis
    c. Fuchs heterochromic iridocyclitis
    d. Reiter syndrome

11. Periocular depot corticosteroid injections should *not* be used in which of the following uveitic syndromes?

    a. pars planitis with cystoid macular edema
    b. sarcoidosis
    c. toxoplasmosis
    d. Reiter syndrome

12. Which of the following is most likely to be positive in an American patient with acute nongranulomatous uveitis?

    a. HLA-B27
    b. HLA-B51
    c. HLA-B5
    d. HLA-B54

13. Reiter syndrome is associated with all *except* which of the following?

    a. nonspecific urethritis
    b. polyarthritis
    c. conjunctivitis
    d. ankylosing spondylitis

14. Behçet syndrome is associated with all *except* which of the following?
    a. aphthous stomatitis
    b. arthritis
    c. genital ulceration
    d. retinal vasculitis

15. Which of the following is usually seen in childhood?
    a. ankylosing spondylitis
    b. Reiter syndrome
    c. Vogt-Koyanagi-Harada syndrome
    d. Kawasaki syndrome

16. Which of the following types of intraocular lenses is most associated with recurrent uveitis?
    a. rigid, closed-loop anterior chamber intraocular lenses
    b. iris plane intraocular lenses
    c. sulcus-placed posterior chamber intraocular lenses
    d. silicone intraocular lenses

17. Risk factors for the development of chronic iridocyclitis in patients with juvenile rheumatoid arthritis include all *except* which of the following?
    a. female gender
    b. positive rheumatoid factor (RF)
    c. pauciarticular arthritis
    d. circulating antinuclear antibody (ANA)

18. Which of the following is least commonly seen in patients with juvenile rheumatoid arthritis (JRA) and uveitis?
    a. cataract
    b. macular edema
    c. glaucoma
    d. band keratopathy

19. Which of the following is *not* characteristic of Fuchs heterochromic iridocyclitis?
    a. unilateral uveitis
    b. mild aqueous cell and flare
    c. iris stromal atrophy
    d. small nongranulomatous keratic precipitates in Arlt's triangle

20. Which of the following is the most common cause of intermediate uveitis?
    a. multiple sclerosis
    b. idiopathic
    c. Lyme disease
    d. syphilis

21. Which of the following is the major cause of visual loss in pars planitis?

    a. band keratopathy

    b. posterior subcapsular cataract

    c. epiretinal membrane

    d. cystoid macular edema

22. Which of the following is least characteristic of acute retinal necrosis (ARN) syndrome?

    a. vitritis

    b. occlusive arteriolitis

    c. extensive retinal hemorrhages

    d. multifocal yellow-white peripheral retinitis

23. Which of the following is commonly associated with an immunocompromised state?

    a. cytomegalovirus retinitis

    b. herpes simplex keratouveitis

    c. acute retinal necrosis syndrome

    d. ocular histoplasmosis syndrome

24. Which of the following is *not* characteristic of ocular histoplasmosis syndrome (OHS)?

    a. peripapillary pigment changes

    b. vitritis

    c. peripheral atrophic chorioretinal ("histo") spots

    d. maculopathy

25. Treatment of visually threatening ocular toxoplasmosis should include which of the following?

    a. amphotericin B

    b. periocular corticosteroid injection

    c. pyrimethamine and sulfonamides

    d. acyclovir

26. Which of the following is the best laboratory test for a newly acquired ocular toxoplasmosis infection?

    a. IgM antibody titer

    b. IgG antibody titer

    c. *Toxoplasma* dye test of Sabin and Feldman

    d. hemagglutination test

27. Ophthalmologic signs of systemic lupus erythematosus include all but which of the following?

    a. vitreous hemorrhage

    b. cotton-wool spots

    c. retinal vascular occlusion

    d. anterior uveitis

28. Which of the following statements is *not* correct about Wegener granulomatosis?
    a. Antineutrophilic cytoplasmic antibodies (ANCA) are present.
    b. There are immune complexes in small vessels.
    c. The main therapeutic agents are prednisone and cyclophosphamide.
    d. Sinusitis and renal disease are common.

29. Characteristics of acute posterior multifocal placoid pigment epitheliopathy (APMPPE) include all *except* which of the following?
    a. It often follows a prodromal influenza-like illness.
    b. It is commonly seen in the fifth or sixth decade of life.
    c. Multiple cream-colored homogenous lesions are seen beneath the retina.
    d. Vitreous cells and disc edema may be present.

30. Which of the following statements about syphilis and uveitis is *not* correct?
    a. A salt-and-pepper fundus may be seen in congenital syphilis.
    b. Uveitis may be seen in secondary-stage syphilis.
    c. Syphilitic uveitis cannot be cured in patients with AIDS syndrome.
    d. A lumbar puncture should be performed in patients with uveitis and syphilis.

31. Which of the following laboratory tests may be negative in a patient with tertiary syphilis?
    a. serum VDRL
    b. serum FTA-ABS
    c. serum MHA-TP
    d. CSF VDRL

32. Which of the following tests is *not* used to diagnose Lyme disease?
    a. ELISA for IgM and IgG
    b. Lyme immunofluorescent antibody (IFA) titer
    c. Western blot testing
    d. culture and antibiotic sensitivity

33. Recommended treatment of Lyme disease includes all but which of the following?
    a. penicillin
    b. erythromycin
    c. cephalosporins
    d. tetracycline

34. Which of the following is *not* used to treat tuberculosis?
    a. ivermectin
    b. isoniazid
    c. rifampin
    d. pyrazinamide

35. Characteristics of sarcoidosis include all but which of the following?
    a. elevated serum angiotensin-converting enzyme (ACE) and lysozyme levels
    b. caseating granuloma on histopathology
    c. pulmonary and liver disease
    d. granulomatous or nongranulomatous uveitis

36. A 41-year-old Japanese man with a remote history of blunt ocular trauma in one eye but good vision and no history of ocular surgery presents with decreased vision and severe pain in both eyes. He has bilateral uveitis, alopecia, vitiligo, and recent cerebrovascular accident. There is an exudative retinal detachment in one eye. Which of the following diagnoses is most likely?
    a. sarcoidosis
    b. sympathetic ophthalmia
    c. Vogt-Koyanagi-Harada syndrome
    d. Behçet syndrome

37. A 67-year-old white female presents with mild uveitis with a mild vitritis and subretinal infiltrates. The condition has been minimally responsive to topical corticosteroid treatment. She has recently experienced weakness and confusion. Which of the following tests would be the most important to obtain at this time?
    a. gallium scan
    b. Westergren sedimentation rate and C-reactive protein
    c. PPD and chest x-ray
    d. CT scan or MRI of the head

38. Which of the following organisms is a frequent cause of endophthalmitis after ocular trauma but is an uncommon cause of endophthalmitis after cataract surgery or in bleb-related endophthalmitis?
    a. *Staphylococcus epidermidis*
    b. *Staphylococcus aureus*
    c. *Haemophilus influenzae*
    d. *Bacillus cereus*

39. Which of the following is the most common cause of endogenous fungal endophthalmitis?
    a. *Candida*
    b. *Aspergillus*
    c. *Rhizopus*
    d. *Cryptococcus*

40. A patient with a previous mitomycin-C trabeculectomy presents with a severe bleb-related endophthalmitis. The visual acuity previously was 20/20 and is now hand movements. Which of the following is *not* correct?
    a. The visual prognosis is poor.
    b. The organism in a bleb-related endophthalmitis is more likely to be *Haemophilus influenzae* or a *Streptococcus* species than it is in a post–cataract surgery endophthalmitis.
    c. Because the visual acuity is better than light perception, a vitreous tap for cultures and injection of antibiotics should be performed.
    d. Endophthalmitis may present months or years after glaucoma filtering surgery.

Study Questions • 277

41. Which intravitreal antibiotic has the greatest potential for causing retinal toxicity?
    a. ceftazidime
    b. vancomycin
    c. gentamicin
    d. penicillin

42. In contrast to the management of acute postoperative endophthalmitis after cataract surgery, the management of *P acnes* chronic endophthalmitis usually requires which of the following?
    a. intravitreal antibiotics
    b. removal of white plaque and capsulectomy
    c. systemic antibiotics
    d. periocular corticosteroids

43. Which of the following organisms usually causes the least virulent endophthalmitis?
    a. *Staphylococcus epidermidis*
    b. *Staphylococcus aureus*
    c. *Streptococcus pyogenes*
    d. *Serratia marcescens*

44. Which of the following glaucoma medications should probably be avoided in a healthy patient with uveitis, cystoid macular edema, and uncontrolled glaucoma?
    a. dorzolamide (Trusopt)
    b. timolol (Timoptic)
    c. brimonidine (Alphagan)
    d. latanoprost (Xalatan)

45. Which procedure is *not* indicated in patients with medically uncontrolled glaucoma associated with uveitis?
    a. laser trabeculoplasty
    b. trabeculectomy
    c. glaucoma implant (aqueous drainage device)
    d. trabeculodialysis

46. The initial management of a patient with uveitis and iris bombé should include which of the following?
    a. laser iridotomy
    b. surgical iridectomy
    c. trabeculectomy
    d. glaucoma implant

47. Management of cystoid macular edema in a patient with uveitis could include all *except* which of the following?
    a. corticosteroids
    b. nonsteroidal anti-inflammatory agents (NSAIDs)
    c. acetazolamide (Diamox)
    d. focal laser retinal treatment

48. Which of the following is the least frequent mode of transmission of HIV infection?

    a. intravenous drug abuse
    b. sexual intercourse
    c. perinatal transmission
    d. blood transfusion

49. Which of the following CD4 count ranges is associated with CMV retinitis?

    a. 250–500 cells/mm^3
    b. 150–200 cells/mm^3
    c. 75–125 cells/mm^3
    d. fewer than 50 cells/mm^3

50. Which of the following is the most common ocular finding in patients with AIDS?

    a. herpes zoster
    b. HIV retinopathy
    c. *Candida*
    d. toxoplasmosis

Answers

1. Answer—b. Innate immunity is genetically preprogrammed and triggered by bacterial toxins and cell debris. Adaptive, not innate, immunity requires recognition, processing, and effector phases, and demonstrates specificity and memory.
2. Answer—c. Eosinophils are commonly seen in local defenses against parasitic infection.
3. Answer—b. Basophils and mast cells are major effectors of IgE-mediated hypersensitivity.
4. Answer—a. IgM is the antibody produced in the effector phase of the first, or primary, effector phase of the immune response.
5. Answer—d. Significant inflammation is usually seen in sympathetic ophthalmia and phacoantigenic endophthalmitis. Milder inflammation is usually seen in *Propionibacterium acnes* endophthalmitis. In phacolytic glaucoma, macrophages engulf leaking lens protein and there is usually little or no intraocular inflammation.
6. Answer—a. Patients with the HLA-B27–associated uveitis may have other immunologic disorders such as Reiter syndrome, ankylosing spondylitis, and psoriatic arthritis. Behçet syndrome, however, is associated with HLA-B51.
7. Answer—a. Patients with rheumatoid arthritis, Behçet syndrome, and Reiter syndrome are more likely to have a nongranulomatous uveitis and patients with sarcoidosis, a granulomatous uveitis.
8. Answer—b. Patients with uveitis associated with Behçet syndrome may present with a hypopyon.
9. Answer—d. Prednisolone acetate 1% (Pred Forte) and prednisolone phosphate 1% (Inflammase Forte) are more effective than loteprednol (Lotemax), fluorometholone 0.25% (FML Forte), and dexamethasone 0.1% (Decadron) in treating intraocular inflammation in uveitis.
10. Answer—c. Fuchs heterochromic iridocyclitis often does not require topical corticosteroid therapy. The others almost always require topical corticosteroid therapy.
11. Answer—c. Periocular corticosteroid injections may benefit patients with uveitis and vitritis or cystoid macular edema. However, periocular corticosteroid injections should not be used in patients with infectious uveitis (eg, toxoplasmosis) and should also be avoided in patients with scleritis.
12. Answer—a. HLA-B27 is most likely to be positive in an American patient with acute nongranulomatous uveitis. Up to 50%–60% of patients with acute iritis may be HLA-B27 positive.
13. Answer—d. Reiter syndrome is associated with nonspecific urethritis, polyarthritis, and conjunctivitis, often accompanied by iritis. Ankylosing spondylitis is not a part of Reiter syndrome.
14. Answer—b. Behçet syndrome is associated with aphthous stomatitis, genital ulceration, erythema nodosum, hypopyon uveitis, and retinal vasculitis. Arthritis is usually not associated with Behçet syndrome.
15. Answer—d. Kawasaki syndrome is usually seen in childhood. Eighty-five percent of patients are less than 5 years old.

16. Answer—a. Rigid, closed-loop anterior chamber intraocular lenses are most associated with recurrent uveitis. Iris plane intraocular lenses occasionally cause inflammation, and, less commonly, a sulcus-placed posterior chamber intraocular lens causes inflammation from iris chafing or uveitis-glaucoma-hyphema (UGH) syndrome. Silicone intraocular lenses have been associated with iritis in the past.

17. Answer—b. Risk factors for the development of chronic iridocyclitis in juvenile rheumatoid arthritis (JRA) patients include female gender, pauciarticular arthritis, and circulating antinuclear antibody (ANA). Most JRA patients are rheumatoid factor (RF) negative.

18. Answer—c. In one series of JRA-associated uveitis cases, cataract was seen in 84%, band keratopathy in 70%, macular edema in 42%, and glaucoma in 26% of patients.

19. Answer—d. Typical characteristics of Fuchs heterochromic iridocyclitis include a unilateral uveitis with mild cell and flare, iris stromal atrophy, cataract, and glaucoma. Small stellate keratic precipitates are scattered diffusely on the corneal endothelium and not just in Arlt's triangle, as usually seen in most other types of uveitis.

20. Answer—b. Intermediate uveitis of unknown etiology, pars planitis, accounts for 85%–90% of cases. Other, less common causes include multiple sclerosis, Lyme disease, syphilis, and tuberculosis.

21. Answer—d. Cystoid macular edema is the major cause of visual loss in pars planitis. Other reasons for visual loss include band keratopathy, cataract, vitreous hemorrhage, epiretinal membrane, and retinal detachment.

22. Answer—c. The classic triad of acute retinal necrosis (ARN) syndrome includes occlusive arteriolitis, vitritis, and a multifocal yellow-white peripheral retinitis. Extensive retinal hemorrhages are usually not present.

23. Answer—a. Cytomegalovirus retinitis is seen in immunocompromised patients with AIDS, as well as in those who have received organ transplants or are receiving chemotherapy. Herpes simplex, ocular histoplasmosis, and acute retinal necrosis syndrome each may be seen in otherwise healthy individuals.

24. Answer—b. Peripapillary pigment changes, peripheral atrophic chorioretinal ("histo") spots, and a maculopathy are all seen in ocular histoplasmosis syndrome; vitritis is not.

25. Answer—c. Treatment of visually threatening ocular toxoplasmosis should include pyrimethamine (Daraprim) and sulfonamides (Bactrim, Septra). Neither amphotericin B, an antifungal agent, nor acyclovir, an antiviral agent, is active against toxoplasmosis, which is caused by a protozoal organism. Periocular corticosteroid injections may cause proliferation of the organism and should be avoided.

26. Answer—a. The IgM antibody titer is the best laboratory test for a newly acquired toxoplasmosis infection. The IgM antibody titer will be elevated early after the infection but will not be detectable 2–6 months after the initial infection.

27. Answer—d. Ophthalmologic signs of systemic lupus erythematosus include cotton-wool spots, retinal arteriolitis and vascular occlusion, vitreous hemorrhage, choroidal infarction, choroiditis, and subretinal exudation. Anterior uveitis is not usually seen with systemic lupus erythematosus.

28. Answer—b. Patients with Wegener granulomatosis may have sinus, pulmonary, and renal disease and usually have antineutrophilic cytoplasmic antibodies (ANCA). Prednisone and cyclophosphamide are the main therapeutic agents for Wegener granulomatosis. The histopathology of Wegener granulomatosis is a necrotizing granulomatous vasculitis, not immune complex deposition, as is seen in polyarteritis nodosa.

29. Answer—b. Characteristics of acute posterior multifocal placoid pigment epitheliopathy (APMPPE) include vitreous cells, optic disc edema, and multiple cream-colored plaquelike homogenous lesions, which are seen beneath the retina. APMPPE often follows a prodromal influenza-like illness. It is commonly seen in adolescents and young adults and not those in the fifth or sixth decade of life.

30. Answer—c. A salt-and-pepper fundus may be seen in congenital syphilis, and uveitis may be seen in secondary syphilis and in other stages. A lumbar puncture should be performed in patients with uveitis and syphilis. Syphilic uveitis can be cured with proper treatment, even in patients with AIDS.

31. Answer—a. In tertiary syphilis, serum FTA-ABS and MHA-TP, and CSF VDRL are positive. However, serum VDRL may be negative in a patient with tertiary syphilis.

32. Answer—d. Lyme immunofluorescent antibody titer, ELISA for IgM and IgG, and Western blot testing have all been used to diagnose Lyme disease, although with a high frequency of both false-positive and false-negative results. Culture and antibiotic sensitivity is not used to diagnose Lyme disease.

33. Answer—c. Recommended treatment of Lyme disease includes penicillin, erythromycin, and tetracycline, but not a cephalosporin.

34. Answer—a. Isoniazid, rifampin, and pyrazinamide are all used in the treatment of tuberculosis. Ivermectin (used to treat onchocerciasis) is not an antitubercular agent.

35. Answer—b. Granulomatous or nongranulomatous uveitis, pulmonary and liver disease, and elevated serum angiotensin-converting enzyme (ACE) and lysozyme levels may all be seen in sarcoidosis. Noncaseating granulomas are seen in sarcoidosis but caseating granulomas are seen in tuberculosis.

36. Answer—c. In the patient described, Vogt-Koyanagi-Harada syndrome is the most likely diagnosis. Sarcoidosis and Behçet syndrome are less likely. Blunt trauma is not likely to incite sympathetic ophthalmia.

37. Answer—d. In an older patient with a nonresponsive uveitis, vitritis, subretinal infiltrates, and neurological signs, a large-cell, non-Hodgkin lymphoma should be suspected. A CT scan or MRI of the head would be the first important step in this patient's management. CSF fluid analysis or vitreous biopsy can confirm the diagnosis. Sarcoidosis, tuberculosis, or giant cell arteritis are possible; however, it is important to rule out the possibility of a large-cell lymphoma.

38. Answer—d. The *Bacillus cereus* organism is frequently (26%–46%) found in traumatic endophthalmitis and may cause a fulminant endophthalmitis. *Staphylococcus epidermidis* and *Staphylococcus aureus* are the most common agents in post–cataract surgery endophthalmitis. *Haemophilus influenzae* and *Streptococcus* species are important causes of late bleb-related endophthalmitis.

39. Answer—a. *Candida albicans* is the most common cause of endogenous fungal endophthalmitis.

40. Answer—c. Bleb-related endophthalmitis may present months or years after glaucoma filtering surgery. The visual prognosis is poor. *Haemophilus influenzae* and a *Streptococcus* species are common causative agents of bleb-related endophthalmitis. In eyes with endophthalmitis after cataract surgery or secondary intraocular lens implantation, a preoperative visual acuity of better than light perception argues for a "tap and inject" rather than vitrectomy (Endophthalmitis Vitrectomy Study). However, the EVS conclusion is not applicable to patients with bleb-related endophthalmitis, and a vitrectomy is usually necessary in severe bleb-related endophthalmitis.

41. Answer—c. Gentamicin and other aminoglycoside antibiotics (tobramycin and amikacin) have a greater potential for retinal toxicity than the other three antibiotics listed.

42. Answer—b. In contrast to the management of acute postoperative endophthalmitis after cataract surgery, the management of *P acnes* chronic endophthalmitis usually requires removal of white plaque and capsulectomy. Both forms of endophthalmitis require intravitreal antibiotics and neither require systemic antibiotics. Periocular corticosteroids are sometimes used in severe acute postoperative endophthalmitis but not in *P acnes* endophthalmitis.

43. Answer—a. *Staphylococcus epidermidis* is the least virulent of the four listed organisms.

44. Answer—d. Latanoprost (Xalatan) should probably be avoided in a patient with uveitis and cystoid macular edema. It may worsen both intraocular inflammation and the cystoid macular edema. The other three agents listed should each pose no problem with respect to uveitis and cystoid macular edema.

45. Answer—a. Laser trabeculoplasty in any form (argon, diode, selective) is not indicated in patients with uveitis and glaucoma. It is ineffective, may exacerbate intraocular inflammation, and may cause severe intraocular pressure elevation in these patients. Trabeculectomy, glaucoma implant (aqueous drainage device), and trabeculodialysis have all been successfully used in surgical management of these patients.

46. Answer—a. The initial management of patients with uveitis and iris bombé should include laser iridotomy, glaucoma medications as needed, and intensive topical corticosteroids. Surgical iridectomy occasionally becomes necessary if a patent laser iridotomy cannot be successfully maintained. A trabeculectomy or glaucoma implant could later become necessary if there is a patent laser iridotomy and medically uncontrolled intraocular pressure.

47. Answer—d. Corticosteroids, nonsteroidal anti-inflammatory agents (NSAIDs), and acetazolamide (Diamox) have all been used in the management of cystoid macular edema in patients with uveitis. Focal retinal laser is not used in these patients.

48. Answer—c. In one study, perinatal transmission was the least frequent (1%) mode of transmission of HIV. Sexual intercourse (70%), intravenous drug abuse (27%), and blood transfusions (2%–3%) were more common causes of HIV transmission.

49. Answer—d. Extremely low CD4 counts, fewer than 50 cells/mm^3, are associated with CMV retinitis.

50. Answer—b. HIV retinopathy is the most common ocular finding in patients with AIDS although many other infections can also affect the eye in AIDS.

Index

(*i* = image; *t* = table)

AA. *See* Arachidonic acid
ACAID. *See* Anterior chamber–associated immune deviation
Accessory molecules, in immune processing, 22
Acetazolamide, for cystoid macular edema in uveitis, 239
Acquired (adaptive) immunity, 9–10. *See also* Adaptive immune response
Acquired immunodeficiency syndrome. *See* HIV infection/AIDS
Activated (stimulated) macrophages, 50, 51*i*, 52–53
Activation
  lymphocyte, 22–24, 23*i*, 25
  macrophage, 14–15, 48–54, 51*i*
  polymorphonuclear leukocyte, 49*i*, 49–50
Acute macular neuroretinopathy, 182
Acute phase reactants, in innate immune response, 47
Acute posterior multifocal placoid pigment epitheliopathy (APMPPE), 177*t*, 178, 179*i*
Acute retinal necrosis, 154–156, 155*i*, 156*i*
Acute retinal pigment epitheliitis (ARPE/Krill disease), 177*t*, 178, 179*i*
Acute zonal occult outer retinopathy (AZOOR), 180
Acyclovir, for acute retinal necrosis, 155
Adaptive immune response, 9–10
  effector reactivities of, 25, 54–74, 55*t*. *See also specific type*
    antibody-mediated, 54–63, 55*t*
    combined antibody and cellular, 55*t*, 70–74
    lymphocyte-mediated, 55*t*, 63–70
  immunization and, 17–31. *See also* Immune response arc
  immunoregulation of, 87–89
  innate immunity and
    differences from, 10–11
    similarities to, 10–11
  mediator systems affecting, 74–86, 75*t*
  triggers of, 9–11
  in viral conjunctivitis, 35
ADCC. *See* Antibody-dependent cellular cytotoxicity
Adenoviruses, ocular infection caused by, immune response to, 35
Adhesion, in neutrophil recruitment and activation, 48, 49*i*
Afferent lymphatic channels, 8, 19
Afferent phase of immune response arc, 17, 18*i*, 19–22, 20*i*, 21*i*
  response to poison ivy and, 29, 30
  response to tuberculosis and, 30–31
Agglutination, antibody, 58, 58*i*
AIDS. *See* HIV infection/AIDS
Alkylating agents, 96
  for uveitis, 119*t*
Alleles, human leukocyte antigen, 91–93. *See also* Human leukocyte (HLA) antigens
Allergens, 74
Allergic conjunctivitis, 74

Allergic reactions
  atopic keratoconjunctivitis, 74
  conjunctivitis, 74
  vernal keratoconjunctivitis, 13
Allografts, corneal, rejection of, 39, 40*i*, 41
Alpha chemokines, 81*t*
Alpha (α)-interferon, 82*t*
Alpha (α)$_2$-macroglobulin, in innate immune response, 47
Amikacin, for endophthalmitis, 217, 217*t*
Aminoglycosides, for endophthalmitis, 217
AMN. *See* Acute macular neuroretinopathy
Amphotericin B
  for coccidioidomycosis, 226–227
  for endophthalmitis, 217*t*, 219
  Aspergillus, 225–226
ANA. *See* Antinuclear (antineutrophil) antibodies
Anaphylactic hypersensitivity (immediate/type I) reaction, 27, 54*t*, 72–73, 73*i*
Anaphylatoxins, 60, 75
  retinal vasculitis in systemic lupus erythematosus and, 61
Anaphylaxis, 73*i*, 73
Anergy, 88
Aneurysms, retinal arterial, in HIV infection/AIDS, 248
Angiography, fluorescein, in uveitis, 113
Angle, in uveitis, 103*t*
Angle-closure glaucoma, pars planitis and, 151
Ankylosing spondylitis, 127*i*, 129–130, 130*i*
  HLA in, 94–95, 125–130
Anterior chamber
  immune response in, 34*t*, 36–39
  Onchocerca volvulus microfilariae in, 196
  in uveitis, 102–105, 103*t*, 104*i*. *See also* Anterior uveitis
Anterior chamber angle, in uveitis, 103*t*
Anterior chamber–associated immune deviation (ACAID), 37–39
  therapeutic potential of immune privilege and, 39
  tolerance to lens crystallins and, 90
Anterior segment
  disorders of, Th1 delayed hypersensitivity and, 68*t*
  immune response in, 34*t*, 36–39
  in uveitis, 102–105, 102*t*, 104*i*, 105*i*. *See also* Anterior uveitis
Anterior synechiae, in sarcoidosis, 198
Anterior uvea. *See* Uvea
Anterior uveitis, 106–107, 127–146. *See also specific cause and* Iridocyclitis; Iritis; Uveitis
  acute, 127–141
  causes of, 112*t*
  in children, juvenile rheumatoid arthritis and, 141–144, 142*i*, 144*t*
  chronic, 141–146
  circulating immune complexes and, 59
  differential diagnosis of, 110*t*
  in herpetic disease, 138–140
  HLA association in, 93, 94*t*, 128–132

283

in inflammatory bowel disease, 131–132
  in onchocerciasis, 185–197
  signs of, 102–105, 103*t*, 104*i*, 105*i*
  Th1 delayed hypersensitivity and, 68*t*
Antibiotics, for endophthalmitis, 215, 217–219, 218*t*, 219
Antibodies, 7, 25. *See also* Immunoglobulins
  definition of, 7
  immune complex formation and, 58–59, 58*i*
  local production of, 63
  monoclonal, 56
  polyclonal, 56
  stimulatory, 62
  structural and functional properties of, 54–55, 56*i*, 57*t*
Antibody-dependent cellular cytotoxicity, 70–72
Antibody isotypes. *See* Isotypes
Antibody-mediated immune effector responses, 54–63, 55*t*
  B-cell tissue infiltration and local antibody production and, 63
  immune complexes in
    circulating, 58–59, 58*i*
      anterior uveitis and, 59
    tissue-bound, 59–62, 60*i*
  immunoglobulin structure and function and, 54–55, 56*i*, 57*t*
  terminology associated with, 56
Antigen-presenting cells, 7, 19–22, 20*i*, 21*i*
  locations of, 34*t*
  in processing, 23*i*
Antigen receptors
  in adaptive immune response, 11
  B- and T-cell, 87
  in innate immune response, 12
Antigens, 7, 19
  adaptive immunity triggered by, 9, 10
  processing of, 22–24, 23*i*
  self, tolerance to, 87–89
  transplantation, 93–94
Anti-idiotypic antibodies, 56
Antimetabolites, 96
  for uveitis, 119*t*
Antinuclear (antineutrophil) antibodies, in juvenile rheumatoid arthritis, 141, 144*t*
Antirecoverin antibodies, cancer-associated retinopathy and, 61
Antitoxoplasma antibodies, 167
Antiviral agents
  for acute retinal necrosis, 155
  for HIV infection/AIDS, 246–248, 247*t*
  for uveitis, 140
APC. *See* Antigen-presenting cells
APMPPE. *See* Acute posterior multifocal placoid pigment epitheliopathy
Apoptosis
  by cytotoxic T lymphocytes, 68, 69*i*
  Fas ligand in, 38, 68, 69*i*
Aqueous cellular reaction, in uveitis, 102
Aqueous flare, in uveitis, 102, 104*i*, 105*i*
Aqueous humor
  immune response and, 36
  specimen collection from, 215–216

Arachidonic acid (arachidonate), in eicosanoid synthesis, 77, 78*i*
Argyll Robertson pupil, in syphilis, 190
Aristocort. *See* Triamcinolone
ARN. *See* Acute retinal necrosis
ARPE. *See* Acute retinal pigment epitheliitis
Arthritis
  juvenile rheumatoid. *See* Juvenile rheumatoid arthritis
  psoriatic, 132, 133*i*
  reactive (Reiter syndrome), 130–131, 131*i*, 132*i*
    HLA association in, 94*t*, 130
Arthus reaction, 60, 60*i*
  acute, 60, 60*i*
  chronic, 63
  retinal vasculitis in systemic lupus erythematosus and, 61
Aspergillus flavus/Aspergillus fumigatus (aspergillosis), endogenous endophthalmitis caused by, 225–226, 225*i*
Assassination (cell), by cytotoxic T lymphocytes, 68, 69*i*
Asteroid bodies, in sarcoidosis, 198
Atopic hypersensitivity (immediate/type I) reaction, 27, 54*t*, 72–73, 73*i*
Atopic keratoconjunctivitis, 74
Atovaquone, for toxoplasmosis, 168
Atropine, for uveitis, 114
Atypical necrotizing retinitis, diagnosis of, 63
Autoantibodies
  retinal vasculitis in systemic lupus erythematosus and, 61, 173–175
  scleritis/retinal vasculitis in Wegener granulomatosis and, 62, 175
Autocrine action, of cytokines, 80
Autoimmune diseases. *See also specific type*
  molecular mimicry and, 91
  tolerance and, 87–89
  uveitis, 91
Azathioprine, for uveitis, 119, 119*t*

B-cell antigen receptors, 87
B cells (B lymphocytes), 15
  activation of, 19–22, 21*i*, 24
  infiltration of into tissues, in antibody-mediated immune response, 63
  maturation of, in bone marrow, 15
Bacille Calmette-Guérin vaccination, PPD test affected by, 195
Bacillus, traumatic endophthalmitis caused by, 208*t*, 212
Bacteria
  endogenous endophthalmitis caused by, 213
  innate immunity triggered by molecules derived from, 43–47, 44*t*
  panuveitis caused by, 187–195
Bacterial cell wall components, in innate immune response, 44
Bactrim. *See* Trimethoprim/sulfamethoxazole
Band keratopathy, in juvenile rheumatoid arthritis, 142, 142*i*, 143
Basophil hypersensitivity, cutaneous, 66
Basophils, 13–14

Baylisascaris procyonis, diffuse unilateral subacute neuroretinitis caused by, 172
Behçet syndrome, 132–135, 134i
   HLA association in, 94t, 134
   hypopyon in, 107, 132, 133, 134i
Berlin nodules, in uveitis, 105, 105i
Beta chemokines, 81t
Betamethasone, for uveitis, 115t
Bilateral diffuse uveal melanocytic proliferation, 233
Birdshot retinochoroidopathy (vitiliginous chorioretinitis), 177t, 180–181, 180i, 181i
   HLA association in, 94t, 181
Bleb-associated endophthalmitis, 207, 208t, 212–213
Blebitis
   bleb-associated endophthalmitis differentiated from, 212–213
   treatment of, 219
Blind spot, prolonged enlargement of, 182
Blindness, river (onchocerciasis), 195–197
Blood–ocular barrier, immune response and
   of retina/retinal pigment epithelium/choroid, 40–41
   of anterior chamber/anterior uvea/vitreous, 36
Blunt trauma, anterior uveitis caused by, 107
Blurred vision/blurring, in uveitis, 101–102, 102t
Bone marrow, as lymphoid tissue, 16
Borrelia burgdorferi, 191. *See also* Lyme disease
Bradykinin, 76
Breaks, retinal. *See* Retinal breaks
Busacca nodules
   in sarcoidosis, 105i, 198, 199i
   in uveitis, 105, 105i

C-reactive protein, in innate immune response, 47
CAM. *See* Cell-adhesion molecules
Cancer, retinopathy associated with, 61
Candida albicans (candidiasis)
   endogenous endophthalmitis caused by, 213–214, 219–220, 223–225
   postoperative endophthalmitis caused by, 210
   retinitis caused by, 163–164, 164i
Candlewax drippings, in sarcoidosis, 199
Capsulorrhexis, in uveitis, 235–236
CAR. *See* Cancer, retinopathy associated with
Carotid endarterectomy, for ocular ischemic syndrome, 222
Carotid occlusive disease, ocular ischemic syndrome and, 221–222
Cataract
   in juvenile rheumatoid arthritis, 142, 142i, 143
   in pars planitis, 151–152
   uveitis and, 235–237
   in Vogt-Koyanagi-Harada syndrome, 205
Cataract surgery
   endophthalmitis after, 207–209, 208t. *See also* Postoperative endophthalmitis
   for Fuchs heterochromic iridocyclitis, 145
   juvenile rheumatoid arthritis–associated iridocyclitis/uveitis and, 143
   in pars planitis, 151–152
   tolerance to lens crystallins and, 90
   in uveitis patient, 235–237
CCR5, in HIV infection/AIDS, 242

CD4 T cells. *See also* T cells
   class II MHC molecules as antigen-presenting platform for, 19–20, 20i
   delayed hypersensitivity, 25, 63–66, 65i
   differentiation of, 22–24, 23i
   in HIV infection/AIDS, 242–243, 244t, 246–248
   in immune processing, 22–24, 23i
CD8 T cells. *See also* T cells
   class I MHC molecules as antigen-presenting platform for, 19–22, 21i
   cytotoxic, 24, 25, 66–70, 69i
      in viral conjunctivitis, 35
   in immune processing, 23i, 24
   suppressor, 23i, 24
CD95 ligand. *See* Fas ligand
Ceftazidime, for endophthalmitis, 217, 218t
Ceftriaxone, for endophthalmitis, 218t
Celestone. *See* Betamethasone
Cell-adhesion molecules
   in homing, 27–28
   in neutrophil recruitment and activation, 48, 49i
Cell death, programmed (PCD/apoptosis)
   by cytotoxic T lymphocytes, 68–70, 69i
   Fas ligand in, 38, 68, 69i
Cell lysis
   complement-mediated, 59, 60i
   by cytotoxic lymphocytes, 68, 69i
CellCept. *See* Mycophenolate mofetil
Cellular immunity (cell-mediated immunity). *See* Lymphocyte-mediated immune effector responses
Cephalosporins, for endophthalmitis, 217
Chamber angle, in uveitis, 103t
Chemokines, 80, 81t
Chemotaxis, 7
   in neutrophil recruitment and activation, 48, 49i
Chickenpox (varicella), iritis/iridocyclitis in, 138
Chlorambucil, for uveitis, 119, 119t
Chloramphenicol, for endophthalmitis, 218t
Chorioretinal biopsy, in uveitis, 113
Chorioretinitis, 107
   in coccidioidomycosis, 163, 226
   differential diagnosis of, 111t
   in ocular histoplasmosis syndrome, 160–163, 160i, 161i, 162i
   in onchocerciasis, 195–197
   in syphilis, 187, 189i, 190
      HIV infection/AIDS and, 189, 255–256
      posterior placoid, 255
   vitiliginous (birdshot retinochoroidopathy), 177t, 180–181, 181i
      HLA association in, 94t, 181
Choroid
   diseases of, Th1 delayed hypersensitivity and, 68t
   immune response in, 34t, 40–41
   in uveitis, 103t
Choroidal neovascularization
   in histoplasmosis, 162i, 163
   in uveitis, 240
   in Vogt-Koyanagi-Harada syndrome, 205, 240
Choroiditis, 107
   geographic (serpiginous/helicoid peripapillary choroidopathy), 177t, 182–183, 184i

in HIV infection/AIDS
Cryptococcus neoformans causing, 257
multifocal, 257–258
Pneumocystis carinii causing, 256–257, 256*i*, 257*i*
multifocal
in HIV infection/AIDS, 257–258
and panuveitis (MCP), 177*t*, 185, 185*i*
in ocular histoplasmosis, 160–161, 161*i*
punctate inner (PIC), 177*t*, 182, 183*i*
Choroidopathy, serpiginous/helicoid peripapillary (geographic choroiditis), 177*t*, 182–183, 184*i*
Cidofovir
for cytomegalovirus retinitis, 252
iritis/hypotony caused by, 252
uveitis caused by, 141, 252
Ciliary body
immunologic microenvironment of, 36–37
in uveitis, 105
Ciliary flush, in uveitis, 102, 103
Ciprofloxacin, for endophthalmitis, 218*t*
Class I major histocompatibility complex molecules, 20–22, 21*i*, 90, 92*t*
Class II major histocompatibility complex molecules, 19, 20*i*, 90, 92*t*
primed macrophages as, 51*i*, 52
Class III major histocompatibility complex molecules, 91
Clindamycin, for toxoplasmosis, 168
Clonal deletion, 88
Clonal inactivation, 88
CMV. *See* Cytomegaloviruses
Coccidioides immitis (coccidioidomycosis), 163, 226–227, 227*i*
Colitis, granulomatous (Crohn disease), 131–132
Collagen vascular diseases, uveitis in, 173–175
Collagenases, 86
Complement, 7, 74–76, 76*i*
in adaptive immune response, 74–76
cell lysis mediated by, 59, 60*i*
in innate immune response, 46–47, 75
receptors for, in phagocytosis, 50
Compromised host, ocular infection in
cytomegalovirus retinitis, 71, 156–157, 249–250
ocular candidiasis, 163–164, 223–224
Congenital rubella syndrome, 158–159, 159*i*
Congenital syphilis, 187–188, 188*i*
Conjunctiva
disorders of, Th1 delayed hypersensitivity and, 68*t*
immune response/immunologic features of, 33–36, 34*t*
mast cells in, 13–14
in uveitis, 103*t*
Conjunctivitis
allergic, 74
in HIV infection/AIDS, 261
in Lyme disease, 191, 192
in reactive arthritis/Reiter syndrome, 131
vernal, 13
viral, immune response to, 35
Connective tissue disorders, uveitis in, 173–175
Connective tissue mast cells, 13–14
Contact hypersensitivity, 66
response to poison ivy as, 29–30
Contact lenses, for trial fitting, disinfection of, 262

Cornea
disorders of, Th1 delayed hypersensitivity and, 68*t*
immune response/immunologic features of, 34*t*, 39, 40*i*
topography of, 39, 40*i*
in uveitis, 103*t*
Corneal allografts. *See* Corneal grafts
Corneal grafts, rejection of, 39, 40*i*, 41
Corticosteroids (steroids)
for endophthalmitis, 217, 218*t*, 219
for juvenile rheumatoid arthritis, 143
for pars planitis, 149–150
for toxoplasmosis, 169
for tuberculous ocular disease, 195, 196*i*
for uveitis, 96, 114, 114*t*, 115–118, 115*t*, 117*i*, 128
before cataract surgery, 235
intraocular pressure elevation and, 238
tuberculous, 195, 196*i*
viral, 140
for Vogt-Koyanagi-Harada syndrome, 205
Cotton-wool spots
in HIV retinopathy, 248, 249*i*
in systemic lupus erythematosus, 173, 173*i*
COX. *See* Cyclo-oxygenase
COX-2 inhibitors, 96
Cranial nerve II (optic nerve). *See* Optic nerve
Crohn disease (granulomatous ileocolitis), 131–132
Cryoretinopexy, for retinal detachment in uveitis, 240
Cryotherapy, for pars planitis, 150
Cryptococcus neoformans (cryptococcosis), 163
in HIV infection/AIDS, 257
Crystallins, lens. *See* Lens proteins
CTLs. *See* Cytotoxic T lymphocytes
Cutaneous basophil hypersensitivity, 66
CXCR4, in HIV infection/AIDS, 242
Cyclitis, chronic (pars planitis). *See* Pars planitis
Cyclogyl. *See* Cyclopentolate
Cyclo-oxygenase (COX-1/COX-2), 79
nonsteroidal anti-inflammatory drugs and, 96
Cyclopentolate, for uveitis, 114, 128
Cyclophosphamide, for uveitis, 119, 119*t*
Cycloplegia/cycloplegics, for uveitis, 114–115, 114*t*, 128
Cyclosporine, 97
for uveitis, 97, 119*t*, 120
for Vogt-Koyanagi-Harada syndrome, 205
Cysticercus cellulosae (cysticercosis), 171, 172*i*
Cystoid macular edema
in pars planitis, 148, 151
prostaglandins and, 79
in uveitis, 239
Cytokines, 7, 80–83, 81–82*t*. *See also specific type*
in delayed hypersensitivity, 63–66, 65*i*
in immune processing, 22, 23*i*
in immunotherapy, 66–70
as inflammatory mediators, 80–83, 81–82*t*
Cytolysis, immune, 59, 60*i*
Cytomegalic inclusion disease, 157
Cytomegaloviruses, 156–157, 157*i*, 249–250
congenital infection caused by, 157
retinitis caused by, 156–157, 157*i*
antiviral immunity in, 71
cidofovir for, 252
fomivirsen for, 252

foscarnet for, 251
ganciclovir for, 155, 250–251
in HIV infection/AIDS, 71, 156–157, 249–253, 251*i*
Cytotoxic drugs, 96
Cytotoxic hypersensitivity (type II) reaction, 54*t*. *See also* Cytotoxic T lymphocytes
Cytotoxic T lymphocytes, 24, 25, 66–70, 69*i*
in viral conjunctivitis, 35
Cytoxan. *See* Cyclophosphamide

Dalen-Fuchs nodules/spots
in sympathetic ophthalmia, 202
in Vogt-Koyanagi-Harada syndrome, 203, 204*i*
Daraprim. *See* Pyrimethamine
DC. *See* Dendritic cells
Delayed hypersensitivity (type IV) reaction, 25, 54*t*, 63–66, 65*i*, 68*t*
in chronic mast cell degranulation, 73
response to poison ivy as, 30
tuberculin form of, 31, 66
Delayed hypersensitivity (DH) T cells, 25, 63–66, 65*i*, 68*t*. *See also* T cells
Dendritic cells, 15
Depo-Medrol. *See* Methylprednisolone
Depot injections, corticosteroid, for uveitis, 116–117, 115*t*, 117*i*
Dexamethasone
for endophthalmitis, 218*t*
for uveitis, 115*t*
DH. *See* Delayed hypersensitivity (type IV) reaction
Diffuse unilateral subacute neuroretinitis (DUSN), 172–173, 172*i*
Diffuse uveitis. *See* Panuveitis
Domains, immunoglobulin, 55, 56*i*
Donor cornea, rejection of, 39, 40*i*, 41
Downregulatory T cells, in suppression, 88
Doxycycline
for syphilis, 190
for toxoplasmosis, 169
Drug-induced uveitis, 141
DUSN. *See* Diffuse unilateral subacute neuroretinitis

E-selectin, in neutrophil rolling, 48, 49*i*
EBV. *See* Epstein-Barr virus
Effector blockade, 38
Effector cells, 11, 25, 26*i*
locations of, 34*t*
lymphocytes as, 11, 15, 25, 26*i*
macrophages as, 14–15
neutrophils as, 13, 48–50, 49*i*
Effector phase of immune response arc, 17–19, 18*i*, 25, 26*i*, 43–86
adaptive immunity and, 27, 54–75, 55*t*
antibody-mediated, 54–63, 55*t*
blockade of, in anterior chamber–associated immune deviation, 38
cells in. *See* Effector cells
combined antibody and cellular, 55*t*, 70–74
innate immunity and, 43–54
lymphocyte-mediated, 55*t*, 63–70
mediator systems and, 74–86
response to poison ivy and, 30

response to tuberculosis and, 31
in viral conjunctivitis, 35
Efferent lymphatic channels, 8
Eicosanoids, as inflammatory mediators, 78–79, 78*i*
Elevated intraocular pressure, in uveitic glaucoma, 237
Endarterectomy, carotid, for ocular ischemic syndrome, 223
Endemic Kaposi sarcoma, 258
Endogenous endophthalmitis/retinitis, 207–209, 209*i*, 213–214, 214*i*
Aspergillus causing, 225–226, 225*i*
fungal, 223–227
nocardial, 223, 223*i*
Endophthalmitis, 207–220
Aspergillus causing, 225–226, 225*i*
bacterial toxins affecting severity of, 46
bleb-associated, 208*t*, 209, 212–213
Candida, 163–164, 213–214, 219, 223–225
diagnosis/differential diagnosis of, 215–216
endogenous, 207, 209*i*, 213–214, 214*i*
fungal, 223–227
exogenous, 207, 208*t*, 209–213, 209*i*
infectious, 207, 208*t*
differential diagnosis of, 215
intraocular specimens for diagnosis of
collection of, 215–216
cultures and laboratory evaluation of, 216
Nocardia asteroides causing, 223, 223*i*
phacoantigenic (lens-induced/phacoanaphylaxis), 64, 135–136, 135*i*, 136*i*
postoperative, 207, 208*t*, 209–211
acute-onset, 210–211, 210*i*, 211*i*
bleb-associated, 207, 208*t*, 212–213
after cataract surgery, 207, 208*t*, 209
chronic (delayed-onset), 211, 212*i*
posttraumatic, 207, 208*t*, 211–212
prophylaxis of, 214–215
Propionibacterium acnes causing, 53, 208*t*, 209, 211, 212*i*
signs and symptoms of, 207
sterile, 207
in toxocariasis, 170, 171*t*
treatment of, 217–220
medical, 217–219, 218*t*
outcomes of, 219–220
surgical, 217
Endophthalmitis Vitrectomy Study (EVS), 217, 220
Endotoxins, microbial, in innate immune response, 43–44, 46
Enteritis, regional (Crohn disease), 131–132
Enterococcus, bleb-associated endophthalmitis caused by, 213
Enucleation, for prevention of sympathetic ophthalmia, 200
Enzyme-linked immunosorbent assay (ELISA)
in HIV infection/AIDS, 245–246
in toxoplasmosis, 167
Eosinophils, 13
Epidemic Kaposi sarcoma, 258
Epitheliitis, acute retinal pigment (ARPE/Krill disease), 177*t*, 178, 179*i*
Epithelioid cells, 15, 52–53. *See also* Macrophages

Epitheliopathy, acute posterior multifocal placoid pigment (APMPPE), 177t, 178, 179i
Epitopes, 7, 11, 19, 56
Epstein-Barr virus, posterior uveitis caused by, 157–158
Equatorial streaks, in histoplasmosis, 160, 161i
Erythema chronicum migrans, in Lyme disease, 191, 192i
Erythromycin, for syphilis, 190
Etanercept, for uveitis, 120
EVS. See Endophthalmitis Vitrectomy Study
Examination, ophthalmic, HIV infection precautions and, 261–262
Exogenous endophthalmitis, 207, 208t, 209–213, 209i
Exotoxins, microbial, in innate immune response, 45–46
External (outer) eye, HIV infection/AIDS affecting, 258–260
Extracapsular cataract extraction (ECCE), in uveitis, 235
Eyedrops (topical medications), corticosteroid, for uveitis, 115–116, 115t
Eyelids, in uveitis, 103t

Fab region (antibody molecule), 55, 56i
Family history/familial factors, in uveitis, 122
Fas ligand, 38, 68, 69i
FasL. See Fas ligand
Fc receptors, 7, 55, 56i
  in antibody-dependent cellular cytotoxicity, 70
  on mast cells, 13–14
  in phagocytosis, 50
Fenton reaction, oxygen radicals produced by, 84
Fibrin, as inflammatory mediator, 76–77
Fibrinogen, 76
Filtering bleb
  endophthalmitis associated with, 207–209, 208t, 212–213
  for uveitic glaucoma, 237
Floaters, in posterior uveitis, 107
Fluconazole, for endophthalmitis, 218t, 219
5-Flucytosine, for endophthalmitis, 219
Fluorescein angiography
  in ocular ischemic syndrome, 222
  in uveitis, 113
Fluorescent treponemal antibody absorption (FTA-ABS) test, 189–190
Fluorometholone, for uveitis, 115t, 116, 238
Fluoroquinolones, for endophthalmitis, 217
FMLP. See N-Formylmethionylleucylphenylalanine
Foldable intraocular lens, in uveitis, 138
Fomivirsen, for cytomegalovirus retinitis, 252
Foreign bodies, retained, endophthalmitis caused by, 212
N-Formylmethionylleucylphenylalanine (FMLP), in innate immunity, 46
Foscarnet, for cytomegalovirus retinitis, 251
Free radicals (oxygen radicals), as inflammatory mediators, 83–85, 84i
FTA-ABS (fluorescent treponemal antibody absorption) test, 189–190
Fuchs heterochromic iridocyclitis/uveitis, 107, 144–146, 145i

Fundus
  salt-and-pepper
    in rubella, 158, 159i
    in syphilis, 188
  sunset-glow, in Vogt-Koyanagi-Harada syndrome, 201i, 203, 204i
Fungi. See also specific type
  endophthalmitis caused by, 208t, 210, 212, 213–214, 214i, 219, 223–227
  posterior uveitis caused by, 160–164

Gamma (γ)-interferon, 82t
  in delayed hypersensitivity, 65i, 66
Ganciclovir, for cytomegalovirus retinitis, 155, 250–252
Gene therapy, retinal, 42
Gentamicin, for endophthalmitis, 217, 218t
Geographic choroiditis (serpiginous/helicoid peripapillary choroidopathy), 177t, 182–183, 184i
German measles. See Rubella
Giant cells, 15, 52–53
Glaucoma
  in herpetic uveitis, 139
  juvenile rheumatoid arthritis–associated iridocyclitis and, 143–144
  lens-induced, 52, 136–137
  pars planitis and, 151
  phacolytic, 52, 136–137
  in sarcoidosis, 198
  uveitis and, 139, 237–239, 238t
  in Vogt-Koyanagi-Harada syndrome, 205
Glaucomatocyclitic crisis (Posner-Schlossman syndrome), 107, 135
Glucocorticoids/glucocorticosteroids, 96
Goldmann-Witmer coefficient, 63
Grafts
  corneal, rejection of, 39, 40i, 41
  retinal/retinal pigment epithelium, 42
  transplantation antigens and, 93–94
Granulomas
  in coccidioidomycosis, 163, 226
  in sarcoidosis, 196–199, 197i, 198i
  in toxocariasis, 170–171, 170i, 171i, 171t
Granulomatosis, Wegener, scleritis/retinal vasculitis and, 62, 175–176, 176i
Granulomatous disease
  ileocolitis (Crohn disease), 131
  uveitis, 104, 108, 197–200
Granulomatous hypersensitivity, 66
Growth factors, 80, 82t
Gummata, syphilitic, 188, 190
GUN syndrome, in primary central nervous system lymphoma, 229

HAART. See Highly active antiretroviral therapy
Haber-Weiss reaction, oxygen radicals produced by, 84, 84i
Haemophilus influenzae, bleb-associated endophthalmitis caused by, 208t, 212–213
Hageman factor, in kinin-forming system, 76
Hapten, 7
  poison ivy toxin as, 29–30
  serum sickness caused by, 59
Heavy chains, immunoglobulin, 54–55, 56i

Helminths
  Panuveitis caused by, 195–197
  posterior uveitis caused by, 170–173
Helper T cells. *See also specific type under T helper*
  class II MHC molecules as antigen-presenting platform for, 19–20, 20*i*
  in delayed hypersensitivity (type IV) reactions, 63–66, 65*i*, 68*t*
  differentiation of, 22–24, 23*i*
  in HIV infection/AIDS, 242–243
  in immune processing, 22–24, 23*i*
Hemorrhages, retinal, in HIV infection/AIDS, 248
Heparin surface modification, intraocular lens, 138
Herpes simplex virus
  acute retinal necrosis caused by, 140, 154–156, 155*i*, 156*i*
  in HIV infection/AIDS, 260
  uveitis caused by, 138–140
Herpes zoster
  acute retinal necrosis caused by, 140, 154–156, 155*i*, 156*i*
  in HIV infection/AIDS, 260
  uveitis and, 138–140, 139*i*
Herpetic uveitis, 138–140, 139*i*
  glaucoma in, 139
Highly active antiretroviral therapy (HAART), 246
  for cytomegalovirus retinitis, 253
Histamine, as inflammatory mediator, 77
Histo spots, 160, 160*i*, 161
Histocompatibility antigens. *See* Human leukocyte (HLA) antigens
Histoplasma capsulatum (histoplasmosis), ocular, 160–163, 160*i*, 161*i*, 162*i*, 177*t*
  histo spots in, 160, 160*i*, 161
  HLA association in, 94*t*, 160
History, in uveitis, 122–126
HIV-1, 242
HIV-2, 242
HIV infection/AIDS, 241–262
  CDC definition of, 243, 244–245*t*
  choroiditis in
    Cryptococcus neoformans, 257
    multifocal, 257–258
    Pneumocystis carinii, 256–257, 256*i*, 257*i*
  classification of, 243–245, 244–245*t*
  cytomegalovirus retinitis in, 71, 156, 249, 251*i*
  diagnosis of, 245–246
    ophthalmologist's role in, 261
  herpes simplex keratitis in, 260, 260*i*
  herpes zoster in, 260
  incidence of, 241
  Kaposi sarcoma in, 258–259, 258*i*, 259*i*
  management of, 246–248, 247*t*
    ophthalmologist's role in, 261
  molluscum contagiosum in, 259
  natural history of, 243–245, 244–245*t*
  occupational exposure to, precautions in health care setting and, 261–262
  ocular infection/manifestations and, 241–262
    external eye manifestations, 258–260
    ophthalmic complications, 248–249
  opportunistic infections associated with, 248, 260, 260*i*
  pathogenesis of, 242–243
  Pneumocystis carinii infections and, 256–257, 256*i*, 257*i*
  progressive outer retinal necrosis in, 155, 253–254, 254*i*
  retinitis in, 71, 140, 154–156, 155*i*, 156, 156*i*, 248–253, 251*i*, 260
  retinopathy associated with, 248, 249*i*
  syphilis/syphilitic chorioretinitis in, 189, 255–256
  systemic conditions associated with, 246
  Toxoplasma retinochoroiditis/toxoplasmosis in, 165–166, 165*i*, 166*i*, 254–255, 255*i*
  transmission of, 245
  tuberculosis and, 193
  virology of, 242
HLA. *See* Human leukocyte (HLA) antigens
Homing, 27–28
  MALT and, 36
Hormonal action, of cytokines, 80
Horror autotoxicus, 87
Human immunodeficiency virus (HIV), 241–242. *See also* HIV infection/AIDS
  testing for antibody to, 245–246
Human leukocyte (HLA) antigens, 90–95, 92*t*. *See also* Major histocompatibility complex
  allelic variations and, 91
  in ankylosing spondylitis, 93, 129
  in anterior uveitis, 93, 94*t*, 129–132
  in Behçet syndrome, 94*t*, 134
  in birdshot retinochoroidopathy, 94*t*, 180–181
  detection and classification of, 91
  disease associations of, 94–95, 94*t*
  in glaucomatocyclitic crisis (Posner-Schlossman syndrome), 135
  in inflammatory bowel disease, 131–132
  in intermediate uveitis/pars planitis, 94*t*, 147
  in juvenile rheumatoid arthritis, 94*t*, 141
  in multiple sclerosis, 94*t*
  normal function of, 90–91
  in ocular histoplasmosis syndrome, 94*t*, 160–161
  in reactive arthritis/Reiter syndrome, 94*t*, 130–131
  in retinal vasculitis, 94*t*
  in sarcoidosis, 94*t*
  in sympathetic ophthalmia, 94*t*
  transplantation and, 93–94
  in Vogt-Koyanagi-Harada syndrome, 94*t*, 205
Humoral immunity. *See* Antibody-mediated immune effector responses
Hutchinson's sign, 138
Hybridomas, monoclonal antibody and, 56
Hydrocortisone sodium succinate, for uveitis, 115*t*
Hydroxyl radical, as inflammatory mediator, 83, 85
Hypersensitivity reactions, 54, 54*t*
  anaphylactic or atopic (immediate/type I), 27, 54*t*, 72–73, 73*i*
  contact, 66
    response to poison ivy as, 29, 30
  cutaneous basophil, 66
  cytotoxic (type II), 54*t*
  delayed (type IV), 54*t*
    in chronic mast cell degranulation, 73
    response to poison ivy as, 29, 30
    tuberculin form of, 31, 65

granulomatous, 66
immediate (type I/anaphylactic/atopic). *See* Hypersensitivity reactions, anaphylactic or atopic
immune-complex (type III), 54*t*. *See also* Immune complexes
stimulatory (type V), 54, 54*t*
Hypopyon
 in Behçet syndrome, 107, 132, 133, 134*i*
 in endophthalmitis, 211, 212, 223–224
 in uveitis, 107, 127, 127*i*
Hypotony, in uveitis, 239

ICAM-1/ICAM-2, in neutrophil rolling, 48
Idiopathic iridocyclitis, 146
Idiotopes, 56
Idiotypes, 56
Ig. *See under Immunoglobulin*
IL. *See* Interleukins
IL-5. *See* Interleukin-5
Ileocolitis, granulomatous (Crohn disease), 131–132
Immediate hypersensitivity (type I) reaction, 27, 54*t*, 72–73, 73*i*
Immune-complex hypersensitivity (type III) reaction, 54*t*. *See also* Immune complexes
Immune complexes
 circulating, 58–59, 58*i*
  anterior uveitis and, 59
 tissue-bound, 59–62, 60*i*
  Arthus reaction and, 60, 60*i*
Immune cytolysis, 59, 60*i*
Immune hypersensitivity reactions. *See* Hypersensitivity reactions
Immune privilege
 in anterior uvea, 37–39
 corneal, 39
 in retina/retinal pigment epithelium/choroid, 41
 therapeutic potential of, 39
 tolerance to lens crystallins and, 90
Immune processing, 22–24, 23*i*
 response to poison ivy and, 29, 30
 response to tuberculosis and, 30–31
Immune response (immunity). *See also* Immune response arc
 adaptive, 9–10. *See also* Adaptive immune response
 definition of, 9
 immunoregulation of, 34*t*, 87–89
 inflammation differentiated from, 12
 innate, 9, 10. *See also* Innate immune response
 mediator systems in, 7, 74–86, 75*t*
 ocular, 33–42
  of anterior chamber/anterior uvea/vitreous, 34*t*, 36–39
  of conjunctiva, 33–36, 34*t*
  of cornea/sclera, 34*t*, 39–41, 40*t*
  of retina/retinal pigment epithelium/choroid, 34*t*, 40–41
 primary
  immune response arc and, 27–28
  secondary response differentiated from, 27
 regional, 28
 secondary
  immune response arc and, 27–28
  primary response differentiated from, 27

Immune response arc, 17–32. *See also* Immune response
 clinical examples of, 29
 immunologic microenvironments and, 28
 overview of, 17, 18*i*
 phases of, 17, 18*i*, 19–25
  afferent, 17, 18*i*, 19–22, 20*i*, 21*i*
   response to poison ivy and, 29, 30
   response to tuberculosis and, 30–31
  effector, 17–19, 18*i*, 25, 26*i*, 43–86. *See also* Effector phase of immune response arc
   response to poison ivy and, 29, 30
   response to tuberculosis and, 30–31
  processing, 22–24, 23*i*
   response to poison ivy and, 29, 30
   response to tuberculosis and, 30–31
 primary or secondary immune responses and, 27–28
 regional immunity and, 28
Immune system. *See also* Immune response; Immune response arc
 components of, 13–16
Immunization, adaptive immunity and, 17–31. *See also* Immune response arc
Immunocompromised host
 cryptococcosis in, 163, 257
 cytomegalovirus retinitis in, 71, 156–157, 249–250
 ocular candidiasis in, 163–164, 223–224
Immunogen, 19
Immunoglobulin A (IgA)
 structural and functional properties of, 57*t*
 in tear film, 33
 in viral conjunctivitis, 35
Immunoglobulin D (IgD), structural and functional properties of, 57*t*
Immunoglobulin E (IgE)
 mast cell degranulation mediated by, 13–14, 72–73, 73*i*
 structural and functional properties of, 57*t*
 in type I hypersensitivity/anaphylactic reactions, 27, 72–73, 73*i*
Immunoglobulin G (IgG), structural and functional properties of, 57*t*
Immunoglobulin M (IgM), structural and functional properties of, 57*t*
Immunoglobulin superfamily molecules, in neutrophil rolling, 48, 49*i*
Immunoglobulins, 25. *See also specific type*
 classes of, 54–55
 isotypes of, 7, 55
  in immunologic tolerance, 89
 structural and functional properties of, 54–55, 56*i*, 57*t*
Immunologic memory, 11, 27–28
Immunologic microenvironments, 28
 of anterior chamber/anterior uvea/vitreous, 34*t*, 36–37
 of conjunctiva, 33, 34*t*
 of cornea/sclera, 34*t*, 39, 40*i*
 of retina/retinal pigment epithelium/choroid, 34*t*, 40–41
Immunologic tolerance, 87–89
 to lens crystallins, 90

Immunology, 7–97. *See also* Immune response; Immune response arc
  basic concepts in, 9–16
  definitions/abbreviations of terms and, 7–8, 9–12
Immunoregulation/immunoregulatory systems, 34t, 87–89
  for anterior uvea, 34t, 37–39
  for conjunctiva, 34t, 36
  for cornea, 34t, 39
  for retina/retinal pigment epithelium/choroid, 34t, 42
  T- and B-cell antigen receptor repertoire and, 87
  tolerance and, 87–89
Immunotherapy/immunosuppression, 95–97
  for pars planitis, 151
  for primary central nervous system lymphoma, 228
  for uveitis, 118–121, 119t
  for Vogt-Koyanagi-Harada syndrome, 205
Imuran. *See* Azathioprine
Indentation tonometry (Schiøtz tonometry), HIV prevention precautions and, 262
INF. *See* Interferons
Infectious disease. *See also specific organism and specific disorder*
  endophthalmitis and, 207–214, 208t
    differential diagnosis of, 215
  panuveitis and, 187–197
  posterior uveitis and, 154–173
Inflammatory bowel disease, 131–132
Inflammatory (stimulated) macrophages, 50, 51i, 52–53
Inflammatory mediators. *See* Mediators
Inflammatory response
  immune response triggering, 11
  immunity differentiated from, 12
  local antibody production and, 63
Infliximab, for uveitis, 120
Innate immune response, 9, 10
  acute phase reactants of, 47
  bacteria-derived molecules in, 43–46, 44t
  complement in, 46–47, 75
  effector reactivities of, 43–54
  macrophage recruitment and activation and, 48–54, 51i
  mediator systems affecting, 74–86, 75t
  neutrophil recruitment and activation and, 48–50, 49t
  triggers of, 11, 43–54, 44t
Integrins, in neutrophil rolling, 48, 49t
Intercellular adhesion molecules, in neutrophil rolling, 48, 49t
Intercrines. *See* Chemokines
Interferons (IFNs), 80, 82t
  α, 82t
  γ, 82t
    in delayed hypersensitivity, 65i, 66
Interleukin-1α, 81t
Interleukin-2, 81t
Interleukin-4, 81t
  in delayed hypersensitivity, 65i, 66
Interleukin-5, 81t
  in delayed hypersensitivity, 65i, 66
Interleukin-6, 81t

Interleukin-8, 81t
Interleukins, 80–83, 81t
Intermediate uveitis (pars planitis/chronic cyclitis), 107, 147–152, 148i
  causes of, 112t
  clinical characteristics of, 147–148, 148i
  complications of, 151–152
  differential diagnosis of, 110t, 148–149
  HLA association in, 94t, 147
  in Lyme disease, 192
  multiple sclerosis and, 152
  prognosis of, 149
  signs of, 105–106
  treatment of, 149–150
Intraocular culture, in postoperative endophthalmitis, 216
Intraocular foreign bodies, retained, endophthalmitis caused by, 212
Intraocular lenses. *See also* Cataract surgery
  foldable, in uveitis, 138
  iritis and, 137
  juvenile rheumatoid arthritis–associated iridocyclitis and, 143
  in uveitis, 235, 236
    postoperative inflammation and, 137–138, 137i
  uveitis-glaucoma-hyphema (UGH) syndrome and, 47, 137–138
Intraocular pressure
  elevated, in uveitic glaucoma, 237
  in uveitis, 103t, 104, 136, 237
    corticosteroids affecting, 238
Intraocular specimens, for endophthalmitis diagnosis, 215–216
Intraocular surgery. *See* Ocular (intraocular) surgery
Intraocular tumors, lymphoma (reticulum cell sarcoma/histiocytic [large-cell] lymphoma/non-Hodgkin lymphoma of CNS), 228–231, 228i, 230i
Intravitreal medications
  corticosteroids
    for pars planitis, 151
    for uveitis, 117–118
  for cytomegalovirus retinitis, 252
Iridocyclitis, 106. *See also* Iritis
  acute, 127–141, 127i, 128i
  in Behçet syndrome, 133
  chronic, 141–146
  in coccidioidomycosis, 163, 226–227
  drug-induced, 141
  Fuchs heterochromic, 107, 144–146, 145i
  in herpetic disease, 138–140
  HLA-associated diseases and, 128–132
  idiopathic, 146
  in inflammatory bowel disease, 131–132
  in juvenile rheumatoid arthritis, 141–144, 142i, 144t
  lens-associated, 135–136, 135i, 136i
  in Lyme disease, 192
  in sarcoidosis, 198, 199i, 200i
  in tuberculosis, 194–195, 194i
  in varicella, 138
  viral, 140
Iridotomy, for iris bombé in uveitis, 237–238

Iris
    atrophy of
        in Fuchs heterochromic iridocyclitis/uveitis, 144–145, 145*i*
        in herpetic inflammation, 139*i*, 140
    coccidioidal granuloma of, 226, 227*i*
    immunologic microenvironment of, 37
    in uveitis, 103*t*, 104
Iris bombé, uveitis and, 237–238
Iris nodosa, in syphilis, 188
Iris nodules
    in sarcoidosis, 105*i*, 198, 199*i*
    in syphilis, 188
    in uveitis, 105, 105*i*
Iris papulosa, in syphilis, 188
Iris roseola, in syphilis, 188
Iritis, 106. *See also* Iridocyclitis
    acute, 127–141, 127*i*, 128*i*
    in ankylosing spondylitis, 129
    in Behçet syndrome, 132, 133, 133*i*
    drug-induced, 141
    in glaucomatocyclitic crisis (Posner-Schlossman syndrome), 135
    in herpetic disease, 138–140
    HLA-associated diseases and, 128–132
    in inflammatory bowel disease, 131–132
    intraocular lenses and, 137
    lens-associated, 135–136, 136*i*
    in psoriatic arthritis, 132
    in reactive arthritis/Reiter syndrome, 131
    in syphilis, 187, 188
    in tuberculosis, 194–195, 194*i*
    in varicella, 138
    viral, 140
        treatment of, 140
Ischemia, ocular (ocular ischemic syndrome), 221–222
Isotypes, 7, 54–55
    in immunologic tolerance, 89
Itraconazole, for endophthalmitis, 218*t*
Ivermectin, for onchocerciasis, 196–197
Ixodes ticks, Lyme disease transmitted by, 191

JRA. *See* Juvenile rheumatoid arthritis
Juvenile rheumatoid arthritis, 141–144, 142*i*, 144*t*
    HLA association in, 94*t*, 141
    iridocyclitis in, 141–144, 142*i*, 144*t*
    management of, 143–144
    pauciarticular, 141, 144*t*
    polyarticular, 141, 144*t*
    systemic onset of (Still disease), 141, 144*t*
    uveitis in, 107, 141–144, 142*i*, 144*t*
Juvenile xanthogranuloma, 233

Kallikrein, 76
Kaposi sarcoma, ocular adnexal, 258–259, 259*i*
Kenalog. *See* Triamcinolone
Keratic precipitates, 104, 105*i*
    in sarcoidosis, 105*i*, 198, 199*i*
    stellate
        in Fuchs heterochromic iridocyclitis/uveitis, 145, 145*i*
        in herpetic ocular infection, 139
    in uveitis, 105*i*, 104, 127
Keratitis
    in congenital syphilis, 188, 188*i*
    herpes simplex, in HIV infection/AIDS, 260, 260*i*
    in HIV infection/AIDS, 260, 260*i*
    interstitial, syphilitic, 187–188, 188*i*
    Microsporida causing, in HIV infection/AIDS, 260, 260*i*
    in reactive arthritis/Reiter syndrome, 131
    syphilitic, 187, 188*i*
Keratoconjunctivitis
    atopic, 74
    vernal, 13
Keratoiritis, in herpetic disease, 138–140
Keratopathy, band, in juvenile rheumatoid arthritis, 142, 142*i*, 143
Keratoplasty, penetrating
    endophthalmitis after, 207
    graft rejection and, 41
Keratouveitis, 107
    in congenital syphilis, 187, 188*i*
Ketoconazole, for endophthalmitis, 218*t*
Khodadoust line, 39, 40*i*
Killer cells
    in antibody-dependent cellular cytotoxicity, 72
    lymphokine-activated, 66–70
    natural, 70
        in viral conjunctivitis, 35
Kininogens, 76
Kinins, 76
Koeppe nodules
    in sarcoidosis, 105*i*, 198, 199*i*
    in uveitis, 105*i*, 105
Krill disease (acute retinal pigment epitheliitis/ARPE), 177*t*, 178, 179*i*

L-selectin, in neutrophil rolling, 48
LAK cells. *See* Lymphokine-activated killer cells
Lamellar bodies, in sarcoidosis, 198
Langerhans cells, 15
Large-cell lymphoma (intraocular lymphoma), 228–231, 230*i*
Laser therapy (laser surgery)
    for iris bombé in uveitis, 237–238
    for ocular histoplasmosis, 161
    for pars planitis, 150
LC. *See* Langerhans cells
Lens (crystalline), uveitis and, 64, 135–136, 135*i*, 136*i*. *See also* Phacoantigenic endophthalmitis
Lens-induced glaucoma, 52, 136
Lens proteins
    in phacoantigenic endophthalmitis, 64, 135, 135*i*, 136*i*
    in phacolytic glaucoma, 52, 136
    tolerance to, 87
    in uveitis, 64, 135, 135*i*, 136*i*
Lensectomy, pars plana, juvenile rheumatoid arthritis–associated uveitis and, 235
Leptospirosis, panuveitis in, 193
Leukemia, neoplastic masquerade syndromes secondary to, 231
Leukeran. *See* Chlorambucil
Leukocoria, in toxocariasis, 170, 170*i*, 171*i*
Leukocyte function–associated antigen 1 (LFA-1), in neutrophil rolling, 48
Leukocytes, 13–16. *See also specific type*

Leukotrienes, 7
  as inflammatory mediators, 80
LFA-1. *See* Leukocyte function–associated antigen 1
Light chains, immunoglobulin, 54, 56*i*
Limbitis, in onchocerciasis, 195–197
Lipids, as inflammatory mediators, 77–79, 78*i*
Lipopolysaccharide, bacterial
  in innate immune response, 43–44, 45
  uveitis caused by, 45
5-Lipoxygenase pathway, eicosanoids produced by, 78–79
Loteprednol, for uveitis, 116
Low-zone tolerance, in anterior chamber–associated immune deviation, 38
LPS. *See* Lipopolysaccharide
Lupus erythematosus, systemic, 61, 173–175, 174*i*
Lyme disease, 191–193, 191*i*, 192*i*
Lymph nodes, 16
Lymphatics, 7, 19
Lymphocyte-mediated immune effector responses, 55*t*, 63–70
  cytotoxic lymphocytes and, 66–70, 69*i*
  delayed hypersensitivity T lymphocytes and, 63–66, 65*i*, 68*t*
Lymphocytes, 15. *See also* B cells; T cells
  activation of, 22–24, 23*i*, 25
  effector, 11, 15, 25, 26*i*
Lymphoid proliferation, uveal tract involvement and, masquerade syndromes secondary to, 231–232
Lymphoid tissues, 16
Lymphokine-activated killer cells, 66–70
Lymphokines, 70, 80
Lymphomas
  intraocular (reticulum cell sarcoma/histiocytic [large-cell] lymphoma/non-Hodgkin lymphoma of CNS), 228–231, 228*i*, 230*i*
  systemic, neoplastic masquerade syndromes secondary to, 231
Lysis, cell
  complement-mediated, 59, 60*i*
  by cytotoxic lymphocytes, 68, 69*i*

M protein, in subacute sclerosing panencephalitis, 159
MAC. *See* Membrane attack complex
Mac-1, in neutrophil rolling, 48
α_2-Macroglobulin, in innate immune response, 47
Macrophage-activating factor, 66
Macrophage chemotactic protein-1, 81*t*
Macrophages, 14–15
  innate mechanisms for recruitment and activation of, 48–54, 51*i*
Macular edema, cystoid
  in pars planitis, 147, 151
  prostaglandins and, 79
  in uveitis, 239
Macular neuroretinopathy, acute, 182
Maculopathies
  in ocular histoplasmosis, 160–161
  in subacute sclerosing panencephalitis, 159
MAGE. *See* Melanoma antigen genes
Major histocompatibility complex (MHC), 90–91, 92*t*. *See also* Human leukocyte (HLA) antigens
  class I molecules of, 19–22, 21*i*, 90, 92*t*

class II molecules of, 19, 20*i*, 90, 92*t*
  primed macrophages as, 51*i*, 52
class III molecules of, 91
transplantation and, 93–94
Malignant melanomas. *See* Melanomas
MALT. *See* Mucosa-associated lymphoid tissue
Masquerade syndromes, 108, 221–233
  neoplastic, 108, 228–233
  nonneoplastic, 221–227
Mast cells, 13–14
  acute IgE-mediated degranulation of, 14, 72–73, 73*i*
  chronic degranulation of plus Th2 delayed hypersensitivity, 73
Mazzotti reaction, 196
MCP. *See* Multifocal choroiditis, and panuveitis syndrome
MCP-1. *See* Macrophage chemotactic protein-1
MDRTB. *See* Multidrug-resistant tuberculosis
Measles (rubeola) virus, 159
  posterior uveitis and, 159
Mediators, 8, 74–86, 75*t*. *See also specific type*
  cytokines, 80–83, 81–82*t*
  lipid, 77–79, 78*i*
  macrophage synthesis of, 52–54
  neutrophil-derived granule products, 86
  plasma-derived enzyme systems, 75–77, 76*i*
  reactive nitrogen products, 85–86
  reactive oxygen intermediates, 83–85, 84*i*
  in uveitis, 102
  vasoactive amines, 77
Melanocytic proliferation, bilateral diffuse uveal, 233
Melanoma antigen genes, 72
Melanomas
  metastatic, 233
  uveal, 72, 232
Membrane attack complex, 59
Memory, immunologic, 11, 27–28
Metastatic eye disease, 233
Methotrexate
  for juvenile rheumatoid arthritis, 143
  for primary central nervous system lymphoma, 230
  for uveitis, 119, 119*t*
Methylprednisolone
  for pars planitis, 149
  for uveitis, 115*t*
MEWDS. *See* Multiple evanescent white dot syndrome
MHA-TP (microhemagglutination assay for *T pallidum*), 189
MHC. *See* Major histocompatibility complex
Microaneurysms, retinal, in HIV infection/AIDS, 248
Microenvironments, immunologic. *See* Immunologic microenvironments
Microhemagglutination assay for *T pallidum* (MHA-TP), 189
Microsporida (microsporidiosis), keratitis/keratoconjunctivitis in HIV infection/AIDS caused by, 260, 260*i*
Mimicry, molecular, 89
  autoimmune uveitis and, 91
  HLA disease associations and, 95
  retinal vasculitis in systemic lupus erythematosus and, 61
Mixed lymphocyte reaction, 94

Molecular mimicry, 89
  autoimmune uveitis and, 91
  HLA disease associations and, 95
  retinal vasculitis in systemic lupus erythematosus and, 61
Molluscum contagiosum, in HIV infection/AIDS, 259
Monoclonal antibodies, 54
Monocytes, 14–15. *See also* Macrophages
Monokines, 80
Moraxella, bleb-associated endophthalmitis caused by, 213
Mucosa-associated lymphoid tissue (MALT), of conjunctiva, 34*t,* 36
Mucosal mast cells, 13
Multidrug-resistant tuberculosis (MDRTB), 195
Multifocal choroiditis
  in HIV infection/AIDS, 257–258
  and panuveitis syndrome (MCP), 177*t,* 185, 185*i*
Multiple evanescent white dot syndrome (MEWDS), 177*t,* 181, 182*i*
Multiple sclerosis
  HLA association in, 94*t*
  intermediate uveitis and, 152
Mutton-fat keratic precipitates, 104, 104*i*
  in sarcoidosis, 104*i,* 198, 199*i*
  in uveitis, 104, 104*i* 136
Mycophenolate mofetil, for uveitis, 119*t*
Mydriasis/mydriatics, for uveitis, 114–115, 128
Myeloma, monoclonal antibody and, 56
Myeloperoxidase, oxygen radicals produced by, 86

Nafcillin, for endophthalmitis, 218*t*
Naming-meshing system, for uveitis differential diagnosis, 109, 110–111*t*
Natural (innate) immunity, 9, 10. *See also* Innate immune response
Natural killer cells, 70
  in viral conjunctivitis, 35
Necrotizing retinitis
  atypical, diagnosis of, 63
  herpetic (acute retinal necrosis), 140, 154–156, 155*i,* 156*i*
Necrotizing scleritis, in Wegener granulomatosis, 62
Neoantigen, 59
Neoplasia. *See also specific type and* Intraocular tumors
  masquerade syndromes and, 228–233
Neoral. *See* Cyclosporine
Neovascularization. *See also* Choroidal neovascularization
  in pars planitis, 148, 151, 240
  in uveitis, 240
Neural reflex arc, immune response arc compared with, 17, 18*i*
Neuropeptides, as inflammatory mediators, 82*t*
Neuroretinitis
  diffuse unilateral subacute (DUSN), 172, 172*i,* 173*i*
  in syphilis, 190
Neuroretinopathy, acute macular, 182
Neutralization, antibody, 58, 58*i*
Neutrophil rolling, 48, 49*i*
Neutrophils (polymorphonuclear leukocytes), 13
  in inflammation, granule products of, 86
  innate mechanisms for recruitment and activation of, 48–50, 49*i*
Nitric oxide, 85–86
Nitric oxide synthase, 85–86
Nitrogen radicals, as inflammatory mediators, 85–86
NK cells. *See* Natural killer cells
NNRTI. *See* Nonnucleoside reverse transcriptase inhibitors
NO. *See* Nitric oxide
Nocardia asteroides, endophthalmitis caused by, 223, 223*i*
Nongranulomatous uveitis, 104, 108, 127–141, 127*i,* 128*i*
Non-Hodgkin lymphomas, of CNS (intraocular lymphoma/reticulum cell sarcoma/histiocytic [large-cell] lymphoma), 228–231, 228*i,* 230*i*
Nonnucleoside reverse transcriptase inhibitors (NNRTIs), 246, 247*t*
Nonsteroidal anti-inflammatory drugs (NSAIDs), 96
  COX-1/COX-2 inhibition by, 96
  for uveitis, 118
Non-T, non-B effector lymphocytes (null cells), 15, 25, 70
NOS. *See* Nitric oxide synthase
NSAIDs. *See* Nonsteroidal anti-inflammatory drugs
Nucleoside analogues, 246, 247*t*
Null cells (non-T, non-B effector lymphocytes), 15, 25, 70

Ocular adnexa, Kaposi sarcoma of, 258–259, 258*i,* 259*i*
Ocular histoplasmosis syndrome, 160–163, 160*i,* 161*i,* 162*i,* 177*t*
  histo spots in, 160, 160*i,* 161
  HLA association in, 94*t,* 160
Ocular immunology. *See* Immune response; Immune response arc; Immunology
Ocular ischemia (ocular ischemic syndrome), 221–222
Ocular (intraocular) surgery
  endophthalmitis after, 207, 208*t,* 209–211
    acute-onset, 210–211, 210*i,* 211*i*
    bleb-associated, 207, 208*t,* 212–213
    chronic (delayed-onset), 211, 212*i*
  for uveitis, 121
OHS. *See* Ocular histoplasmosis syndrome
Onchocerca volvulus (onchocerciasis), 195–197
Opacities, vitreous
  in toxoplasmosis, 166, 166*i,* 239
  in uveitis, 239
Open-angle glaucoma
  pars planitis and, 151
  uveitis and, 237
Ophthalmia, sympathetic, 67–68, 200–203, 200*i,* 201*i,* 202*t*
  HLA association in, 94*t*
  surgical procedures/injuries leading to, 202*t*
Opportunistic infections. *See also specific type*
  in HIV infection/AIDS, 248, 260, 260*i*
Opsonization, antibody, 58, 58*i*
Optic atrophy, in onchocerciasis, 196
Optic nerve (cranial nerve II), in uveitis, 103*t*
Orbit, disorders of, Th1 delayed hypersensitivity and, 68*t*

Oxygen radicals (free radicals), as inflammatory mediators, 83–85, 84*i*

P-selectin, in neutrophil rolling, 48, 49*i*
P24 antigen testing, in HIV infection/AIDS, 246
PAF. *See* Platelet-activating factors
Pain, in uveitis, 102, 102*t*, 127
PAN. *See* Polyarteritis nodosa
Panencephalitis, subacute sclerosing, posterior uveitis caused by, 159–160
Panuveitis, 107, 187–204. *See also specific cause and* Uveitis
  in Behçet syndrome, 132–133
  causes of, 112*t*
    immunologic and granulomatous diseases, 197–206
    infectious diseases, 187–197
  differential diagnosis of, 109*t*
  multifocal choroiditis and (MCP), 177*t*, 185, 185*i*
  signs of, 106
  subretinal fibrosis and uveitis syndrome (SFU), 177*t*, 184, 184*i*, 185*i*
  sympathetic ophthalmia and, 67–68, 200–203, 200*i*, 201*i*, 202*t*
  in Vogt-Koyanagi-Harada syndrome, 203–205, 204*i*, 205*i*, 206*i*
Paracrine actions, of cytokines, 80
Pars plana
  cryoablation of, for pars planitis, 150
  in uveitis, 103*t*
Pars plana lensectomy, juvenile rheumatoid arthritis–associated uveitis and, 235
Pars plana vitrectomy
  for endophthalmitis, 217, 219, 226
  endophthalmitis after, 207
  for pars planitis, 150
  for retinal detachment, in cytomegalovirus retinitis, 253
  for specimen collection, 216
  for vitritis, 121
Pars planitis, 147–152, 148*i*. *See also* Intermediate uveitis
  clinical characteristics of, 147–148, 148*i*
  complications of, 151–152
  diagnosis/differential diagnosis of, 148–149
  prognosis of, 149
  treatment of, 149–150
PCNSL. *See* Primary central nervous system lymphomas
PCR. *See* Polymerase chain reaction
PDGF. *See* Platelet-derived growth factors
Penetrating injuries, endophthalmitis after, 212
Penetrating keratoplasty
  endophthalmitis after, 207
  rejection of corneal allograft and, 41
Penicillins, for syphilis, 190
Pentamidine, for *Pneumocystis carinii* choroiditis, 257
Perforin, 68, 69*i*
Periocular drug administration
  for pars planitis, 149–150
  for toxoplasmosis, 168
  for uveitis, 115*t*, 116–117, 117*i*
Peripheral lymphoid structures, 16

Peripheral uveitis. *See* Pars planitis
Periphlebitis
  in multiple sclerosis, 152
  in sarcoidosis, 199
PG. *See* Prostaglandins
PGH synthase (prostaglandin G/H synthase). *See* Cyclo-oxygenase
Phacoantigenic endophthalmitis (lens-induced granulomatous/phacoanaphylactic endophthalmitis/phacoanaphylaxis), 64, 135–136, 136*i*
Phacoemulsification, in uveitis, 135*i*, 235–237
Phacolytic glaucoma, 52, 136
Phacotoxic uveitis, 135
Phagocytosis, 50
Phospholipase A$_2$, 80
Photocoagulation
  for ocular histoplasmosis, 161
  for pars planitis, 150
  prophylactic, in acute retinal necrosis, 155–156
Photophobia, in uveitis, 127
PIC. *See* Punctate inner choroiditis
Platelet-activating factors, 77, 78*i*, 79–80
Platelet-derived growth factors, 82*t*
PMN. *See* Polymorphonuclear leukocytes
Pneumocystis carinii infections
  choroiditis, 256–257, 256*i*, 257*i*
  pneumonia, 247, 256
Poison ivy toxin, immune response arc in response to, 29–30
Poliosis, in Vogt-Koyanagi-Harada syndrome, 203, 204*i*
Polyarteritis nodosa, 175, 176*i*
Polyclonal antibodies, 56
Polymerase chain reaction (PCR), in HIV infection/AIDS, 245
Polymorphonuclear leukocytes (neutrophils), 13
  in inflammation, granule products of, 86
  innate mechanisms for recruitment and activation of, 48–50, 49*i*
PORN. *See* Progressive outer retinal necrosis
PORT. *See* Punctate outer retinal toxoplasmosis
Posner-Schlossman syndrome (glaucomatocyclitic crisis), 107, 135
Posterior chamber, in uveitis, 103*t*, 106. *See also* Posterior uveitis
Posterior synechiae
  in sarcoidosis, 198
  in uveitis, 104*i*, 105*i*
Posterior uveitis, 107, 153–185. *See also specific cause and* Choroiditis; Retinitis; Uveitis
  causes of, 112*t*
  differential diagnosis of, 111*t*
  immunologic, 175–185
  infectious, 154–173
  signs of, 103*t*, 106
Postoperative endophthalmitis, 207, 208*t*, 209–211
  acute-onset, 210–211, 210*i*, 211*i*
  bleb-associated, 207, 208*t*, 212–213
  after cataract surgery, 207, 208*t*, 209
  chronic (delayed-onset), 211, 212
Posttraumatic endophthalmitis, 207, 208*t*, 211–212
PPD test. *See* Purified protein derivative (PPD) test
Precursor cytotoxic T lymphocytes, 68, 69*i*

Prednisolone
  for endophthalmitis, 218*t*
  for uveitis, 115*t*, 116
Prednisone
  for endophthalmitis, 218*t*
  for uveitis, 115*t*
Pregnancy, toxoplasmosis during, 165, 167, 168, 168*i*
Primary central nervous system lymphomas, 228–231, 228*i*
Priming
  of effector lymphocytes, 25
  of macrophages, 51*i*, 52
Processing phase of immune response arc, 22–24, 23*i*
  response to poison ivy and, 29, 30
  response to tuberculosis and, 30–31
Prograf. *See* Tacrolimus
Programmed cell death (PCD/apoptosis)
  by cytotoxic T lymphocytes, 68, 69*i*
  Fas ligand in, 38, 68, 69*i*
Progressive outer retinal necrosis (PORN), 155, 156*i*
  in HIV infection/AIDS, 155, 253–254, 254*i*
Propionibacterium acnes, in postoperative endophthalmitis, 53, 208*t*, 209, 210–211, 212*i*
Prostaglandin G/H synthase. *See* Cyclo-oxygenase
Prostaglandins
  as inflammatory mediators, 78–79, 78*i*
  nonsteroidal anti-inflammatory drugs and, 96
Protease inhibitors, 246, 247*t*
Proteases, PMN-derived, 86
Proteinase-3, scleritis/retinal vasculitis in Wegener granulomatosis and, 62
Proteus, postoperative endophthalmitis caused by, 211
Protozoa, ocular infection/inflammation caused by, 164–169
Pseudomonas, postoperative endophthalmitis caused by, 211
Psoriatic arthritis, 132, 133*i*
Punctate inner choroiditis/choroidopathy (PIC), 177*t*, 182, 183*i*
Punctate outer retinal toxoplasmosis (PORT), 166, 167*i*
Purified protein derivative (PPD) test, 194–195
  immune response arc and, 31
Pyrimethamine, for toxoplasmosis, 168

Rapid plasma reagin (RPR) test, 189–190
Reactive arthritis (Reiter syndrome), 130–131, 131*i*, 132*i*
  HLA association in, 94*t*, 129
Reactive nitrogen products, as inflammatory mediators, 85
Reactive oxygen intermediates, as inflammatory mediators, 83–85, 84*i*
Receptor activation, in immune response, adaptive versus innate immunity and, 10
Recognition receptors, in immune response, adaptive versus innate immunity and, 10, 11
Recombination, T- and B-cell antigen receptor diversity and, 87
Recoverin, cancer-associated retinopathy and, 61
Reflex arc, neural, immune response arc compared with, 17–19, 18*i*
Regional enteritis (Crohn disease), 131–132
Regional immunity, 28

Reiter syndrome (reactive arthritis), 130–131, 131*i*, 132*i*
  HLA association in, 94*t*, 130
Rejection (graft)
  corneal allograft, 39, 40*i*, 41
  transplantation antigens and, 93–94
Remodeling pathway, platelet-activating factors in, 80
Reparative (stimulated) macrophages, 50, 51*i*, 52–53
Restimulation, of effector lymphocytes, 25
Resting macrophages, 51–52, 51*i*
Resting neutrophils, 48
Reticulum cell sarcoma (intraocular lymphoma), 228–231, 228*i*, 230*i*
Retina
  diseases of, Th1 delayed hypersensitivity and, 68*t*
  immune response in, 34*t*, 40–41
  necrosis of
    acute (necrotizing herpetic retinitis), 140, 154–156, 155*i*, 156*i*
    progressive, 155, 156*i*
      in HIV infection/AIDS, 155, 253–254, 254*i*
  in primary central nervous system lymphoma, 228, 228*i*, 230*i*
  in systemic lupus erythematosus, 61, 173–175, 174*i*
  transplantation of, 42
  in uveitis, 103*t*
Retinal artery, microaneurysms of, in HIV infection/AIDS, 248
Retinal breaks, in acute retinal necrosis (herpetic necrotizing retinitis), 155, 156*i*
Retinal detachment
  in acute retinal necrosis (herpetic necrotizing retinitis), 155, 156*i*
  in cytomegalovirus retinitis, 157, 157*i*, 253
  in pars planitis, 148, 151
  rhegmatogenous, 222
  in uveitis, 240
  in Vogt-Koyanagi-Harada syndrome, 203, 204*i*
Retinal gene therapy, 42
Retinal hemorrhages, in HIV infection/AIDS, 248
Retinal pigment epithelium (RPE)
  immune response in, 34*t*, 40–41
  inflammation of (acute retinal epitheliitis/ARPE/Krill disease), 177*t*, 178, 179*i*
  in primary central nervous system lymphoma, 229
  transplantation of, 42
Retinal sheathing, in sarcoidosis, 199, 200*i*
Retinal vasculitis
  in Behçet syndrome, 133, 134*i*
  differential diagnosis of, 111*t*
  in herpetic disease, 140
  HLA association in, 94*t*
  in polyarteritis nodosa, 175, 176*i*
  in systemic lupus erythematosus, 61, 173–175, 174*i*
  in Wegener granulomatosis, 62, 175–176, 176*i*
Retinitis, 107
  atypical necrotizing, diagnosis of, 63
  Candida, 163–164, 164*i*, 223–225, 223*i*
  cytomegalovirus, 156–158, 157*i*
    antiviral immunity in, 71
    cidofovir for, 252
    fomivirsen for, 252
    foscarnet for, 251

ganciclovir for, 155, 250–252
  in HIV infection/AIDS, 71, 156, 249–253, 251*i*
  herpetic necrotizing (acute retinal necrosis), 140, 154–156, 155*i*, 156*i*
  measles, 159
  pigmentosa, 221
  rubella, 158–159, 159*i*
  in syphilis, 188, 189*i*, 190, 190*i*
  in toxoplasmosis, 165–166, 166*i*, 167*i*, 254–255, 255*i*
  in Wegener granulomatosis, 62, 175, 176*i*
Retinoblastoma, 232
Retinochoroiditis, 107
  Toxoplasma causing, 164–169
    in HIV infection/AIDS, 254–255, 255*i*
Retinochoroidopathies, 176–185, 177*t*. *See also specific disorder*
  birdshot (vitiliginous chorioretinitis), 177*t*, 180–181, 180*i*, 181*i*
    HLA association in, 94*t*, 180–181
Retinopathy
  acute zonal occult outer (AZOOR), 180
  cancer-associated, 61
  HIV, 248, 249*i*
Reverse transcriptase inhibitors, nonnucleoside (NNRTIs), 246, 247*t*
Rhegmatogenous retinal detachment. *See* Retinal detachment
Rheumatoid arthritis, juvenile. *See* Juvenile rheumatoid arthritis
Rheumatrex. *See* Methotrexate
Rifabutin, uveitis caused by, 141
Rimexolone, for uveitis, 115*t*, 116, 238
River blindness (onchocerciasis), 195–197
RPE. *See* Retinal pigment epithelium
RPR (rapid plasma reagin) test, 189
Rubella, 158–159, 159*i*
  congenital, 158–159, 159*i*
  posterior uveitis in, 158, 159*i*
Rubeola (measles) virus, 159
  posterior uveitis and, 159

Sabin-Feldman dye test, for toxoplasmosis, 166–167
Salt-and-pepper fundus/retinopathy
  rubella and, 158, 159*i*
  syphilis and, 188
Sandimmune. *See* Cyclosporine
Sarcoidosis, 197–200, 197*i*, 198*i*, 199*i*, 200*i*
  HLA association in, 94*t*
  panuveitis in, 107, 197–200, 197*i*, 198*i*, 199*i*, 200*i*
Scavenging, 51
Scavenging macrophages, 51–52, 51*i*
Schaumann's bodies, in sarcoidosis, 198
Schiøtz (indentation) tonometry, HIV prevention precautions and, 262
Schwartz syndrome, 222
Sclera
  disorders of, Th1 delayed hypersensitivity and, 68*t*
  immunologic response/features of, 34*t*
Scleral buckle, for retinal detachment in uveitis, 240
Scleritis, in Wegener granulomatosis, 62, 175
Sclerouveitis, 106
  in inflammatory bowel disease, 132

Secondary glaucoma. *See* Angle-closure glaucoma; Glaucoma, uveitis and
Selectins, in neutrophil rolling, 48, 49*i*
Self-antigens, tolerance to, 87–89
Sensitization, lymphocyte, 22–24, 23*i*. *See also* Activation
Septra. *See* Trimethoprim/sulfamethoxazole
Seronegative spondyloarthropathies, uveitis in, 129–132
Serotonin, as inflammatory mediator, 77
Serpiginous choroidopathy (geographic choroiditis/helicoid peripapillary choroidopathy), 177*t*, 182–184, 184*i*
Serratia marcescens, postoperative endophthalmitis caused by, 211, 211*i*
Serum sickness, 59
SFU. *See* Subretinal fibrosis and uveitis syndrome
Sheathing, retinal vascular, in sarcoidosis, 199, 200*i*
SLE. *See* Systemic lupus erythematosus
Snowballs
  in intermediate uveitis/pars planitis, 105, 147, 148*i*
  in sarcoidosis, 198
Snowbank formation, in intermediate uveitis/pars planitis, 106, 147
Snowmen, in intermediate uveitis/pars planitis, 147
SO. *See* Sympathetic ophthalmia
Social history, in uveitis, 122
Solu-Cortef. *See* Hydrocortisone sodium succinate
Specific (adaptive) immunity, 9–10. *See also* Adaptive immune response
Specificity, immunologic, 11
Spiramycin, for toxoplasmosis, 168
Spleen, 16
Spondylitis, ankylosing, 127*i*, 129–130, 130*i*
  HLA in, 94–95, 129
Spondyloarthropathies, seronegative, uveitis in, 129–130
SSPE. *See* Subacute sclerosing panencephalitis
Staphylococcus
  aureus
    postoperative endophthalmitis caused by, 208*t*, 210–211
    posttraumatic endophthalmitis caused by, 208*t*, 212
    in bleb-associated endophthalmitis, 212–213
  epidermidis
    bleb-associated endophthalmitis caused by, 213
    postoperative endophthalmitis caused by, 208*t*, 210, 210*i*
    posttraumatic endophthalmitis caused by, 208*t*, 211
  in postoperative endophthalmitis, 208*t*, 209–211, 210*i*
  in posttraumatic endophthalmitis, 208*t*, 212
Steroids. *See* Corticosteroids
Still disease, 141
Stimulated macrophages, 50, 51*i*, 52–53
Stimulatory antibodies, 62
Stimulatory hypersensitivity (type V) reaction, 54, 54*t*
Streptococcus
  in bleb-associated endophthalmitis, 208*t*, 212–213
  in postoperative endophthalmitis, 208*t*, 211
  in posttraumatic endophthalmitis, 212

Subacute sclerosing panencephalitis, posterior uveitis caused by, 159–160
Subretinal fibrosis and uveitis syndrome (SFU), 177t, 184, 184i, 185i
Substance P, as inflammatory mediator, 82t
Substantia propria, immunologic and inflammatory cells in, 33
Sub-Tenon's approach, for periocular corticosteroid injection, 116–117, 117i
　in pars planitis, 150
Sugiura's sign, 203, 204i
Suicide induction (cell), by cytotoxic T lymphocytes, 68, 69i
Sulfonamides, for toxoplasmosis, 168
Sunset-glow fundus, in Vogt-Koyanagi-Harada syndrome, 203, 204i
Superoxide, as inflammatory mediator, 83
Superoxide dismutase, as inflammatory mediator, 83
Suppression (immunologic), in development of tolerance, 88–89
Suppressor T cells. *See also* T cells
　class I MHC molecules as antigen-presenting platform for, 19–22, 21i
　in immune processing, 23i, 24
Surface markers, lymphocyte, 15
Surgery
　endophthalmitis after, 207, 208t, 209–211
　　acute-onset, 210–211, 210i, 211i
　　bleb-associated, 207, 208t, 212–213
　　chronic (delayed-onset), 211, 212i
　for uveitis, 121
Sympathetic ophthalmia, 67–68, 200–203, 200i, 201i, 202t
　HLA association in, 94t
　surgical procedures/injuries leading to, 202t
Syndrome of prolonged enlargement of blind spot, 182
Synechiae
　in sarcoidosis, 198
　in uveitis, 104i, 105i
Syphilis, 187–191
　chorioretinitis in, 188, 189i
　　in HIV infection/AIDS, 189, 255
　　posterior placoid, 255
　congenital/intrauterine, 187–188, 188i
　in HIV infection/AIDS, 189, 255–256
　secondary, 188, 189i
　uveitis and, 107, 187–191
Syphilitic posterior placoid chorioretinitis, 255
Systemic drug therapy, corticosteroid, for uveitis, 115t, 117
Systemic lupus erythematosus, 61, 173, 174i

T-cell antigen receptors, 87
　HLA disease associations and, 95
T-cell signaling inhibitors, for uveitis, 119t, 120
T cells (T lymphocytes), 15. *See also specific type*
　activation of, 19–22, 21i, 25
　class I MHC molecules as antigen-presenting platform for, 19–22, 21i
　class II MHC molecules as antigen-presenting platform for, 19, 20i
　cytotoxic, 24, 25, 66–70, 69i
　delayed hypersensitivity (DH), 25, 63–66, 65i, 68t
　differentiation of, 22–24, 23i
　downregulatory, 88
　effector, 25
　helper, 22–24, 23i
　in HIV infection/AIDS, 242–243, 244t, 246–248
　in immune processing, 22–24, 23i
　maturation of, in thymus, 16
　suppressor, 23i, 24
　in viral conjunctivitis, 35
T helper 0 cells, 22
T helper 1 cells, 22–24, 23i
　in delayed hypersensitivity (type IV) reactions, 63–66, 65i, 68t
　in sympathetic ophthalmia, 67–68
T helper 2 cells, 22–24, 23i
　in chronic mast cell degranulation, 73
　in delayed hypersensitivity (type IV) reactions, 63–66, 65i
　in *Toxocara* granuloma, 67
Taches de bougie, in sarcoidosis, 199
Tacrolimus, for uveitis, 119t
Taenia solium, 171
Tapeworms, eye invaded by, 171, 172i
TGF. *See* Transforming growth factor–β
Th0 cells. *See* T helper 0 cells
Th1 cells. *See* T helper 1 cells
Th2 cells. *See* T helper 2 cells
Thymus
　clonal deletion in, 88
　as lymphoid tissue, 16
Ticks, Lyme disease transmitted by, 191
Tissue-bound immune complexes, 60–62, 60i
TNF. *See* Tumor necrosis factor
Tobramycin, for endophthalmitis, 217
Tolerance (immunologic), 87–89
　to lens crystallins, 90
Tonometry (tonometer), HIV prevention precautions and, 262
Toxocara (toxocariasis), 170–171, 170i, 171i, 171t
　canis, 67, 172
　granuloma caused by, 67, 170–171, 170i, 171i, 171t
Toxoplasma (toxoplasmosis), 164–169
　congenital, 165, 167, 168i
　gondii, 164–165, 165i
　in HIV infection/AIDS, 165, 165i, 166i, 254–255, 256i
　during pregnancy, 165, 167, 168, 168i
　punctate outer retinal (PORT), 166, 167i
　uveitis in, 164–169
Toxoplasma dye test, 166–167
Trabecular meshwork, in uveitis, 105
Trabeculitis, 105
Transforming growth factor–β, 82t
Transmigration, in neutrophil recruitment and activation, 48–50, 49i
Transplant rejection. *See* Rejection (graft)
Transplantation
　corneal, graft rejection and, 39, 40i, 41
　histocompatibility antigens and, 93–94
　retinal/retinal pigment epithelium, 42
Transplantation antigens, 93–94
Trauma
　anterior uveitis caused by, 107

endophthalmitis after, 207, 208t, 211–212
innate immune response and, 47
sympathetic ophthalmia and, 200–203, 200i, 201i, 202t
Treponema pallidum, 187. *See also* Syphilis
Triamcinolone
for pars planitis, 149, 150
for uveitis, 115t
Trimethoprim/sulfamethoxazole
for *Pneumocystis carinii* choroiditis, 257
for *Pneumocystis carinii* pneumonia, 247
for toxoplasmosis, 168, 169
Tropicamide, for uveitis, 115, 128
Tubercles, in sarcoidosis, 197–199, 197i, 198i
Tuberculin hypersensitivity, 31, 66
Tuberculin skin test, 31, 195
in HIV infection/AIDS, 245
immune response arc and, 31
Tuberculosis, 193–195, 194i, 196i
choroidal involvement and, 194, 194i
in HIV infection/AIDS, 193
immune response arc in, 30–31
multidrug-resistant, 195
treatment of, 195
uveitis in, 193–195, 194i, 196i
Tumor necrosis factor
α, 81t
in apoptosis, 68
β, 81t
in delayed hypersensitivity, 65i, 66

UGH syndrome. *See* Uveitis-glaucoma-hyphema (UGH) syndrome
Ulcerative colitis, 131–132
Ultrasonography/ultrasound, in uveitis, 113
Unilateral wipe-out syndrome (diffuse unilateral subacute neuroretinitis), 172–173, 172i, 173i
Universal precautions, 261
Urushiol. *See* Poison ivy toxin
Uvea (uveal tract), 101
bilateral diffuse uveal melanocytic proliferation of, 233
disorders of, Th1 delayed hypersensitivity and, 68t
immune response in, 34t, 36–39
inflammation of. *See* Uveitis
lymphoid proliferation and, masquerade syndromes secondary to, 231–232
melanomas of, 72, 232
Uveitis, 101–121. *See also specific type*
acute, 108
anterior. *See* Anterior uveitis
associated factors in, 108–109, 109t, 122–126
autoimmune, molecular mimicry and, 89
cataracts and, 235–237
causes of, 109–112, 110–111t, 112t
chronic, 108
circulating immune complexes and, 57
classification of, 106–107
clinical approach to, 101–126
complications of, 235–240
cystoid macular edema and, 239
diagnostic survey for, 122–126
differential diagnosis of, 109–112, 110–111t, 112t

diffuse. *See* Panuveitis
drug-induced, 141
experimental, oxygen-mediated damage in, 85
Fuchs, 107, 144–146, 145i
glaucoma and, 135, 237–238, 238t
granulomatous, 104, 108
herpetic, 138–140, 139i
glaucoma in, 139
HLA association in, 93, 94t, 128–132
hypotony and, 239
intermediate. *See* Intermediate uveitis
intraocular lenses and, 235, 236
postoperative inflammation and, 137–138, 137i
in juvenile rheumatoid arthritis, 141–144, 142i, 144t
laboratory and medical evaluation of, 110–111t, 113
lens-associated, 64, 135–136, 136i. *See also* Phacoantigenic endophthalmitis; Phacolytic glaucoma
lipopolysaccharide-induced, 45
nongranulomatous, 104, 108, 127–141, 127i, 128i
in onchocerciasis, 195–197
peripheral. *See* Pars planitis
phacotoxic, 135
posterior. *See* Posterior uveitis
prevalence of, 109–112, 112t
Propionibacterium acnes causing, 53
retinal detachment and, 240
signs of, 102–106, 103t, 104i, 105i
subretinal fibrosis and (SFU), 177t, 184, 184i, 185i
sympathetic ophthalmia and, 67–68, 200–203, 200i, 201i, 202t
symptoms of, 101–102, 102t
syphilitic, 106, 187–191
systemic disease associations and, 108, 109
Th1 delayed hypersensitivity and, 68t
treatment of, 114t
medical, 114–121, 114t
antiviral agents in, 140
surgical, 114t, 121
in tuberculosis, 193–195, 194i, 196i
vitreous opacification and vitritis and, 239
in Vogt-Koyanagi-Harada syndrome, 203–205, 204i, 205i, 206i
Uveitis-glaucoma-hyphema (UGH) syndrome, 47
intraocular lens implantation and, 47, 137–138

Valganciclovir, 252
Vancomycin, for endophthalmitis, 217, 218t, 219
Varicella (chickenpox), iritis/iridocyclitis in, 138
Varicella-zoster virus
acute retinal necrosis caused by, 140, 154–156, 155i, 156i
uveitis caused by, 138–140, 139i
Vasculitis, retinal
in Behçet syndrome, 133, 134i
differential diagnosis of, 111t
in herpetic disease, 140
HLA association in, 94t
in polyarteritis nodosa, 175, 176i
in systemic lupus erythematosus, 61, 173–175, 174i
in Wegener granulomatosis, 62, 175, 176
Vasoactive amines, as inflammatory mediators, 77

Vasoactive intestinal peptide (VIP), as inflammatory mediator, 82*t*
Venereal Disease Research Laboratory (VDRL) test, 189–190
Vernal conjunctivitis/keratoconjunctivitis, mast cells in, 13
VIP. *See* Vasoactive intestinal peptide
Viruses
  conjunctivitis caused by, immune response to, 35
  uveitis and, 140, 154–160
Visual loss/impairment, in endophthalmitis, 207, 211, 219–220
Vitiliginous chorioretinitis (birdshot retinochoroidopathy), 177*t*, 180–181, 180*i*, 181*i*
  HLA association in, 94*t*, 180
Vitiligo, in Vogt-Koyanagi-Harada syndrome, 203, 204*i*
Vitravene. *See* Fomivirsen
Vitrectomy
  for acute retinal necrosis, 155
  for endophthalmitis, 217, 219, 226
  endophthalmitis after, 207
  for pars planitis, 150
  for primary central nervous system lymphoma, 228
  for retinal detachment, in cytomegalovirus retinitis, 253
  for specimen collection, 216
  for vitritis, 121
Vitreous
  immune response in, 34*t*, 36–39
  inflammation of. *See* Endophthalmitis; Vitritis
  opacification of
    in toxoplasmosis, 166, 166*i*, 239
    in uveitis, 239
  specimen collection from, 215–216
  in uveitis, 103*t*
Vitreous biopsy
  for specimen collection, 216
  in uveitis, 109
Vitreous cellular reaction, in uveitis, 102
Vitreous tap, for specimen collection, 216
Vitritis. *See also* Endophthalmitis
  chorioretinitis with/without, differential diagnosis of, 111*t*
  in Lyme disease, 191, 192, 192*i*
  in pars planitis, 148, 152
  in primary central nervous system lymphoma, 228
  in uveitis, 111*t*
Vogt-Koyanagi-Harada (VKH) syndrome, 203–205, 204*i*, 205*i*, 206*i*
  HLA association in, 94*t*, 205

Wegener granulomatosis, 62, 175–176, 176*i*
Western blot analysis, in HIV infection/AIDS, 245–246
White blood cells, 13–16. *See also specific type*
White dot syndromes, 176–185, 177*t*. *See also* Retinochoroidopathies
  multiple evanescent (MEWDS), 177*t*, 181–182, 182*i*
Wreath sign, in multiple evanescent white dot syndrome, 182*i*

Xanthogranuloma, juvenile, 233

Yeasts, *Candida albicans,* 163–164